CANCER ETIOLOGY, DIAGNOSIS AND TREATMENTS

PARANEOPLASTIC SYNDROMES

SYMPTOMS, DIAGNOSIS AND TREATMENT

Cancer Etiology, Diagnosis and Treatments

Additional books in this series can be found on Nova's website under the Series tab.

Additional e-books in this series can be found on Nova's website under the e-book tab.

CANCER ETIOLOGY, DIAGNOSIS AND TREATMENTS

PARANEOPLASTIC SYNDROMES

SYMPTOMS, DIAGNOSIS AND TREATMENT

LORA H. WINTER
EDITOR

NOVA BIOMEDICAL

New York

For permission to use material from this book please contact us:
Telephone 631-231-7269; Fax 631-231-8175
Web Site: http://www.novapublishers.com

Library of Congress Cataloging-in-Publication Data

ISBN: 978-1-63117-878-8

LCCN: 2014938430

Published by Nova Science Publishers, Inc. † New York

Contents

Preface		**vii**
Chapter I	Current Concepts in Common Paraneoplastic Syndromes: Symptoms, Diagnosis and Treatment *Candace Mainor, Ashiq Masood, Muddassir Shahdhar and Heather D. Mannuel*	**1**
Chapter II	Cutaneous Paraneoplastic Syndromes and Skin Features of Internal Malignancy: Symptoms, Diagnosis and Treatment *M. Yuste Chaves and M. González de Arriba*	**23**
Chapter III	Paraneoplastic Syndromes in Patients with Malignancies of the Genitourinary Tract *Emilio Sacco, Ph.D. and Riccardo Bientinesi, M.D.*	**107**
Chapter IV	Paraneoplastic Polyneuropathies: Searching in the Mist *Antonios Kerasnoudis, M.D.*	**149**
Chapter V	Correction of Cancer-Related Anemia with Oxyresveratrol *G. I. Solyanik, O. N. Pyaskovskaya and N. K. Rodionova*	**163**

Chapter VI Paraneoplastic Syndromes Associated with Lung Cancer **201**
Neven Z. Rakusic and Nevena Rakusic

Index **225**

Preface

Paraneoplastic Syndromes (PNS) are a group of disorders that cause endocrinologic, hematologic, neurologic, and dermatologic manifestations of cancer. These conditions are not directly caused by tumor metastasis, but rather the malignancies produce hormones and other proteins which act to disrupt the body's homeostasis, thereby causing symptoms. The neurological complications of PNS are the result of an immune response to tumor antigens. PNS have been associated with a variety of cancers, such as genitourinary, ovarian, and breast, but are most commonly associated with neuroendocrine tumors. These syndromes can even occur before the primary tumor is identified. Historically, these conditions were considered rare, but given the difficulties with diagnosis, the exact prevalence is unknown. This book focuses on the symptoms, diagnosis, and treatment of PNS. More specifically, it discusses current concepts in common PNS; cutaneous PNS and skin features of internal malignancy; PNS in patients with malignancies of the genitourinary tract; PNS polyneuropathies; the correction of cancer-related anemai with oxyresveratrol; and PNS associated with lung cancer.

Chapter I – Paraneoplastic Syndromes (PNS) are a group of disorders that cause endocrinologic, hematologic, neurologic, and dermatologic manifestations of cancer. These conditions are not directly caused by tumor metastasis, but rather the malignancies produce hormones and other proteins which act to disrupt the body's homeostasis, thereby causing symptoms. The neurological complications of PNS are the result of an immune response to tumor antigens. PNS have been associated with a variety of cancers, such as genitourinary, ovarian, and breast, but are most commonly associated with neuroendocrine tumors. These syndromes can even occur before the primary tumor is identified. Historically, these conditions were considered rare, but given the difficulties with diagnosis, the exact prevalence is unknown. The clinical signs and symptoms are often general or non-focal: nausea, vomiting, fatigue, weakness, mental status changes, neuropathy, hypertension, and rashes. These symptoms, even in an individual with a malignancy, can occur in a wide variety of diseases, thus making the diagnosis difficult. The diagnosis requires taking a careful history and physical, laboratory data, imaging, and often times will still be a diagnosis of exclusion. Even though diagnosis may be difficult, it is important as the clinician to maintain a high suspicion for PNS because in addition to the medical management of symptoms, the treatment of PNS often involves immunosuppression and treating the underlying malignancy. This chapter will focus on the symptoms, diagnosis and treatment of PNS and offer a review of the literature.

Chapter II – The skin plays a critical role in the detection of internal malignances and cutaneous lesions may represent the tip of the iceberg. The cutaneous features that can occur are numerous and heterogeneous, and many different etiologic mechanisms are represented, from direct tumor invasion of skin or distant metastases to a wide variety of inflammatory dermatoses that may occur as paraneoplastic phenomena.

Paraneoplastic syndromes are a group of clinical manifestations associated with a malignancy, but not directly related to the primary tumor itself or to its metastases.

Generally, the onset and course of the disease will closely correlate with the malignancy, as described in Curth's original criteria, although this is not always the case. Characteristically, they resolve with successful treatment of the primary tumor, and tend to recur with its relapse or the onset of metastases.

A uniform etiology for paraneoplastic cutaneous syndromes is unlikely, given the diversity of paraneoplastic manifestations. The pathogenesis is poorly understood, but may be related to the production of bioactive substances by or in response to the tumor, such as polypeptide hormones, hormone-like peptides, antibodies or immune complexes, cytokines, or growth factors.

In addition, there are a number of inherited syndromes that carry an increased risk of cutaneous as well as internal malignancies. Furthermore, there are another cutaneous signs and symptoms not included as paraneoplastic syndromes that could warning us in some particular situations. Increased clinician awareness and education regarding the associations between these lesions and internal malignancy will facilitate screening and early diagnosis.

This chapter reviews this wide range of cutaneous manifestations of internal malignancy, discusses their associations with neoplastic, and recommends appropriate evaluation in this setting.

Chapter III – Paraneoplastic syndromes may represent a major clinical problem also in patients with malignancies of the genitourinary tract. In this context, some paraneoplastic syndromes are of particular interest because of their clinically relevant incidence, such as endocrine paraneoplastic syndromes caused by inappropriate release of hormonal peptides, syndromes caused by inappropriate release of biologic amines, syndromes caused by inappropriate release of growth factors and renal cell carcinoma-related syndromes. The neuroendocrine differentiation of the tumour is often associated with paraneoplastic syndromes, especially endocrine syndromes.

Although with a low incidence, neurological paraneoplastic syndromes have been also reported in the published literature in association with genitourinary tumours. However, neurological syndromes are of clinical relevance because they may dominate the clinical picture in some patients and the diagnosis is often difficult due to the high index of suspicion needed to be recognized.

Renal cell carcinoma is the most frequent urological malignancy involved in paraneoplastic syndromes of urological interest. Prostate cancer is the second urological tumour associated with these syndromes. Bladder and testicular cancers, on the other hand, are less commonly associated with paraneoplastic manifestations.

Important technical advances in diagnostic tools have sensibly improved our ability to detect the primary tumours.

Generally, the radical therapy of the underlying cancer represent the most effective treatment strategy, although specific therapeutic options are available in particular clinical situations.

Chapter IV – Paraneoplastic neurologic syndromes are a heterogeneous group of neurologic disorders associated with systemic cancer and caused by mechanisms other than metastases, metabolic and nutritional deficits, infections, coagulopathy, or side effects of cancer treatment. These syndromes may affect any part of the nervous system from cerebral cortex to neuromuscular junction and muscle, either damaging one area or multiple areas.

The clinical importance of paraneoplastic polyneuropathies is high, as in most patients the neurologic symptoms are the presenting feature of an otherwise undiagnosed tumor. In addition, paraneoplastic polyneuropathies often cause severe and permanent neurologic morbidity. On the other hand, prompt recognition of this disorder may maximize the likelihood of successful tumor treatment and a favorable neurologic outcome.

For patients without a known neoplasm who present with a peripheral neuropathy, the likelihood of a paraneoplastic etiology is difficult to quantitate and depends on the particular clinical syndrome. For example, severe rapidly progressive sensory neuronopathy is much more likely to be paraneoplastic than a mild, distal, slowly progressive axonal polyneuropathy. Among the most common paraneoplastic polyneuropathies are included: a) subacute sensory neuronopathy, b) demyelinating polyneuropathies, c) autonomic insufficiency, d) motor neuronopathy, e) vasculitic neuropathy.

This review provides an update on the clinical, paraclinical and electrophysiological presentation of the most common paraneoplastic polyneuropathies and fresh insight to the pathomechanism of peripheral nerve injury.

Chapter V – It is well-known that malignant tumor exerts nonmetastatic systemic effects on organism caused the development of paraneoplastic syndrome (PNS). The symptomatic manifestations of PNS may pose the most troublesome and life threatening problems for cancer patients. Treatments of paraneoplastic conditions are frequently based on beneficial anti-cancer therapy. Unfortunately such therapy can not be carried out against resistant form of tumors and also in case of serious symptoms of PNS (paraneoplastic disorders of hemapoiesis, liver and kidney). Development of tumor-specific and/or tumor non-specific therapeutics against organism disorder PNS symptoms is of great importance to improve qualify of life, and in some cases, prolong life of cancer patients.

Despite the onrush of molecular biology and chemistry providing fast escalation of synthesized *de novo* drugs, plants still remain traditional sources of medicinal compounds. Widely distributed plant polyphenols are today among the most studied classes of phytochemicals.

In recent years stilbenes, naturally occurring polyphenolic com-pounds, have come to the attention because of their potential use as prophylactic and therapeutic agents in many diseases. The most well-known stilbenes are resveratrol and oxyresveratrol (OXY). Resveratrol, a representative of this group, has been widely investigated for its protecting and therapeutic effects against a number of pathological processes including cancer. Although OXY is characterized by better water solubility, higher bioavailability and less cytotoxicity (as compared to resveratrol) yet it is pharmacologically less investigated and the most study of OXY are applied to non-cancer diseases.

In this chapter the data concerning the pharmacological activity of OXY against both cancer-related anemia and tumor growth and metastasis are presented and discussed.

In order to evaluate an ability of OXY to correct cancer-related anemia without increasing risk of tumor progression the research was carried out using highly angiogenic and metastatic variant of Lewis lung carcinoma which growth in tumor-bearing mice is accompanied by an extensive manifestation of anemia and thrombopenia. Metronomic administration of OXY resulted in considerable elevation of erythrocyte counts, hemoglobin content and number of platelets.

At the same time the efficacy of OXY to inhibit tumor growth and metastasis has been revealed.

Chapter VI – A spectrum of paraneoplastic syndromes occur in 10-20% of patients with lung cancer, ranging from mild to severe manifestations including cutaneous, skeletal, neuromuscular, endocrine, hematological, renal, vascular, collagenous, metabolic and systemic features.

A paraneoplastic symptoms and signs occur distant from the primary tumor or metastasis, and are caused by the underlying pathogenic mechanisms which include immunologic cross-reaction of tumor associated antigens with normal tissue directed by antibody, or cellular cytotoxic response. Besides, production of systemic factors by the tumor, such as hormones, hormone-like peptides, cytokines and prostaglandins cause variety of paraneoplastic spectrum. However, all pathogenic mechanisms and some new paraneoplastic features associated with lung cancer are not yet fully understood and recognized.

Paraneoplastic extent of symptoms and signs may precede the diagnosis and be the first sign of underlying lung cancer, as well as the first sign of its recurrence; or may occur in the later phase of disease irrespectively of tumor mass.

The understanding and early recognition of paraneoplastic symptoms may speed-up the proper diagnosis and in some cases correspond with the therapy effect in the follow-up.

In: Paraneoplastic Syndromes
Editor: Lora H. Winter
ISBN: 978-1-63117-878-8

Chapter I

Current Concepts in Common Paraneoplastic Syndromes: Symptoms, Diagnosis and Treatment

*Candace Mainor, Ashiq Masood, Muddassir Shahdhar and Heather D. Mannuel**

Abstract

Paraneoplastic Syndromes (PNS) are a group of disorders that cause endocrinologic, hematologic, neurologic, and dermatologic manifestations of cancer. These conditions are not directly caused by tumor metastasis, but rather the malignancies produce hormones and other proteins which act to disrupt the body's homeostasis, thereby causing symptoms. The neurological complications of PNS are the result of an immune response to tumor antigens. PNS have been associated with a variety of cancers, such as genitourinary, ovarian, and breast, but are most commonly associated with neuroendocrine tumors. These syndromes can even occur before the primary tumor is identified.

* Corresponding Author: Heather D. Mannuel, MD, MBA, Assistant Professor of Medicine, Program Director, Oncology/ Hematology program, University of Maryland Greenebaum Cancer Center, 22. S Greene Street, Baltimore, MD 21201, Email: hmannuel@umm.edu, Phone: (410)328-2567.

Historically, these conditions were considered rare, but given the difficulties with diagnosis, the exact prevalence is unknown. The clinical signs and symptoms are often general or non-focal: nausea, vomiting, fatigue, weakness, mental status changes, neuropathy, hypertension, and rashes. These symptoms, even in an individual with a malignancy, can occur in a wide variety of diseases, thus making the diagnosis difficult. The diagnosis requires taking a careful history and physical, laboratory data, imaging, and often times will still be a diagnosis of exclusion. Even though diagnosis may be difficult, it is important as the clinician to maintain a high suspicion for PNS because in addition to the medical management of symptoms, the treatment of PNS often involves immunosuppression and treating the underlying malignancy. This chapter will focus on the symptoms, diagnosis and treatment of PNS and offer a review of the literature.

Introduction

Paraneoplastic Syndromes (PNS) are a group of disorders that cause endocrinologic, hematologic, neurologic, and dermatologic manifestations of cancer [1]. These conditions are not directly caused by tumor metastasis or by invasion of the tumor, but rather the malignancies produce hormones and other proteins which act to disrupt the body's homeostasis, thereby causing symptoms. PNS occurs in 7%-15% of people diagnosed with cancer [2], although this is up for debate depending on what clinical syndromes are considered PNS. There is no data on whether PNS affect gender or ethnic groups differently. PNS have been associated with a variety of cancers, such as genitourinary, ovarian, and breast, but are most commonly associated with neuroendocrine tumors. These syndromes can even occur before the primary tumor is identified, and thus it is important to recognize these disorders so that the patient can be evaluated for a malignancy.

Endocrinologic Manifestations of PNS

The endocrinologic manifestations of PNS are the result of the ectopic production of molecules in an unregulated manner. In addition, PNS may result from tissues producing molecules that they may have been producing at an early cellular stage [1]. Examples which result in clinically significant diseases are the ectopic production of parathyroid hormone-related protein

(PTHrp) which results in hypercalcemia, vasopressin which results in SIADH, ACTH which results in Cushing's disease and IGF-II which results in hypoglycemia. These diseases result in significant morbidity and mortality and thus prompt recognition of these syndromes will allow for early evaluation and diagnosis of a malignancy. It is equally important to recognize that these syndromes can occur with other disease processes, and thus will necessitate a thorough history, physical and laboratory evaluation.

Hypercalcemia

Hypercalcemia is defined as serum calcium level greater than 10.5mg/dL. It can be caused by a variety of medical conditions including, but not limited to, primary hyperparathyroidism, sarcoidosis, vitamin D intoxication, and medications. In cancer patients, hypercalcemia is typically caused by increased bone resorption [3], although it may also be caused by the overproduction of PTHrp produced by the tumor cells. PTHrp, which is structurally similar to PTH, binds to the PTH receptor[i] and causes expression of RANK ligand, which in turnbinds to the RANK receptor which causes osteoclast differentiation and bone resorption. [3] Hypercalcemia is typically associated with squamous cell carcinomas of the head and neck, lung, breast [4, 5] gastroenterological (GI), and genitourinary (GU) cancers[i] and this diagnosis can precede the diagnosis of the malignancy. Most patients do not experience symptoms unless the serum calcium level is over 12.0mg/dL. Patients may experience lethargy, dehydration, and changes in mental status. The diagnosis is typically made when a patient has a serum calcium level greater than 14mg/dL in the setting of a known malignancy, and after other causes have been excluded. Additionally, other laboratory data may aid in the diagnosis such as ionized calcium [5]. Hypercalcemia is usually accompanied with hypercalciuria. Patients will also present with hypophosphatemia, low serum PTH levels, and high serum PTHrP levels (although this only needs to be measured if the clinical presentation is not clear [6]), and normal or low serum calcitriol levels [4]. The ultimate goal of treatment is to remove calcium from the body [1, 6] but temporizing measures may be needed. In the short term, intravenous fluids can be given to dilute the calcium [1]. These patients should also receive phosphorus repletion. Once the patient has been given intravenous fluids, loop diuretics can be used to aid in the excretion of calcium in urine [1, 6]. If a patient has severe hypercalcemia and/or is symptomatic (e.g., altered mental status), bisphosphonates or prednisone may be given to further reduce calcium levels. If these measures fail, dialysis is another treatment possibility. The only long-term solution is to treat the underlying malignancy [1].

Syndrome of Inappropriate Antidiuretic Hormone Secretion (SIADH)

Tumor associated SIADH is characterized by euvolemic, hypotonic hypnonatremia caused by increased free-water resorption by the kidney[1]. SIADH is caused by excess production of vasopressin or ADH from the tumors. Tumors normally associated with this condition are lung cancer, particularly small cell lung cancer, as well as GI, GU and ovarian cancers. Patients will often experience vague symptoms like fatigue, headache, nausea, weakness, mental status changes or confusion. More severe hypnonatremia may cause coma, seizures, and death [7, 8]. Many patients with hyponatremia are asymptomatic because it develops slowly over time, giving the body time to compensate. The diagnosis involves documenting hyponatremia in a euvolemic patient with a known malignancy. It is important to recognize that even in patients with known malignancy, other medical problems can cause hyponatremia such as pneumonia and medications [1]. Other lab values may aide in the diagnosis, including low serum osmolality and increased urine osmolality. The optimal treatment for this condition is to treat the underlying malignancy. Until then, the goal should be to correct the hyponatremia. Initially, the patient can be placed on fluid restriction. It is important to correct the serum hyponatremia in a slow manner to avoid adverse events such as central pontine myelinolysis [1]. Typically, sodium should be corrected by 1 mmol/L per hour [9, 10]. In severe cases where patients are extremely symptomatic, they may require transfer to an intensive care unit for hypertonic saline administration. If patients have failed fluid restriction and if they are not symptomatic, other agents can be used to correct the hyponatremia. Available agents include vasopressin receptor antagonists (available in parenteral and oral formulations) and demeclocycline [7]. Unfortunately, it is not possible to estimate how fast these agents will correct the sodium, so they should be administered in a hospital with frequent monitoring of the basic metabolic panel [7].

Cushing Disease

Cushing disease is caused by hypercortisolism. Hypercortisolism is caused by excess production of ACTH from tumor cells. In this disease, the tumor produces excess proopiomelanocortin (POMC) which is then cleaved to ACTH [3].

This disease is most commonly associated with small cell lung cancer, but also with pancreatic islet tumors, thymic, and medullary thyroid carcinomas [1]. Patients present with hypertension, hypokalemia, fluid retention, metabolic alkalosis, easy bruising, and glucose intolerance. It is important to rule out other causes of hypercortisolism as elevated ACTH levels can be associated with other disease processes such as pituitary tumors or adrenal disease [3]. The diagnosis is made by measuring a urine free-cortisol level which will be greater than two times normal, and/or elevated serum ACTH levels, typically greater than 100pg/ml [3]. Lastly, a dexamethasone suppression test can be helpful in making this diagnosis because in a patient with ectopic production of ACTH, the serum cortisol will not be suppressed. The treatment for this condition involves treating the underlying malignancy with surgery and/or chemotherapy [3]. The physician will have to also manage the associated symptoms such as hypertension and diabetes.

Hypoglycemia

Hypoglycemia is defined as blood glucose less than 60mg/dL. This is a dangerous condition and can result in death. Hypoglycemia can be caused by many medical problems such as islet cell tumors producing insulin [3], impaired gluconeogenesis, and by ectopic production of IGF-II [11]. Insulin produced by islet cell tumors is only significant when the tumor burden is high. Similarly, impaired gluconeogenesis only occurs when the tumor burden in the liver is high [3]. Excess IGF-II activates the insulin receptor which leads to hypoglycemia. The ectopic production of IGF-II is associated with sarcomas, liver, kidney, GI, prostate, and mesenchymal tumors. Symptoms of hypoglycemia include nausea, vomiting, tremors, and confusion. The diagnosis of this condition involves documenting low serum glucose levels and low serum IGF-I levels. Additionally, there will be low to normal levels of insulin, proinsulin, and C-peptide. It is important to monitor glucose levels carefully and replete glucose as needed to prevent adverse events. In certain circumstances, glucagon can be administered[3]. The ultimate goal of therapy is to treat the underlying malignancy.

Hematologic Manifestations of PNS

The Hematologic manifestations of PNS are less common then endocrinologic manifestations and often do not result in clinically significant symptoms. They are usually diagnosed on routine lab work after the initial diagnosis of the malignancy. These syndromes are not associated with significant morbidity or mortality and usually do not require treatment.

Anemia

Anemia is defined as hemoglobin level less than 12.5g/dL in adults. The most common manifestation associated with malignancy is anemia. This anemia tends to be normochromic and normocytic and is usually caused by tumor cells infiltrating the bone marrow, causing decreased red blood cell production. Alternatively, anemia can occur secondary to red cell aplasia, which is defined as decreased maturation of red blood cells. This has been associated with the diagnosis of thymoma, but can also be associated with leukemias and lymphomas [7]. The mechanism of action is thought to be secondary to an autoimmune attack on the red blood cell [7, 12]. There are many non-paraneoplastic causes of anemia, including blood loss and destruction of red blood cells, and it is important to rule those out before making this diagnosis. Patients can present with no symptoms or complain of fatigue and in extreme cases, shortness of breath. The diagnosis is made when a complete blood count reveals anemia in the absence of other causes to explain the anemia. In addition, a bone marrow biopsy will reveal very low levels of erythroblasts [7]. Therapy involves treating the underlying malignancy, and in some cases, using immunosuppressive therapy [7, 12, 13].

Erythrocytosis

Erythrocytosis is an increase in the hematocrit to greater than 52% in men and 48% in women. In the setting of a malignancy, it is caused by tumor production of erythropoietin [1, 7]. It is associated with several malignancies, but renal cell carcinoma is the most common. Patients are usually asymptomatic, but symptoms can be vague and include headache, shortness of breath, and dizziness. Diagnosis is made by increased hematocrit, increase in red cell mass, and elevated levels of erythropoietin [1]. Treatment, as with most PNS syndromes, involves treating the underlying malignancy [1]. In the interim, or if the malignancy is unable to be treated, another option is to use phlebotomy to control the erythrocytosis [1, 13].

Granulocytosis

Granulocytosis is an increase in the white blood cell count, typically 12x10^9/L to up to 50x10^9/L [7, 14]. This condition is thought to result from tumor production of G-CSF and IL-6. This is associated with lung cancer, typically large cell lung cancer [7, 15], GI, GU, and ovarian cancers. This is largely a clinical diagnosis, because although serum blood tests are helpful, other causes of leukocytesis such as infection must first be ruled out. This is not a clinically significant problem, as most mature white blood cells are unlikely to cause leukostasis and hence most patients are asymptomatic. The treatment for granulocytosis is to treat the underlying malignancy[1].

Thrombocytosis

Thrombocytosis is an increased production of platelets, typically to values greater than 400 x 10^9/L [1, 7]. The etiology is not been completely elucidated[1], but is thought to be secondary to tumor secretion of IL-6 [7, 16]. Thrombocytosis is associated with lung cancer, GI, and breast cancer [1]. Patients are typically asymptomatic. Although certain serum blood tests such as IL-5 levels may be useful, this is usually a diagnosis of exclusion as other causes such as infection must first be ruled out. The therapy for thrombocytosis is to treat the underlying malignancy, and in the short term, this condition does not require temporizing measures [1, 7].

Eosinophilia

Eosinophilia is an increased production of eosinophils detected in the serum. Increased production of eosinophils is likely caused by production of

IL-3, IL-5 and CM-CSF [17, 18]. Eosinophilia is associated with leukemias and lymphomas. These patients may present with shortness of breath and wheezing, and may display eosinophilia on blood tests [7]. The treatment for this PNS is treating the underlying malignancy and symptomatic treatment of the side effects, with steroids [7, 1, 13].

Thrombosis

Thrombosis is inflammation of a vein secondary to a clot. Cancer patients typically develop this problem because they are immobilized and they are in a hypercoagulable state [1]. This can present before, during, or after the diagnosis of the malignancy. Symptoms can include erythematous, swollen, and painful extremities. If the patient subsequently develops a pulmonary embolism, they can present with tachycardia, shortness of breath, and pleuritic chest pain [1]. The diagnosis is made after venous duplex ultrasound detects a clot. Pulmonary embolism can be detected by computed tomography angiography (CTA). Thrombosis is treated with anticoagulation, typically a low molecular weight heparin LMWH,[1] as the CLOT Trial revealed that LMWH was superior to warfarin in preventing recurrent venous thromboembolism events [19].

The Neurologic Manifestations of PNS

The neurological complications of PNS are the result of an immune response to tumor antigens, and they involve a complicated interaction between the humoral and cellular immune systems [20]. This results in antibodies secreted by the tumor against neural antigens. The most common antibodies are anti-Hu, anti-Yo and anti CV2/CRMP5 [21, 22], but there are other antibodies against receptors on the synaptic cell membrane [21], that are also associated with PNS. The most common one in that category is anti-N-methy-D-aspartic acid (NMDA) [21]. Historically, these conditions were considered rare, but given the difficulties with diagnosis, the exact prevalence is unknown. It is thought that PNS that involves the neurologic system may only occur in 0.01% of patients [23]. More often than not, in PNS of the neurological system, the symptoms are often clinically significant, even before the diagnosis of cancer [21]. The symptoms vary and affect any part of the neurological system. In 2004, Graus et al. recommended the development of more defined diagnostic criteria for PNS [24]. They suggested that PNS should be defined as "definite" or "possible", but while still recognizing classic PNS syndromes (sub acute cerebellar degeneration, encephalitis, limbic encephalitis, opsoclonus-myoclonus, sensory neuronopathy, Lambert-Eaton mysthenic syndrome, and Dermatomyositis) and non-classical PNS [24]. The criteria for "definite PNS" include: " 1. A classic syndrome and cancer within five years of neurologic disorder, 2. Non-classical syndrome that resolves/improves after cancer treatment, but without immunotherapy, 3. Non-classical syndrome with onconeural antibodies and cancer within five years of diagnosis, and 4. No cancer, but neurological syndrome well characterized with onconueral antibodies" [24]. "Possible PNS" is defined as: "1. Classical syndrome, but no antibodies, and no cancer, 2. Neurological syndrome with partially characterized onconeural antibodies and no cancer, and 3. A non-classical syndrome, no onconeural antibodies, and cancer within two years of diagnosis" [24].

Neurological PNS can cause a wide variety of symptoms that can be attributed to other diagnoses, such as CNS infection, medication overdoses, and electrolyte abnormalities. To diagnose this condition, it is imperative to gather a good history/physical and initial laboratory data. These patients often receive an MRI and lumbar puncture to rule out other disease processes. Usually, the MRI will be normal and the cerebral spinal fluid analysis will be non-specific, often revealing pleocytosis and increased protein [21, 25]. Most often the CSF is normal, but at times antibodies will be detected. If a patient is diagnosed with one of the syndromes below, then a thorough investigation for a malignancy must take place.

Treatment and response are largely dependent on whether the syndromes are associated with onconeural antibodies or neuronal cell antibodies. Generally, syndromes secondary to neuronal cell antibodies respond better to treatment [21] as compared to antibodies against anti-Hu. The mainstay of therapy is to treat the malignancy, either with surgery or chemotherapy. Immunosuppressive therapy may have to be used as well [26]. Therapies used include steroids, IVIG, plasmapheresis [27], and cyclophosphamide as a second line agents [21]. The neurologic manifestations of PNS discussed in greater detail below.

Paraneoplastic Encephalomyelitis (EM)

Paraneoplastic encephalomyelitis is characterized by diffuse dysfunction in many parts of the nervous system [23] and is the result of inflammation in the brain [22]. It presents in a subacute manner and patients can present with a wide range of symptoms including, but not limited to, confusion, seizures, autonomic dysfunction, myoclonus, gait dysfunction, dysarthria, and dysphagia [20]. Paraneoplastic EM is most commonly secondary to small cell lung cancer (SCLC), but it has been found in other malignancies such as breast, ovarian, esophageal, and kidney cancer [22] and it is associated with anti-Hu, anti-CV2, anti-Ma1 antibodies [28, 29]. It has been observed that treatment of the tumor helps to stabilize the disease [30]. Patient with this condition have been treated with immunotherapy, with varying results.

Limbic Encephalitis

Paraneoplastic Limbic encephalitis is characterized by memory problems, personality changes/behavior problems and/or depression [21] caused by an inflammatory condition in the limbic system [22]. The onset of symptoms can occur within days or up to three months [24]. It is associated with SCLC, testicular cancer, Hodgkin's lymphoma and thymoma [31]. The diagnosis should involve a thorough history and physical and MRI that reveals intensity in the temporal lobes on T1 and FLAIR [32]. The antibodies associated with it are anti-Hu, anti-MA2, anti-amphiphysin, Anti CV2/CRMP5 [22], and anti-NMDA. In patients with disease associated with NMDA, patients may also present with fever, nausea, vomiting, and headache [32, 33]. Additionally, patients with neuronal cell surface antibodies, may have a less severe encephalitis but may present with symptoms such as hyponatremia and monoclonus [21].

Paraneoplastic Cerebella Ataxia (PCA)

Cerebellar degeneration from PNS is characterized by loss of purkinje neurons which lead to cerebellar dysfunction [34]. The symptoms that can accompany this disease include double vision, dizziness, nausea, ataxia, dysarthria and dysphagia [20]. The malignancies associated with this are ovarian, breast, Hodgkin's and SCLC [20]. The diagnosis is largely clinical and includes development of symptoms in less than 12 weeks in the setting of a normal MRI [23]. In later stages of the disease, a MRI may reveal cerebellar atrophy [34]. This diagnosis is associated with certain autoantibodies, including Anti-Yo and anti-Tr. CV2-ab, Zic4-Ab, Ma2-Ab and VGCC-Ab are also associated [34, 35, 36]. Unfortunately, the treatment is not well elucidated [20].

Opsoclonus-Myoclonus (OM)

Paraneoplastic opsoclonus-myoclonus syndrome is characterized by large amplitude, fast eye movements in all directions [20]. This is often accompanied by myoclonus in the torso and extremities [34]. The symptoms that patients present with include ataxia, hypotonia, and behavioral changes. The cancers associated with this disease include neuroblastoma [34, 37], breast cancer [34, 38] and SCLC [34]. The diagnosis involves attaining a thorough history and physical, and identifying antibodies (although these do not have to be present to make the diagnosis [34]). The treatment for this syndrome is to treat the underlying malignancy [22], but often even after treatment, the patient will need immunosuppressive therapies. Therapies that have been tried include steroids, plasma exchange, IVIG, and rituximab [20].

Sensory Neuronopathy (PSN)

PNS sensory neuronopathy is characterized by sensory deficits, specifically decreased proprioception with painful paresthesias in the extremities [21], and choreoathetotic-like movements [21]. It is caused by inflammatory infiltrates. [22] The diagnosis includes: subacute onset, asymmetry of symptoms, symptoms in upper extremities, and loss of proprioception, electrophysiological studies showing involvement of sensory fibers and no sensory action potentials [23]. It is associated with SCLC and anti-Hu, anti-amphiphysin, and anti-CV2/CRMP5 [21]. This usually does not improve after treating the underlying malignancy and immunotherapy may stabilize the disease [22].

Lambert-Eaton Myasthenic Syndrome (LEMS)

Lambert-Eaton Myasthenic syndrome is an autoimmune disease in which there is impaired release of acetylcholine (Ach) from the presynaptic motor nerve resulting in autonomic dysfunction, decrease in reflexes [22], and muscle weakness [34]. The patients usually present with muscle weakness, proximal greater than distal [22] It is usually associated with SCLC, and often precedes the diagnosis [34]. This is diagnosed by demonstrating the presence of autoantibodies to the voltage-gated calcium channel and electromyographic findings of decreased muscle potential amplitudes [22]. The treatment involves treating the underlying malignancy; in cases of severe weakness, immunotherapy can be used [39].

The Dermatologic Manifestations of PNS

When a patient presents with these manifestations, it is important to gather enough clinical information to discern if the presentation is a benign dermatologic disease or a result of a malignancy, in which case further work up and diagnostic testing will have to be completed.

Malignant Acanthosis Nigricans (AN)

The clinical characteristics of this disease include velvety, hyperpigmented plaques that appear on the skin in the neck, axillary, umbilical, and genitals [40]. Oral papillomatous areas can also develop on the mucosal surfaces of the body [40, 41]. This is most commonly associated with GI cancers [41], but can be present in other conditions. Similarly, Tripe palms, characterized by thickening of the epidermal layers of the palms of the hands with mesh-like appearance and deep sulci, are a feature of acanthosis nigricans [40, 41, 42]. Tripe palms are associated with lung cancer [40], but tripe palms with AN are associated with squamous cell carcinoma and gastric adenocarcinoma [40]. The etiology is not well elucidated, but it is thought that a ligand binds to epidermal growth factor to produce the disease [40, 42, 43]. The diagnosis is made largely on clinical appearance and skin biopsy. The skin biopsy of this lesion will reveal hyperkeratosis and hypergranulosis [40]. The treatment is largely symptomatic and topical retinoids are often used [40].

Acquired Ichthyosis

Acquired Ichthyosis is characterized by an erythematous, pruritic plate-like symmetric scaling rash on the body. It usually spares the face and neck, and preferentially affects the lower limbs compared to the upper limbs [44, 45]. It is largely a clinical diagnosis based on a thorough history, but a skin biopsy can be helpful. It will reveal acanthosis with laminated hyperkeratosis, and no inflammatory infiltrates in the dermis or epidermis [46]. It is associated with lymphoma and other malignancies [46] like multiple myeloma (MM), Kaposi's sarcoma, Leiomosarcoma, and gynecological cancers [44, 47]. Treatment involves treating the underlying malignancy and symptomatic relief with topical agents.

Acrokeratosis Paraneoplastica

Acrokeratosis paraneoplastica is a skin manifestation of a malignancy that is characterized by psoriasis-like erythematous plaques on the acral surfaces of the hands, feet, elbows, knees and ears [41]. It can also progress to the extremities [40]. The nails can be discolored with ridges and onycholysis [40, 48]. This is associated with squamous cell carcinoma of the lung and GI systems. The diagnosis is largely clinical, but skin biopsy can reveal perivascular lymphohistiocytic infiltration, hyperkeratosis, and acanthosis [40], which are nonspecific findings. Treatment involves identifying the underlying malignancy and treating that appropriately. Retinoid therapy can be used if the malignancy cannot be treated.

Extramammary Paget Disease

Extramammary Paget disease is an intraepithelial adenocarcinoma usually characterized by a pruritic eczema like lesion around the anus [40]. The patient may complain of problems with defecation, discharge or a mass near the anus [40, 49]. The diagnosis is made by skin biopsy which will show large round cells with a large nucleus and vacuolated cytoplasm [40, 49, 50]. This is associated with anorectal carcinoma, although this can present in the absence of another malignancy. Treatment involves resection of the anal lesion. If the lesion is associated with an anorectal carcinoma, that will have to be treated as well [49].

Florid Cutaneous Papillomatosis

Florid cutaneous papillomatosis is characterized by skin-colored papillomas, or "wart-like" lesions in the groin, perianal, and axillary regions [51]. The diagnosis is largely based on the clinical presentation and is associated with gastric adenocarcinoma, gynecological malignancies, GU malignancies, and lung cancer. The skin biopsy may reveal acathosis orpapillomatosis [52]. The pathophysiology is not well elucidated, but it is thought to arise as a result of the malignancy secreting growth factors [52]. Treatment involves treating the underlying malignancy. These lesion also respond to retinoid therapy and topical agents [52, 53].

Leser-Trelat Sign

Leser-Trelat is characterized by seborrheic keratosis on the chest and back that eventually progresses to cover the whole body [40, 65]. This is associated with adenocarcinomas of the GI tract, but can also be associated with breast cancer and AML [40, 54]. The diagnosis is largely clinical, but if a patient has a sudden onset of severe seborrheic keratosis, then the physician should evaluate for a malignancy. A skin biopsy will show EGFR staining in the upper epidermal layer and the keratinocytes [40]. Usually treating the underlying malignancy will result in resolution of the lesions [55].

Dermatomyositis

Dermatomyositis is an inflammatory myopathy which results in proximal muscle weakness and skin lesions [40]. The skin lesions are erythematous maculo-papular lesions [41, 56, 57]. It usually appears on the face, and may present as edema of the periorbital areas. The diagnostic criteria include skin lesions in the presence of proximal muscle weakness, inflammatory infiltrates present on muscle biopsy, elevation in skeletal muscle enzyme levels, abnormal electromyography study, and autoantibodies including Jo-1, Mi2, PL-7, OJ PL-12, or SRP [41, 58]. It is often associated with adenocarcinomas of the colon, lung, and stomach.

Multicentric Reticulohistiocytosis

Multicentric reticulohistiocytosis is a syndrome that is characterized by painful flesh-colored nodules on the skin, bones, and mucosa [59, 60]. These nodules grow together to form a "cobblestone" pattern [59]. It is associated with gynecological cancers, AML, MDS, thyroid cancer, GI adenocarcinoma, lung squamous cell carcinoma, and GU carcinoma [59], as well as other benign medical conditions. The exact pathophysiology is unknown, but this disease might be a manifestation of a macrophage disorder [59]. Typically, patients first present with constitutional symptoms and joint problems, such as erosive arthritis, and then go on to develop skin nodules. In addition, the patient may have other systemic involvement such as pulmonary fibrosis [59, 61]. This is extremely rare, but has been described in a case report. The diagnosis is based on the clinical presentation. Biopsy of the nodules may reveal histiocytes with multinucleated giant cells and eosinphilic cytoplasm which is periodic acid Schiff positive [59]. Treatment includes treating the underlying malignancy/medical condition. Other agents such as oral steroids and non-steroidal anti-inflammatory drugs can be used [59, 62]. There is other data to support the use of DMARDS and TNF-alpha inhibitors [59].

Necrolytic Migratory Erythema

Necrolytic migratory erythema is characterized by erythematous, painful, pruritic lesions with blisters which eventually crust over and cause hyperpigmentation [40]. They mostly occur in the groin, abdomen, perineum, and around the mouth. Other associated symptoms include angular chelitis and alopecia [40]. It is associated with a glucagon-secreting pancreatic alpha cell tumor, but often precedes the diagnosis. The etiology is unknown. The diagnosis is largely clinical, but biopsy may be helpful. The histology will reveal necrosis, keratinocytes with vacuolar degeneration, neutrophils, and parakeratosis [40]. Also present in the dermis are histiocytic and perivascular lymphocytic infiltration [40]. Although these skin manifestations can be associated with benign diseases, the presence of this skin finding should alert the physician to evaluate for malignancy. The treatment for this involves treating the underlying malignancy or medical problem.

Sweet's Syndrome

Sweet's syndrome is characterized by erythematous and painful nodules on the upper extremities, head and neck [55]. In addition to the cutaneous signs, the patients may present with fever. It is largely a clinical diagnosis but skin biopsy may reveals neutrophilic infiltrates in the dermis [55]. It is associated with AML and myelodysplastic syndrome (MDS), but has been observed in solid malignancies [55]. This is usually treated with corticosteroids [63, 55].

Paraneoplastic Pemphigus

Paraneoplastic pemphigus is a bullous disease secondary to autoantibodies against proteins in the keratinocytes [41]. Clinically, patients can have papules, vesicles, or pruritic plaques. Patients may experience oral inflammation or stomatitis that may also affect the esophagus [64]. The other cutaneous manifestations vary greatly. Diagnostic criteria include IgG and C3 deposition in the intraepidermal and or the basal membrane, bullous eruption on skin and mucous membranes (including the mouth, eye, and genital region), intraepidermal acanthyolysis and dyskeratosis with vacuolar changes observed on histopathological examination, and autoantibodies against 190, 210, 230, and 250 kDa antigens [41]. This has been associated with CLL, lymphoma, and sarcomas.

Carcinoid Syndrome

The symptoms of carcinoid syndrome are a result of tumor secretion of serotonin [55]. Typical symptoms associated with this include flushing of the skin, which can be limited to face, or more extensive and involve the entire body [40]. This continued flushing may lead to rosacea [65]. Diarrhea and shortness of breath may also be present in these patients [55]. Different types of tumors are associated with a different degree of flushing. Other cutaneous manifestations of carcinoid tumors can be scleroderma. It is diagnosed with a 24 hour 5-hydroxyindoleacetic acid test [55]. The treatment includes treating the underlying malignancy/surgical removal of the tumor [55], niacin supplementation, subcutaneous octreotide and steroids [40].

Hypertrichosis Lanuginosa

Hypertrichosis lanuginose is characterized by the formation of thin, unpigmented hairs on the skin, mainly the ears and face [41], but may also progress to the whole body. Associated symptoms include: diarrhea, weight loss, inflammation in the corners of the mouth [55, 64]. It often precedes the diagnosis of the malignancy and is associated with colorectal cancer, breast cancer, and lung cancer. It affects women greater than men [41], but thus far the exact pathophysiology has not been defined.

Peutz-Jeghers Syndrome

Peutz-Jeghers syndrome is an autosomal dominant disease defined by mucocutaneous hyperpigmented lesions and hamartomatouspolyposis in the GI tract [40]. The cutaneous lesions are characterized by pigmented macules that occur on the lips, labia, eyes and anus [41]. It is associated with gastric and breast cancers. The diagnosis requires having hamartomatous polyps, a family history of the disease, and skin lesions [40]. If a patient presents to his clinician with the hyperpigmented skin lesions, they should be screened for cancer because they are at increased risk [66].

References

[1] Jameson JL, Longo DL. Chapter 100. Paraneoplastic Syndromes: Endocrinologic/Hematologic. In: Fauci AS, Jameson JL, Longo DL, Hauser SL, eds. *Harrison's Principles of Internal Medicine*. 18th ed. New York: McGraw-Hill; 2012. http://www.accesspharmacy.com/content.aspx?aID=9116875. Accessed November 18, 2013.

[2] Richardson GE, Johnson BE. Paraneoplastic syndromes in lung cancer. *Curr Opin Oncol*. 1992;4(2):323-333.

[3] Yeung SCJ GR. Endocrine paraneoplastic syndromes ("ectopic" hormone production). In: Kufe DW, Pollock RE, Weichselbaum RR, et al., ed. *Holland-frei cancer medicine*. 6th ed. BC Decker; 2003.

[4] Mundy GR, Edwards JR. PTH-related peptide (PTHrP) in hypercalcemia. *J Am Soc Nephrol*. 2008;19(4):672-675

[5] Powell GJ, Southby J, Danks JA, et al. Localization of parathyroid hormone-related protein in breast cancer metastases: Increased incidence in bone compared with other sites. *Cancer Res.* 1991;51(11):3059-3061.
[6] Stewart AF. Clinical practice. hypercalcemia associated with cancer. *N Engl J Med.* 2005;352(4):373-379.
[7] Pelosof LC, Gerber DE. Paraneoplastic syndromes: An approach to diagnosis and treatment. *Mayo Clin. Proc.* 2010;85(9):838-854.
[8] Raftopoulos H. Diagnosis and management of hyponatremia in cancer patients. *Support Care Cancer.* 2007;15(12):1341-1347.
[9] Ellison DH, Berl T. Clinical practice. the syndrome of inappropriate antidiuresis. *N. Engl. J. Med.* 2007;356(20):2064-2072.
[10] Adrogué HJ, Madias NE. Hyponatremia. *N. Engl. J. Med.* 2000;342(21):1581-1589.
[11] Rikhof B, de Jong S, Suurmeijer AJ, Meijer C, van der Graaf WT. The insulin-like growth factor system and sarcomas. *J. Pathol.* 2009;217(4):469-482.
[12] Sawada K, Hirokawa M, Fujishima N. Diagnosis and management of acquired pure red cell aplasia. *Hematol. Oncol. Clin. North Am.* 2009;23(2):249-259.
[13] DeVita V, Lawrence T, Rosenberg S. Hematologic manifestations of cancer. In: *DeVita hellmanand rosenberg's cancer: Principles & practice of oncology.* Lippincott Williams & Wilkins; Lippincott Williams & Wilkins:2346-2348.
[14] Shoenfeld Y, Tal A, Berliner S, Pinkhas J. Leukocytosis in non hematological malignancies--a possible tumor-associated marker. *J. Cancer Res. Clin. Oncol.* 1986;111(1):54-58.
[15] Ascensao JL, Oken MM, Ewing SL, Goldberg RJ, Kaplan ME. Leukocytosis and large cell lung cancer. A frequent association. *Cancer.* 1987;60(4):903-905
[16] Blay JY, Favrot M, Rossi JF, Wijdenes J. Role of interleukin-6 in paraneoplastic thrombocytosis. *Blood.* 1993;82(7):2261-2262.
[17] Walter R, Joller-Jemelka HI, Salomon F. Metastatic squamous cell carcinoma with marked blood eosinophilia and elevated serum interleukin-5 levels. *Exp. Hematol.* 2002;30(1):1-2.
[18] Anagnostopoulos GK, Sakorafas GH, Kostopoulos P, et al. Disseminated colon cancer with severe peripheral blood eosinophilia and elevated serum levels of interleukine-2, interleukine-3, interleukine-5, and GM-CSF. *J. Surg. Oncol.* 2005;89(4):273-275.

[19] Lee AY, Levine MN, Baker RI, et al. Low-molecular-weight heparin versus a coumarin for the prevention of recurrent venous thromboembolism in patients with cancer. *N. Engl. J. Med.* 2003;349(2):146-153.
[20] Dalmau J, Rosenfeld MR. Chapter 101. Paraneoplastic Neurologic Syndromes. In: Fauci AS, Jameson JL, Longo DL, Hauser SL, eds. *Harrison's Principles of Internal Medicine.* 18th ed. New York: McGraw-Hill; 2012. http://www.accesspharmacy.com/content.aspx?aID=9116986. Accessed November 18, 2013.
[21] Leypoldt F, Wandinger KP. Paraneoplastic neurological syndromes. *Clin. Exp. Immunol.* 2013.
[22] Braik T, Evans AT, Telfer M, McDunn S. Paraneoplastic neurological syndromes: Unusual presentations of cancer. A practical review. *Am. J. Med. Sci.* 2010;340(4):301-308.
[23] Darnell RB, Posner JB. Paraneoplastic syndromes involving the nervous system. *N. Engl. J. Med.* 2003;349(16):1543-1554.
[24] Graus F, Delattre JY, Antoine JC, et al. Recommended diagnostic criteria for paraneoplastic neurological syndromes. *J Neurol Neurosurg Psychiatry.* 2004;75(8):1135-1140.
[25] Psimaras D, Carpentier AF, Rossi C, PNS Euronetwork. Cerebrospinal fluid study in paraneoplastic syndromes. *J Neurol Neurosurg Psychiatry.* 2010;81(1):42-45. doi: 10.1136/jnnp.2008.159483; 10.1136/jnnp.2008.159483.
[26] Goldman L, Schafer A. Neurologic paraneoplastic syndromes. In: *Goldman;s cecil medicine.* 24th ed. Elsevier; 2012.
[27] Rosenfeld MR, Dalmau J. Diagnosis and management of paraneoplastic neurologic disorders. *Curr. Treat Options Oncol.* 2013;14(4):528-538.
[28] Graus F, Keime-Guibert F, Rene R, et al. Anti-hu-associated paraneoplastic encephalomyelitis: Analysis of 200 patients. *Brain.* 2001;124(Pt 6):1138-1148.
[29] Grisold W, Giometto B, Vitaliani R, Oberndorfer S. Current approaches to the treatment of paraneoplastic encephalitis. *Ther Adv. Neurol. Disord.* 2011;4(4):237-248.
[30] Keime-Guibert F, Graus F, Broet P, et al. Clinical outcome of patients with anti-hu-associated encephalomyelitis after treatment of the tumor. *Neurology.* 1999;53(8):1719-1723.
[31] Dalmau J, Rosenfeld MR. Paraneoplastic syndromes of the CNS. *Lancet Neurol.* 2008;7(4):327-340.

[32] McKeon A. Paraneoplastic and other autoimmune disorders of the central nervous system. *Neurohospitalist.* 2013;3(2):53-64.

[33] Grisold W, Giometto B, Vitaliani R, Oberndorfer S. Current approaches to the treatment of paraneoplastic encephalitis. *Ther Adv Neurol Disord.* 2011;4(4):237-248.

[34] Honnorat J, Antoine JC. Paraneoplastic neurological syndromes. *Orphanet J. Rare Dis.* 2007;2:22.

[35] Bataller L, Wade DF, Graus F, Stacey HD, Rosenfeld MR, Dalmau J. Antibodies to Zic4 in paraneoplastic neurologic disorders and small-cell lung cancer. *Neurology.* 2004;62(5):778-782.

[36] Shams'ili S, Grefkens J, de Leeuw B, et al. Paraneoplastic cerebellar degeneration associated with antineuronal antibodies: Analysis of 50 patients. *Brain.* 2003;126(Pt 6):1409-1418.

[37] Gambini C, Conte M, Bernini G, et al. Neuroblastic tumors associated with opsoclonus-myoclonus syndrome: Histological, immunohistochemical and molecular features of 15 italian cases. *Virchows Arch.* 2003;442(6):555-562.

[38] Luque FA, Furneaux HM, Ferziger R, et al. Anti-ri: An antibody associated with paraneoplastic opsoclonus and breast cancer. *Ann. Neurol.* 1991;29(3):241-251.

[39] Sanders DB. Lambert-eaton myasthenic syndrome: Diagnosis and treatment. *Ann N Y Acad Sci.* 2003;998:500-508.

[40] Shah KR, Boland CR, Patel M, Thrash B, Menter A. Cutaneous manifestations of gastrointestinal disease: Part I. *J. Am. Acad. Dermatol.* 2013;68(2):189.e1-21; quiz 210.

[41] Dourmishev LA, Draganov PV. Paraneoplastic dermatological manifestation of gastrointestinal malignancies. *World J. Gastroenterol.* 2009;15(35):4372-4379.

[42] Pentenero M, Carrozzo M, Pagano M, Gandolfo S. Oral acanthosis nigricans, tripe palms and sign of leser-trelat in a patient with gastric adenocarcinoma. *Int. J. Dermatol.* 2004;43(7):530-532.

[43] Stone SP, Buescher LS. Life-threatening paraneoplastic cutaneous syndromes. *Clin. Dermatol.* 2005;23(3):301-306.

[44] Patel N, Spencer LA, English JC,3rd, Zirwas MJ. Acquired ichthyosis. *J. Am. Acad. Dermatol.* 2006;55(4):647-656. doi: 10.1016/j.jaad.2006.04.047.

[45] Okulicz JF, Schwartz RA. Hereditary and acquired ichthyosis vulgaris. *Int. J. Dermatol.* 2003;42(2):95-98.

[46] Word AP, Cayce R, Pandya AG. Beware of underlying malignancy: Acquired ichthyosis. *Am. J. Med.* 2013.

[47] Flint GL, Flam M, Soter NA. Acquired ichthyosis. A sign of nonlymphoproliferative malignant disorders. *Arch. Dermatol.* 1975;111(11):1446-1447.

[48] Pecora AL, Landsman L, Imgrund SP, Lambert WC. Acrokeratosis paraneoplastica (bazex' syndrome). report of a case and review of the literature. *Arch. Dermatol.* 1983;119(10):820-826.

[49] Jabbar AS. Perianal extramammary paget's disease. *Eur. J. Surg. Oncol.* 2000;26(6):612-614.

[50] Stone SP, Buescher LS. Life-threatening paraneoplastic cutaneous syndromes. *Clin. Dermatol.* 2005;23(3):301-306.

[51] Csete B, Moezzi M, Lengyel Z, Hodosi B, Zombai E, Battyani Z. Florid cutaneous papillomatosis leading to social exclusion. *Br. J. Dermatol.* 2005;153(3):667-669.

[52] Klieb HB, Avon SL, Gilbert J, Sade S, Enepekides D. Florid cutaneous and mucosal papillomatosis: Mucocutaneous markers of an underlying gastric malignancy. *J. Clin. Oncol.* 2013;31(13):e218-9.

[53] Janniger EJ, Schwartz RA. Florid cutaneous papillomatosis. *J. Surg. Oncol.* 2010;102(6):709-712.

[54] Yavasoglu I, Kadikoylu G, Bolaman Z. The leser-trelat sign is a associated with acute myeloid leukemia. *Ann. Hematol.* 2011;90(3):363-010-1041 y.

[55] Pipkin CA, Lio PA. Cutaneous manifestations of internal malignancies: An overview. *Dermatol. Clin.* 2008;26(1):1-15, vii.

[56] Santmyire-Rosenberger B, Dugan EM. Skin involvement in dermatomyositis. *Curr. Opin. Rheumatol.* 2003;15(6):714-722.

[57] Dourmishev LA, Dourmishev AL, Schwartz RA. Dermatomyositis: Cutaneous manifestations of its variants. *Int. J. Dermatol.* 2002;41(10):625-630.

[58] Targoff IN, Miller FW, Medsger TA, Jr, Oddis CV. Classification criteria for the idiopathic inflammatory myopathies. *Curr. Opin Rheumatol.* 1997;9(6):527-535.

[59] Islam AD, Naguwa SM, Cheema GS, Hunter JC, Gershwin ME. Multicentric reticulohistiocytosis: A rare yet challenging disease. *Clin. Rev. Allergy Immunol.* 2013;45(2):281-289.

[60] Rao AG, Lakshmi TS, Vani V. Multicentric reticulohistiocytosis. *Indian J. Dermatol. Venereol. Leprol.* 2003;69(1):35-36.

[61] West KL, Sporn T, Puri PK. Multicentric reticulohistiocytosis: A unique case with pulmonary fibrosis. *Arch Dermatol.* 2012;148(2):228-232.

[62] Kaul A, Tolat SN, Belgaumkar V, Mhaske CB. Multicentric reticulohistiocytosis. *Indian J. Dermatol. Venereol. Leprol.* 2010; 76(4):404-407.

[63] Fett DL, Gibson LE, Su WP. Sweet's syndrome: Systemic signs and symptoms and associated disorders. *Mayo Clin. Proc.* 1995;70(3):234-240.

[64] Silva JA, Mesquita Kde C, Igreja AC, et al. Paraneoplastic cutaneous manifestations: Concepts and updates. *An. Bras. Dermatol.* 2013;88(1):9-22.

[65] Kleyn CE, Lai-Cheong JE, Bell HK. Cutaneous manifestations of internal malignancy: Diagnosis and management. *Am. J. Clin. Dermatol.* 2006;7(2):71-84.

[66] Taheri D, Afshar-Moghadam N, Mahzoni P, et al. Cancer problem in peutz-jeghers syndrome. *Adv. Biomed. Res.* 2013;2:35-9175.109721.

In: Paraneoplastic Syndromes
Editor: Lora H. Winter
ISBN: 978-1-63117-878-8

Chapter II

Cutaneous Paraneoplastic Syndromes and Skin Features of Internal Malignancy: Symptoms, Diagnosis and Treatment

*M. Yuste Chaves and M. González de Arriba**
Servicio de Dermatología
Hospital Clínico Universitario de Salamanca. España

Abstract

The skin plays a critical role in the detection of internal malignances and cutaneous lesions may represent the tip of the iceberg. The cutaneous features that can occur are numerous and heterogeneous, and many different etiologic mechanisms are represented, from direct tumor invasion of skin or distant metastases to a wide variety of inflammatory dermatoses that may occur as paraneoplastic phenomena.

Paraneoplastic syndromes are a group of clinical manifestations associated with a malignancy, but not directly related to the primary tumor itself or to its metastases.

* Correspondencia: Manuela Yuste Chaves y Marta González de Arriba, Servicio de Dermatología; Hospital Clínico Universitario de Salamanca; Paseo se San Vicente s/n, 37007 Salamanca; Correo electrónico: manuelayuste@hotmail.com y mgdearriba@yahoo.es

Generally, the onset and course of the disease will closely correlate with the malignancy, as described in Curth's original criteria, although this is not always the case. Characteristically, they resolve with successful treatment of the primary tumor, and tend to recur with its relapse or the onset of metastases.

A uniform etiology for paraneoplastic cutaneous syndromes is unlikely, given the diversity of paraneoplastic manifestations. The pathogenesis is poorly understood, but may be related to the production of bioactive substances by or in response to the tumor, such as polypeptide hormones, hormone-like peptides, antibodies or immune complexes, cytokines, or growth factors.

In addition, there are a number of inherited syndromes that carry an increased risk of cutaneous as well as internal malignancies. Furthermore, there are another cutaneous signs and symptoms not included as paraneoplastic syndromes that could warning us in some particular situations. Increased clinician awareness and education regarding the associations between these lesions and internal malignancy will facilitate screening and early diagnosis.

This chapter reviews this wide range of cutaneous manifestations of internal malignancy, discusses their associations with neoplastic, and recommends appropriate evaluation in this setting.

1. Introduction

The skin should never be overlooked in systemic diseases, as it is perhaps the most accessible organ in the body and his examination has the advantage of revealing important information about the patient's condition without requiring the use of invasive techniques. Furthermore, it can provide the first clues to a diagnosis in 1% of internal malignancies [1].

The cutaneous features that can occur are numerous and heterogeneous, and many different etiologic mechanisms are represented, from direct tumor invasion of skin or distant metastases to a wide variety of inflammatory dermatoses that may occur as paraneoplastic phenomena.

In the literature, most discussions of cutaneous manifestations of internal malignancy refer to classic paraneoplastic syndromes. However, there is a wide variety of skin conditions not strictly paraneoplastic that may indicate the presence of malignancy or an increased risk of developing cancer later in life, in certain contexts.

The aim of this review is to familiarize dermatologists and clinicians in general with cutaneous signs and symptoms that can help to lead an early diagnosis of an underlying malignancy.

2. Paraneoplastic Syndromes

In 1976, Curth [2] proposed a set of criteria for establishing a link between skin conditions and internal malignancies. Cutaneous manifestations are a reflection of the interaction between tumor cells (from the primary tumor or its metastases) and the host.

Paraneoplastic syndromes are a group of clinical manifestations associated with a malignancy, but not directly related to the primary tumor itself or to its metastases.

The current definition is a condition that precedes, occurs with, or develops after a malignancy in the absence of evident tumor cells (the tumor may be present but not yet diagnosed). The onset and course of the disease will closely correlate with the malignancy [3].

The pathogenesis is poorly understood, but may be related to the production of bioactive substances by or in response to the tumor, such as polypeptide hormones, hormone-like peptides, antibodies or immune complexes, cytokines, or growth factors [4].

Paraneoplastic syndromes are estimated to occur in 7% to 15% of malignancies [5]. Increased clinician awareness and education regarding the associations between these lesions and internal malignancy will facilitate screening and early diagnosis.

2.1. Autoimmune/Connective Tissue Disorders

Dermatomyositis

Approximately 15 to 50% of adult patients with dermatomyositis have an associated malignancy [6], which can appear before, during, or after diagnosis of the muscle disease, resulting in weakness of the proximal muscles.

Dermatomyositis presents as a scaly erythematous to violaceous eruption affecting photoexposed areas of the face, V of the neck, upper eyelids (heliotrope rash) with or without periorbital edema, extensor surfaces of the forearms, dorsum of the hands and knuckles (Figure 1), as well as interphalangeal areas of the fingers in addition to characteristic poikiloderma, and nail-fold telangiectasias. The development of vesiculobullous lesions [7] and associated cutaneous necrosis [8, 9] are closely associated with malignancy. Response to treatment with corticosteroids is poor and immunosuppressive therapy is necessary in these situations.

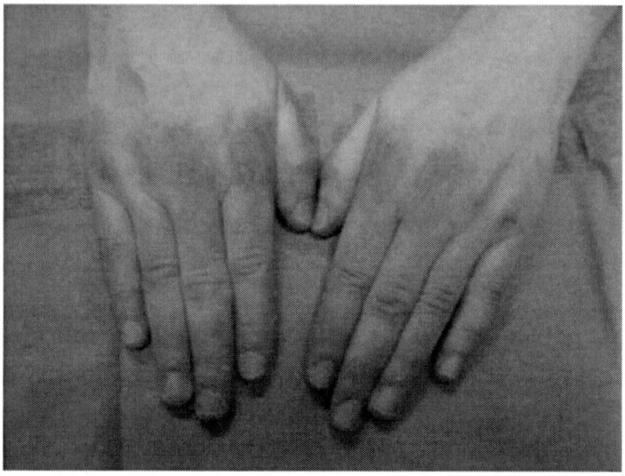

Figure 1. Dermatomyositis: erythematosquamous lesions on knuckels and finguers. Note hyperkeratotic nail-folds and periungueal telangiectasias.

The most common malignancies associated are ovarian and breast cancer in women [15] and lung and prostate cancer in men, although gastrointestinal, ureteral tumors [10], and nasopharyngeal carcinomas [11] are also seen, specially in chinese patients [12].

In paraneoplastic dermatomyositis, the cutaneous features tend to predominate over the myositis, female preponderance is seen and frequency increases with age. Adults diagnosed with dermatomyositis should undergo screening for an occult malignancy at least once a year for 3 years. This should include a thorough history and physical examination, standard laboratory investigations (biochemistry, liver function tests, full blood count with differential, urinalysis), chest x-ray, mamography and complete gynecologic examination in women, an age-appropiate cancer sreening (prostate-specific antigen test, fecal occult blood test) and any test directed toward abnormal symptoms or results [13-16]. In recent years, two new dermatomyositis-specific antibodies have been identified: CADM-140 in clinically amyopathic dermatomyositis (CADM), and anti-p155/p140, in cancer-associated dermatomyositis [17].

Juvenile dermatomyositis is rarely associated with an underlying malignancy [18, 19].

Paraneoplastic Autoinmune Multiorgan Syndrome/ Paraneoplastic Pemphigus

Paraneoplastic autoimmune multiorgan syndrome, first described as paraneoplastic pemphigus in 1990 [20], is an autoimmune blistering disease associated with neoplasia. Multiorgan system involvement, particularly of the bronchopulmonary tree, resulting on the substantial mortality associated [21].

Certain skin features differs from pemphigus vulgaris, namely persistent severe and painful stomatitis (Figure 2), involvement of other mucosa and the presence of polymorphous, vesicular or lichenoid skin eruptions that mimicking erythema multiforme exudativum, toxic epidermal necrolysis, erythroderma, or lichen planus. Acral lesions affecting the palms and soles and paronychia are common in paraneoplastic pemphigus but rarely observed in pemphigus vulgaris.

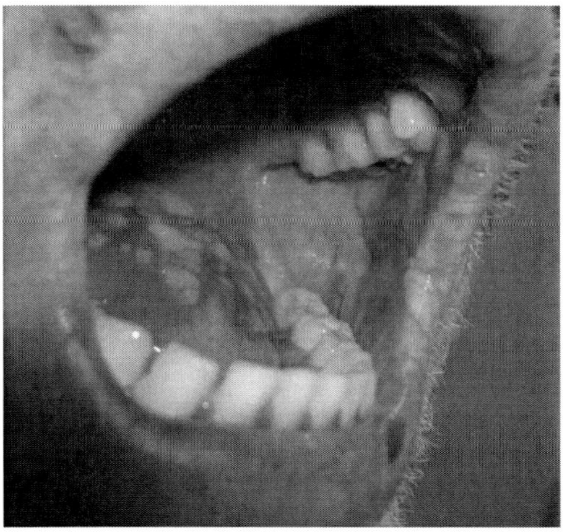

Figure 2. Severe stomatitis in paraneoplastic pemphigus.

Histopathology of skin lesions is as varied as the clinical features of the disease, showing interface dermatitis, vacuolization of the basement membrane, necrotic keratinocytes, suprabasal clefting, and acantholysis. The lichenoid inflammatory infiltrate may also be more predominant than in pemphigus vulgaris. Direct immu- nofluorescence testing reveals immunoglobulin G and C3 deposits in intercellular epidermal spaces and at the dermal-epidermal junction, but negative results are also a characteristic feature of paraneoplastic pemphigus [22]. Antigens targeted in paraneoplastic pemphigus include desmoplakin 1 (250 kDa), BP Ag1 (230 kDa), desmoplakin II (210 kDa), and periplakin (190 kDa) [6].

Pulmonary involvement is seen in approximately 30% of cases, manifesting as obstructive lung disease, progresses to bronchiolitis obliterans, and almost always results in death [3].

In two-thirds of cases, the underlying neoplasm is diagnosed before the onset of pemphigus. The most commonly associated malignancies are non-Hodgkin lymphoma, chronic lymphoid leukemia, and Castleman disease (which is more common in children). Less common malignancies are thymoma, Waldenström macroglobulinemia, lung adenocarcinoma, follicular lymphoma, retroperitoneal liposarcoma, and on occasions, hepatocellular carcinoma. Paraneoplastic autoimmune multiorgan syndrome has also been described in patients with cutaneous malignancies such as mycosis fungoides [3, 21, 23-25]. In the remaining one-third of cases, the neoplasm appears after the pemphigus lesions, hence the importance of screening for occult disease in patients with persistent mucosal lesions that are refractory to treatment.

Evaluation should include a detailed history and physical examination, as well as a complete blood count, serum protein electrophoresis, and computed tomography of the chest, abdomen, and pelvis. Complete dermatologic evaluation includes skin biopsies for routine histologic examination, DIF, serum testing for IIF, and immunoprecipitation studies.

There are no treatment guidelines for Paraneoplastic autoimmune multiorgan syndrome, but theoretically three treatment strategies are available. These options include: treatment of the underlying malignancy, treatment of the autoimmune process by reducing serum levels of autoantibodies, and suppression of the immune system [3].

Vasculitis

Vasculitis is associated with malignancies in between 3% and 8% of cases. Underlying infections, drugs, and rheumatologic disorders may also be associated. The clinical presentation is heterogeneous, with palpable purpura (Figure 3), papules, nodules, urticaria, necrosis, and ulceration. The presence of cutaneous vasculitis does not necessarily indicate a poor prognosis, and cutaneous lesions usually improve with treatment of the primary tumor [1, 13].

As paraneoplastic syndrome, 80% of patients have an associated hematological malignancy, while the remaining 20% have a solid tumor or an unknown origin neoplasia. The hematologic malignancies associated with vasculitis include hairy cell leukemia, chronic lymphoid leukemia, myeloma, Hodgkin and non-Hodgkin lymphoma, acute myeloblastic leukemia, malignant histiocytosis, and myelodysplastic syndromes [26]. The most common solid tumor associated with this paraneoplastic presentation is lung cancer, followed by gastrointestinal, renal, urinary, prostate, and breast cancer [27].

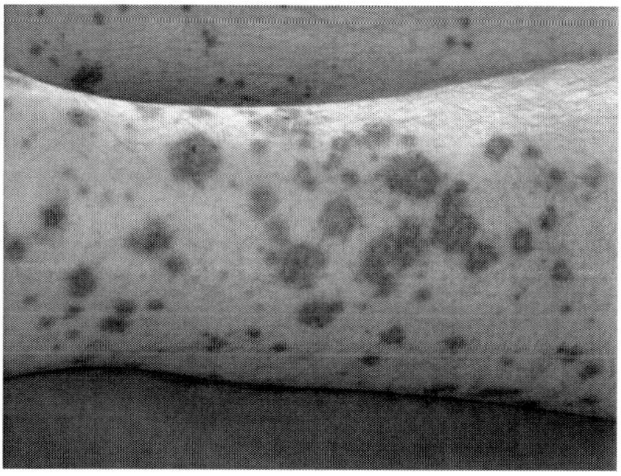

Figure 3. Leukocytoclastic vasculitis: erythemotous and purple macules and papules in lower extremities.

However, some tumors are more common in patients with certain subtypes of vasculitis. Solid tumors are more frequently associated with Henoch-Schönlein purpura or temporal arteritis, while lymphoma and leukemia are more frequently associated with leukocytoclastic cutaneous vasculitis and polyarteritis nodosa. The later was also described associated with hepatocellular carcinoma, gastric adenocarcinoma and hypopharyngeal carcinoma [16]. Urticarial vasculitis (Figure 4) has been associated with multiple myeloma, metastatic adenocarcinoma of the colon, metastatic teratoma from a testicular tumor, non-Hodgkin lymphoma, and renal carcinoma [28, 29].

There are several hypotheses regarding the pathogenesis of vasculitis in such cases, including the formation of antigen-antibody immune complexes associated with the tumor, direct vascular damage to endothelial cells due to a cross reaction with antigens on the tumor cells, and a direct effect of leukemic cells (hairy cells) on the vascular wall [30-33].

Vasculitis can predate the diagnosis of the malignant condition by 2 to 4 years. It is therefore important to monitor at risk patients, like elderly individuals with chronic or persistent and refractary lesions [1, 27]. A thorough history, physical examination, and routine laboratory investigations (biochemistry, full blood count with differential and ESR) should be sufficient for screening [13].

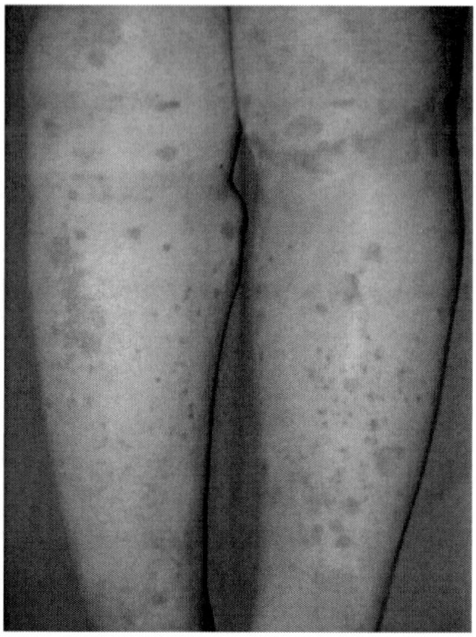

Figure 4. Urticarial vasculitis: persistent erythamatoedematous plaques in legs. Note a purpuric appearance on rims.

Others

Systemic Sclerosis or Scleroderma

Systemic sclerosis, or systemic scleroderma, is a chronic inflammatory autoimmune condition characterized by vascular changes, immune system activation, and fibrosis of the skin and other organs. One of the cutaneous manifestations is progressive hardening of the skin, tipically on acral sites (Figure 5). The first symptom tends to be Raynaud phenomenon, which reflects the involvement of the small blood vessels.

Retrospective studies have shown that systemic sclerosis is associated with an increased risk of malignancy. A recent report indicates a strong association between scleroderma and lung and haematological cancers [34]. Less often breast cancer. Altered B-cell function, which can give rise to lymphoid malignancies, has been implicated in the pathogenesis of this autoimmune disorder [35-38].

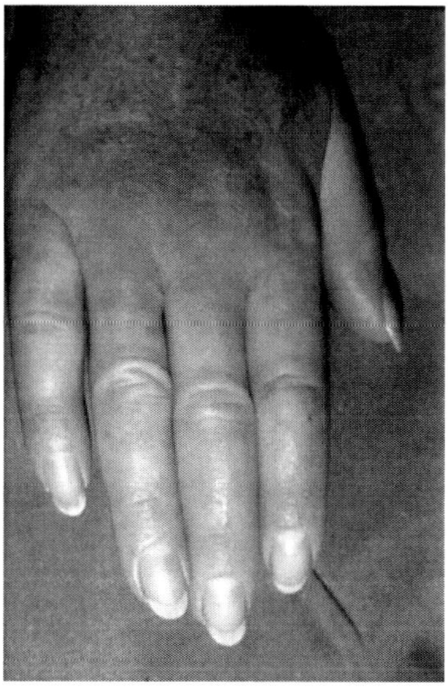

Figure 5. Systemic sclerosis in Lymphoma.

Other associated neoplasms are hepatocellular carcinoma, skin cancer non-melanoma, non-Hodgkin lymphoma and oral cavity carcinoma. The relative risk of cancer in patients with scleroderma is 2.31, in males and 1.64, in women [39].

When the scleroderma is associated with malignancies, debuted tardily, at an average age of 54 years, almost 15 years later that the idiopathic cases, and presents a quickly development, with appearance of systemic manifestations in less than 1 year. Early onset of specific complications are common, as severe and refractory renal hypertensive crises or pulmonary fibrosis [40].

Our attention being paid to those patients upper 60 years, with a rapid evolution, an assymmetrical skin involvement, an early systemic manifestations or poor response to treatment.

Lupus Erythematosus

Systemic lupus erythematosus is an autoimmune disorder with mucocutaneous and systemic features: "butterfly-shaped" malar erythema, discoid plaques, alopecia, oral erosions, together with arthritis, renal or another systemic involvement and laboratory abnormalities. In subacute cutaneous lupus erythematosus, there may be annular or psoriasiform plaques (Figure 6).

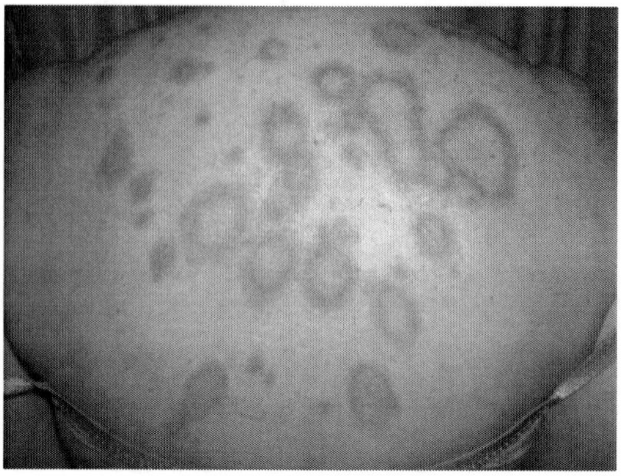

Figure 6. Erythematous annular plaques with superficial scaling presents on the back of a patient with subacute lupus erythematosus.

Cancers develop in patients with systemic lupus erythematosus, and the reported frequency of malignancy in these patients ranges between 2.5% and 13.8% [41]. Specifically, the most significant association of cancer in systemic lupus erythematosus patients is the development of non-Hodgkin's lymphoma, Hodgkin's disease, myeloma and leukemia. Several studies have also described the conccurrence of solid tumors in this patients as breast, cervix, liver, lung, larynx, stomach, soft tissue sarcoma, prostate, ovary, vulva and vagina tumors [41-45]. However, a recent report estimates only a small increased risk in systemic lupus erythematosus patients (versus the general population) for cancer over-all, although there is clearly an increased risk of non-Hodgkin's lymphoma, and cancers of the vulva, lung, thyroid, and possibly liver [46].

Paraneoplastic subacute cutaneous lupus erythematosus has been described in association with solid tumors: breast, lung [47], stomach, and uterus. In these patients, subacute cutaneous lupus erythematosus skin lesions either appeared within 8 months prior to cancer discovery or resolved within hours to 6 months after the initiation of tumor-directed therapy [41].

However, Paraneoplastic systemic lupus erythematosus is seldom described as such in the literature [48-50]. Doubts still remain about the paraneoplastic nature of lupus erythematosus and may be considered in cases with a parallel course, and screening studies are an option in refractory patients.

2.2. Neutrophilic Disorders

Sweet´s Syndrome

Sweet syndrome affect adults in their third to fifth decades and is characterized by the sudden onset of asymmetric skin lesions on the face, the extremities, and the upper part of the trunk. The lesions include multiple erythematous or violaceous papules, indurated plaques, and painful inflammatory nodules that are typically accompanied by fever, neutrophilia, and systemic alterations. Intense plaque edema can give the appearance of pseudovesiculation (Figure 7). In some cases, the lesions are distributed mainly on the hands: neutrophilic dermatosis of the palms (NDP) and neutrophilic dermatosis of the dorsal hands (NDDH) [51].

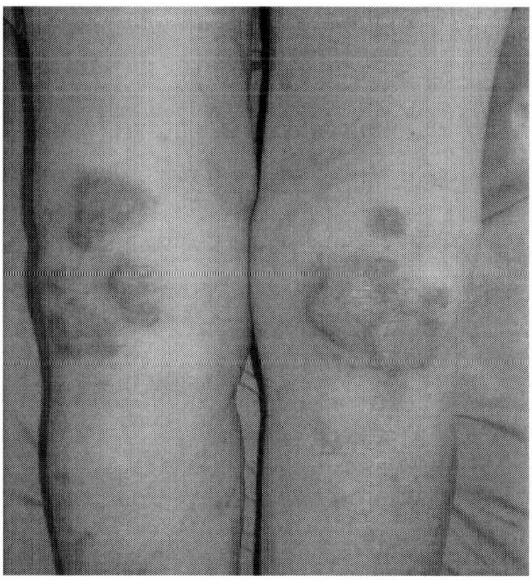

Figure 7. Sweet´s Syndrome: erythematous and edematous plaques on the Knees. Note the pseudovesiculation appearance.

Skin biopsy shows a dense neutrophilic infiltrate in the papillary dermis, with a variable degree of edema and absence of vasculitis. However, vascular damage was frequently observed in the neutrophilic dermatosis of the dorsal hands (NDDH) [51].

Sweet´s syndrome may be idiopathic or induced by other factors such as infections (predominantly upper respiratory and gastrointestinal), inflammatory bowel disease (both Crohn disease and ulcerative colitis), pregnancy, medications (most commonly granulocyte colony-stimulating factor), and cancer [52].

Between 10% and 40% of patients have an associated malignancy, which can precede or arise at the same time as the skin lesions. The most common malignancies are acute myeloid leukemia and other hematological disorders. Solid tumors (genitourinary, breast, lung, and gastrointestinal cancer) are less common [13].

Malignancies must ruled out in elderly patients and children without or low leukocytosis or neutrophilia but with concomitant anemia and thrombopenia. These patients are generally afebrile and have painful lesions on the head, the neck, and the arms. These lesions often take the form of vesicles, pustules, blood-filled blisters, or ulcers, and tend to affect the mucous membranes [14, 53-56].

The NDDH cases were strongly associated with malignant disorders, whereas the neutrophilic NDP cases were not. The latter showed a typical dermal neutrophilic infiltrate with neither vasculitis nor fibrinoid necrosis, whereas vascular damage was frequently observed in the NDDH cases. Bullous lesions may occur and the lesions may resemble superficial pydoerma gangrenosum [51] (Figure 8).

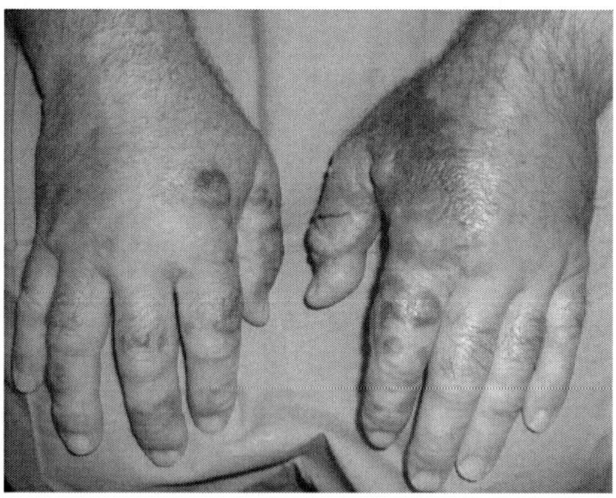

Figure 8. Sweet´s syndrome: bullous lesions on the dorsum of the hands reminding superficial pyoderma gangrenosum, in a patient with lung cancer.

Pyoderma Gangrenosum

Classic or ulcerative pyoderma gangrenosum consists in painful, enlarging necrotic ulcers with bluish undermined borders surrounded by advancing zones of erythema (Figure 9). Several variants of the condition have subsequently been observed as pustular, bullous, vegetative or peristomal types.

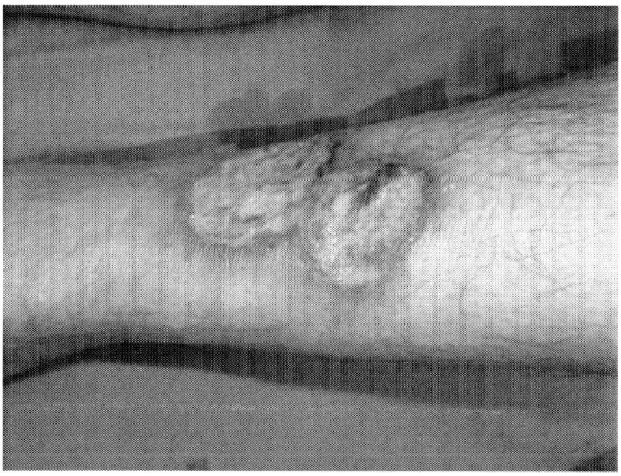

Figure 9. Pyoderma gangrenosum: necrotic ulcers with surrounding erythema.

Pyoderma gangrenosum can be idiopathic. However, the most commonly associated conditions are inflammatory bowel disease and rheumatoid arthritis. Cancer has also been associated with the development of pyoderma gangrenosum: most frequently hematologic malignancies (leukemia, lymphoma, myeloma, myelodysplastic syndromes, and monoclonal gammopathies) and less often solid tumors [57].

It has been suggested that pyoderma gangrenosum and Sweet syndrome may be part of the same spectrum. In fact, atypical pyoderma gangrenosum, which is an ulcerative neutrophilic dermatosis, is more closely associated with hematological malignancies similar to those seen in Sweet syndrome than classical pyoderma gangrenosum. This is the bullous type characterized by painful bullous lesions that form superficial ulcers and are typically located on the hands, head and neck, although they can affect other parts of the body [13, 14, 55, 58].

Subcorneal Pustular Dermatosis

Subcorneal pustular dermatosis is a rare, relapsing, symmetric pustular eruption, more frequently in middle-aged women, that involves intertriginous areas and also the flexural sites of the trunk and extremities, first described by Sneddon and Wilkinson in 1956.

Sweet syndrome, pyoderma gangrenosum, and subcorneal pustular dermatosis usually occur as the only neutrophilic dermatosis in an individual.

Subcorneal pustular dermatosis is frequently associated with monoclonal gammopathies, multiple myeloma, and other lymphoproliferative disorders and solid tumors such as metastatic thymoma, and epidermoid carcinoma of the lung [57].

2.3. Annular Erythemas

Erythema Gyratum Repens

Erythema gyratum repens is the most common type of erythema associated with cancer. It was described by Gammel in 1952 and the prevalence of internal malignancy in patients with erythema gyratum repens is currently estimated to be between 77% and 82% [59].

Erythema gyratum repens is a rare condition characterized by erythematous, pruritic, serpiginous, concentric rings that advance at a rate of 1cm a day, producing a wood-grain effect on the skin (Figure 10). It occurs on the trunk and proximal parts of the extremities. Accompanying skin manifestations include palmoplantar hyperkeratosis, nail dystrophy, and ichthyosis [60-62]. It is associated with cancer of the lung (32%-40% of cases), the esophagus (8%), and the breast (6%), as well as with cancers of the digestive tract, bladder, uterus, prostate, anus, and oral cavity and pharynx, and with multiple myeloma and malignant melanoma [63].

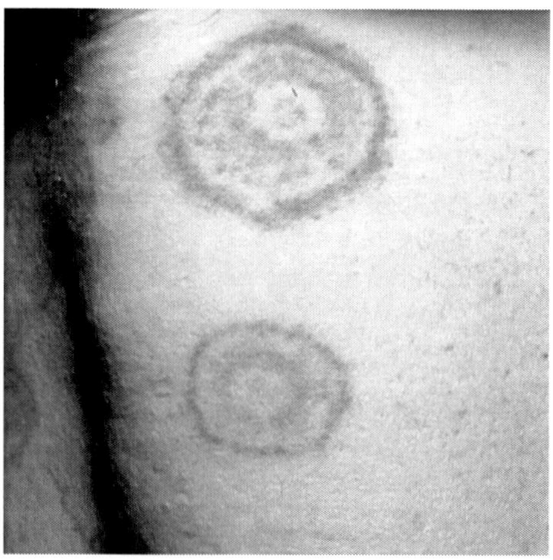

Figure 10. Erythema gyratum repens: appearance.

It generally appears between a month and 6 years before the malignancy is diagnosed, but it can also appear at the same time or even later.

On rare occasions, erythema gyratum repens has also been observed in benign conditions, such as tuberculosis, calcinosis, and CREST (Calcinosis, Raynaud phenomenon, Esophageal dysmotility, Sclerodactily, and Telangiectasia) syndrome or rheumatoid arthritis [64], even in a healthy individuals [65].

Histologic features include moderate spongiosis, parakeratosis, and a perivascular lymphohistiocytic infiltrate. As also occurs with pemphigus, deposits of immunoglobulin G and/or C3 may be seen in the basal membrane, so immune mechanisms are probably involved [13].

Erythema gyratum repens responds to treatment of the underlying tumor, and when this is not possible, systemic corticosteroids are useful [6, 13, 14, 18, 55, 62, 66].

Patients with erythema gyratum repens should undergo a routine malignancy screen and there should be a low threshold for bronchoscopy in at-risk individuals [67].

Necrolytic Migratory Erythema

Migratory necrolytic erythema is typically associated with glucagon-secreting alpha-islet cell tumors of the pancreas, which cause glucagonoma syndrome. It is characterized by erythematous annular or arciform lesions that tend to coalesce into plaques, adopting a polycyclic pattern. The lesions are distributed in the perioral or periorifice regions, and areas subject to friction and pressure as the distal parts of the extremities, abdomen, perineum, thighs, buttocks, and groin. Blisters, erosions, and crusts are seen at the active, serpiginous borders of lesions. The skin has a dry, cracked appearance that is reminiscent of staphylococcal scalded skin syndrome and acrodermatitis enteropathica (which is due to zinc deficiency). Mucosal involvement causes glossitis and excess glucagon leads to weight loss, glucose intolerance, anemia, diarrhea, alopecia, thromboembolic disease, and psychiatric disorders. Hyperglucagonemia greater than 1000 pg/mL are highly suggestive of glucagonoma. Migratory necrolytic erythema and weight loss are the most prevalent symptoms of glucagonoma, which can occur in about 65 -70% of patients [63].

Migratory necrolytic erythema has also been reported in association with myelodysplastic syndrome without glucagonoma, hepatocellular carcinoma, bronchial carcinoma, and jejunal adenocarcinoma [61, 62, 68].

Glucagon induces proinflammatory mediators, and generalized malabsorption. Deficient levels of zinc, amino acids, and essential fatty acids have been implicated in the pathogenesis of migratory necrolytic erythema, explaining why this eruption is seen in malabsorption syndromes, liver failure, inflammatory bowel disease, and celiac disease in the absence of glucagonoma. This condition is referred to as pseudoglucagonoma [6].

Histologic features include psoriasiform hyperplasia or vacuolization and epidermal necrosis, depending on the stage of disease at the time of biopsy.

Treatment is targeted at the underlying condition, and patients do not respond to zinc supplements. Surgical treatment of glucagonoma has resulted in rapid improvement of migratory necrolytic erythema. There have been recent reports of the use of octreotide, a somatostatin analog that inhibits glucagon production, but does not stop tumor growth. Patients with unresectable tumors have shown improvement in skin lesions after the administration of intravenous amino acids [6, 13, 14, 55, 62, 66, 70].

Presence of migratory necrolytic erythema, new onset diabetes mellitus, and unexplained weight loss strongly suggest the diagnosis of glucagonoma.

3.4. Papulosquamous and Hyperkeratosis Disorders

Bazex Syndrome

Acrokeratosis paraneoplastica of Bazex (Bazex syndrome) [72], which was first described in 1965 as a skin marker for supradiaphragmatic neoplasia. Probably, Gougerot and Grupper described the same entity, 40 years before [73].

This is a psoriasiform condition that affects men between 60 and 70 years of age. It presents with acral, symmetric, erythematous and scaling lesions that affect hands, feet, elbows, and knees. As the condition progresses, patients develop palmoplantar keratoderma (Figure 11) with a violaceous color and marked nail dystrophy (Figure 12), followed by psoriasiform lesions on the ears, nose, trunk, and scalp. The lesions do not respond to conventional treatment.

Psoriasis must be considered in the differential diagnosis. The lesions have a psoriasiform appearance, but they are poorly circumscribed and have a fine pityriasiform scale and a blue color; vesicles and blisters may also develop. Palmoplantar hyperkeratosis is more common at the pressure points of the palm and does not affect the central area. Histologic features differ to those seen in psoriasis, and consist of hyperkeratosis with focal parakeratosis, acanthosis, dyskeratotic keratinocytes, and a lymphocytic perivascular infiltrate. Other differential diagnoses include recalcitrant eczema, mycosis fungoides, drug-induced psoriasiform eruptions, and superficial fungal infections.

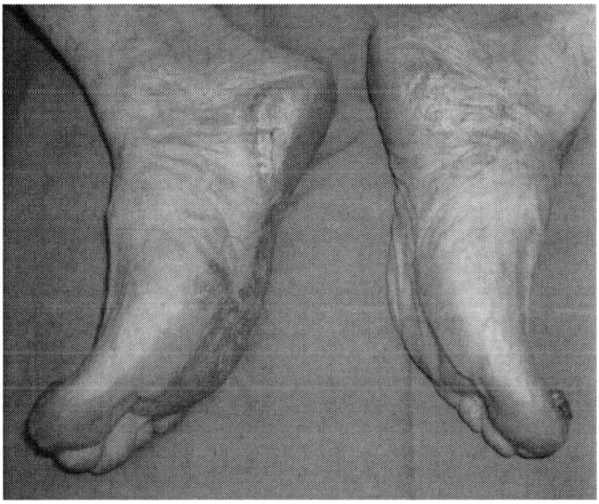

Figure 11. Bazex´s syndrome: plantar keratoderma.

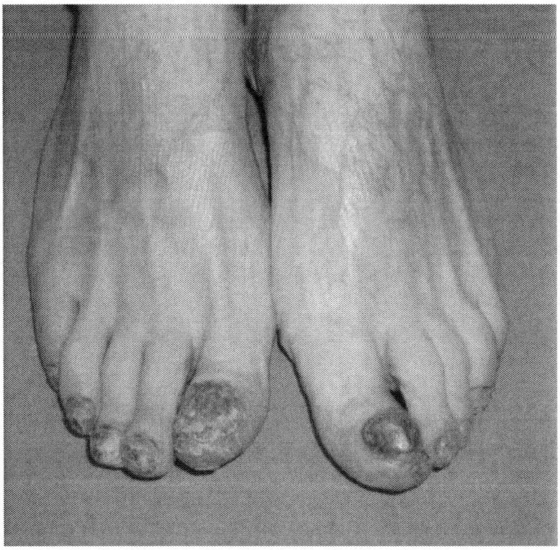

Figure 12. Bazex´s syndrome: nails disthrophy.

About 80% of cases are associated with tumors of the upper aerodigestive tract. The lesions can precede the detection of the underlying malignancy by a year. Commonly associated malignancies are squamous cell carcinomas of the larynx, lung [74, 75] and esophagus, so this disorder mainly affects males aged upper 40 years. Some cases have been reported in other malignancies, including ductal breast adenocarcinoma, cholangiocarcinoma, adenocarcinoma of the colon and prostate [76], lymph node metastasis in the neck, and liposarcoma [77].

Several factors have been implicated in the pathogenesis of acrokeratosis paraneoplastica of Bazex, including antigen cross-reactivity between the tumor and the skin, production of a keratinocyte growth factor, vitamin A deficiency, and genetic susceptibility. Prognosis can be improved by conducting an exhaustive investigation for an occult malignancy [13, 14, 18, 55, 66].

Treatment is aimed at eradication of the underlying malignancy with appropriate surgery, chemotherapy, or radiotherapy. Systemic retinoid therapy should be considered if the tumor is unresectable or treatment resistant.

Acquired Ichthyosis

Ichthyosis acquisita is a more severe form of eczema craquelé characterized by small white or brownish rhomboid scales on the extensor surfaces of the extremities and on the trunk, mainly in pretibial (Figure 13) regions and back. The palms, soles, and flexures are spared.

Ichthyosis acquisita is mostly seen in association with Hodgkin lymphoma, but it can also occur in association with other lymphoproliferative diseases (mycosis fungoides, reticulolymphosarcoma, multiple myeloma) and non lymphoproliferative diseases (ovarian dysgerminoma, leiomyosarcoma, transitional cell cancer of the kidney, hepatocellular carcinoma, breast cancer, and Kaposi sarcoma). Other causes include benign conditions such as medications, infections such as leprosy and acquired immunodeficiency syndrome, sarcoidosis, malnutrition [16] and endocrine, autoinmune and renal disorders [13].

One characteristic feature of ichthyosis acquisita is that it typically appears several weeks or months after diagnosis of the tumor. Its pathogenesis is attributed to reduced synthesis of lipids or to an abnormal immune response [14, 78-80].

Skin biopsy, demonstrates hyperkeratosis with a decreased or absent granular layer, similar to what is seen in inherited forms of ichthyosis vulgaris.

Topical lubricating agents and keratolytics are generally only helpful with symptom control and not with lesion regression [3].

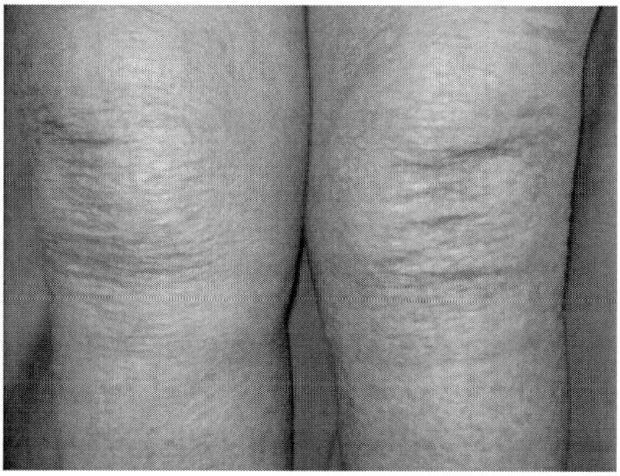

Figure 13. Acquired ichthyosis: xerosis and scaling skin on lower extremities.

Acquired Palmoplantar Keratoderma

Palmoplantar Keratoderma is characterized by abnormal thickening of the skin on the palms and soles, which punctate or focal pattern, or diffuse spreading (Figure 14). Hyperhidrosis may or not may be present.

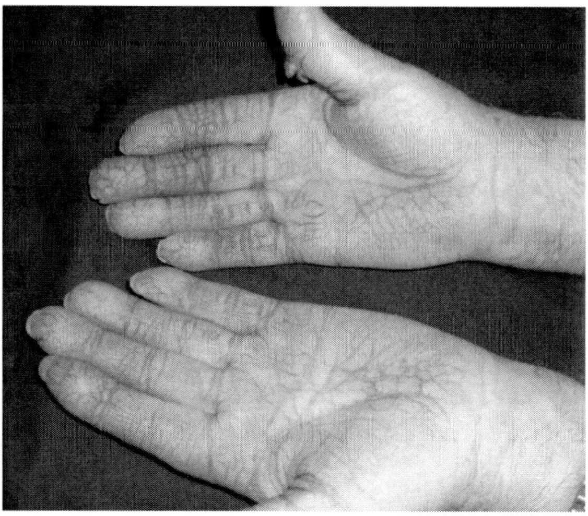

Figure 14. Thickening skin in palmar keratoderma.

There is a hereditary form known as Howell- Evans syndrome, that is associated with a higher incidence of oral and esophageal cancer. Skin lesions usually begin in childhood, although neoplastic involvement occurs on average at 61 years of age. The pathogenesis of the syndrome has been linked to chromosome 17q24, a site of keratin [63].

Acquired Palmoplantar keratoderma is seen in benign conditions, such as psoriasis, pityriasis rubra pilaris and climacteric, or to be a paraneoplastic syndrome like Bazex syndrome, erythema gyratum repens, and as mentioned later, acanthosis nigricans (tripe palms). Palmoplantar keratosis may also occur in chronic arsenic poisoning, which is a risk factor for several cancers.

The sudden onset of palmoplantar keratoderma in the absence of other findings should prompt investigation of an underlying malignancy. Prognosis is poor and the condition can indicate lung or esophageal cancer, or less commonly, breast or pancreatic cancer or myeloma [13, 18, 78, 81].

Acanthosis Nigricans. Tripe Palms. Leser-Trélat

Malignant Acanthosis Nigricans

Hyperpigmentation of the skinfolds is generally the first sign of acanthosis nigricans. Subsequently, the skin acquires a velvety appearance with verrucous lesions affecting the axillae, neck (Figure 15), and inguinal region.

Benign acanthosis nigricans is associated with endocrinopathies, such as obesity and insulin-resistant diabetes mellitus or drug-induced (nicotinic acid and corticosteroid). It is normally limited at that body areas and it appears in childhood or puberty [14, 18, 55, 66].

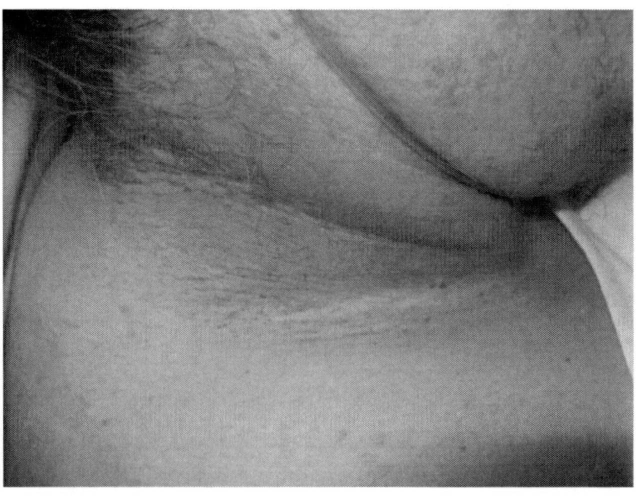

Figure 15. Acanthosis nigricans.

In contrast, malignant acanthosis nigricans is often extensive and severe and it progresses rapidly: papillomatous plaques appears on the oral mucosa, lips, areola, and on areas subject to friction. Palmoplantar keratoderma is seen in more advanced cases, like tripe palms pattern.

Malignant acanthosis nigricans is a classic paraneoplastic dermatologic disorder associated with gastrointestinal malignancy, most frequently gastric adenocarcinoma, which may not be diagnosed until several years later. In fact, malignant acantosis nigricans is often associated with unresectable abdominal adenocarcinomas. Less commonly, the condition may also be seen in uterus, liver, bowel, ovary, kidney, breast, thyroid, and lung malignancies. Growth factors secretting by tumoral cells could be the origin [6, 56, 82].

Malignant acanthosis nigricans is also occasionally observed in association with other paraneoplastic conditions, such as eruptive seborrheic keratosis or sign of Lesar-Trélat (see later) and florid cutaneous papillomatosis [83, 84].

Cutaneous florid papillomatosis consists of the development of multiple wartlike lesions on the trunk, face, and extremities. With an identical appearance to that of viral warts. These lesions multiply rapidly and become confluent, occasionally causing unsightly growths and disfigurement of the hands and feet. It is a paraneoplastic disorder that in the opinion of some authors is a clinical variant of malignant acanthosis nigricans [78]. It has been described in association with gastric, breast, lung, and ovarian cancer [84-87].

Tripe Palms

Tripe palms are similar in appearance to the lining of bovine, porcine, or sheep stomach. It is characterized by a rough velvety appearance with exaggerated dermato- glyphics. The condition is also known as acanthosis palmaris and acanthosis nigricans of the palms and may be considered as a variant of malignant acanthosis nigricans rather than a separate entity [88].

In over 90% of the published cases, tripe palms occurred in patients with an underlying malignancyand together with acanthosis nigricans. When these two paraneoplastic skin manifestations are associated, gastric carcinoma is the most common underlying neoplasm. Tripe palms alone are classically associated with lung cancer [89]. However, a wide variety of other solid tumors have also been observed, including renal origin [90].

Sign of Leser-Trélat

Seborrheic keratosis are a noncancerous benign skin growth that originates in keratinocytes. The lesions are round or oval keratotic papules, flat or slightly elevated and light tan to black colour. They can resemble warts though they have no viral origins.

Seborrheic keratoses are very common in elderly patients, but a sudden eruption or increase in number and size, accompanied by intense itching, may be indicative of malignancy. This phenomenon is known as the sign of Leser-Trélat.

However, the paraneoplastic nature of these lesions has long been subject of debate as seborrheic keratoses and neoplasms are relatively common in elderly individuals. The sign of Leser-Trélat has been linked to malignant acanthosis nigricans as they sometimes occur together [83]. In such cases, the lesions are most often located on the back and can follow a Christmas tree-like pattern (Figure 16).

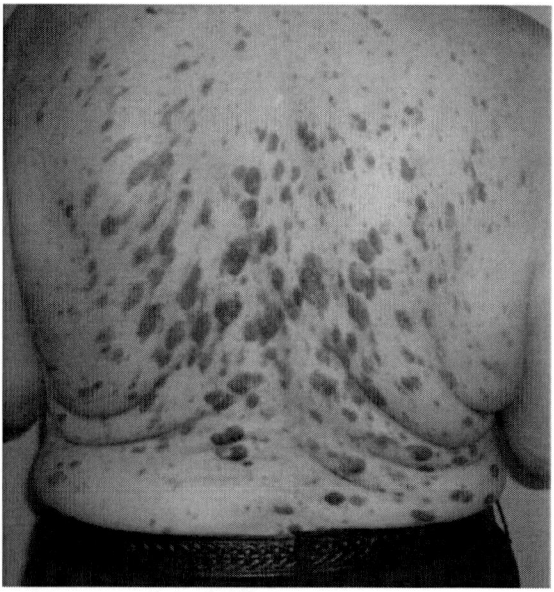

Figure 16. Multiple seborreic keratosis with a Chritsmas-tree pattern.

The sign of Leser-Trélat has been associated with gastrointestinal adenocarcinomas and lymphoproliferative diseases, and less commonly, with lung, bladder, renal, ovarian, and breast cancer [14, 56, 66, 91].

The associated malignancy is typically aggressive and carries a poor prognosis [92].

A similar condition named dermatosis papulosa nigra affects black individuals and has occasionally been linked to malignancy [93].

2.5. Reactive Erythemas

Erythroderma and Exfoliative Dermatitis

Erythroderma is characterized by diffuse erythema and scaling involving at least 90% of the body. The patients frequently also have alopecia, nail dystrophy, generalized lymphadenopathy, hypothermia, hypoalbuminemia, and heart failure. Pruritis, fever, eosinophilia, and leukocytosis are also associated.

Erythroderma and exfoliative dermatitis is associated with malignancy in 8% to 23% of cases [71]. In most cases, the condition is associated with direct invasion by a cutaneous T-cell lymphoma, but more rarely, it can occur in association with other lymphomas and leukemias or solid tumors as cancers of the uterus, cervix, lung, colon, stomach, prostate, thyroid, liver and larynx [94-96].

Skin changes are typically seen prior to the diagnosis of malignancy. Repeat skin biopsies are likely, since the findings are frequently nonspecific.

It is thought that the interactions of cytokines with cellular adhesion molecules are related to the formation of erythroderma [97].

Treatment is targeted at the underlying malignancy, since the course of erythroderma parallels the course of the malignancy. Narrow-band ultraviolet B (UVB) phototherapy, topical emollients and corticosteroids, as well as antihistamines, are also indicated [3].

Erythromelalgia

Erythromelalgia is a rare disorder characterized by recurrent bouts of burning pain, redness, and warmth of the distal extremities. It has been described with concomitant Raynaud's phenomenon that can be relieved by cold exposure and/or elevation of the extremities [98].

Mostly idiopathic when starting in childhood, erythromelalgia could be another paraneoplastic reactive erythema in adults. It may be associated with polycythemia vera, essential thrombocythemia, or another myeloproliferative disorders in adults in 20% to 40% of patients, and its onset is generally several months prior to the diagnosis of malignancy [3, 16].

This condition often precedes the diagnosis of malignancy by a period of 2.5 years. It is recommendably that all patients who have erythromelalgia be screened with a regular peripheral blood count [99].

As a consequence of intravascular platelet activation and aggregation, the distal arterioles become occluded, which is why a daily 500-mg dose of acetylsalicylic acid can alleviate symptoms [100].

Palmar Erythema

Palmar erythema (Figure 17) is an acral vascular syndrome whose main causes are pregnancy, liver failure, rheumatoid arthritis, and hyperthyroidism although it can also occur in healthy individuals. It is attributed to vasodilatation.

Associations have been reported for lung cancer, Hodgkin lymphoma, myeloproliferative syndrome, gastric adenocarcinoma, and brain tumors. There is a correlation between the intensity of the erythema and the vascularity of the brain tumor [101].

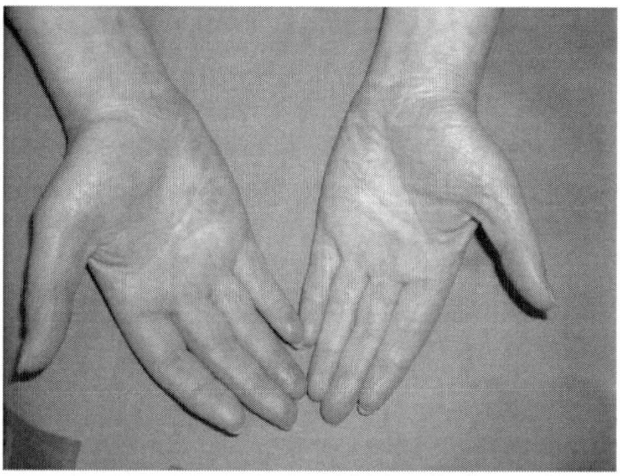

Figure 17. Palmar erythema.

Facial Redding, Swelling and Flushing

Furthermore carcinoid syndrome or mastocytosis which are described later, facial redding, swelling and flushing may be seen in:

Pheochromocytoma

Pheochromocytoma is a catecholamine-secreting neuroendocrine tumor derived from chromaffin cells. In 80% of cases, it originates in the adrenal marrow, but ectopic tumors can also occur.

Flushing appears after episodes of hypertension, tachycardia, palpitations, chest pain, throbbing headache, excessive sweating, and facial pallor. Another cutaneous feature is Addison-like hyperpigmentation, which is caused by the ectopic secretion of adrenocorticotropic hormone and the production of melanocyte stimulating hormone. The pigmentation fades after surgical removal of the tumor [102].

Pheochromocytoma is more common in patients with neurofibromatosis type 1, which is not always malignant.

The detection of high levels of vanylmandelic acid and catecholamine in urine, confirms the diagnosis.

Others Conditions

Less commonly, facial reddening and swelling can be a sign of a brain tumor, medullary thyroid cancer (secretion of vasoactive aminas ond others bioactive substances that causes widespread flushing affecting face and up extremities, in association with diarrhea and bone metastasis), renal carcinoma (secretion of prostaglandines and hormonal substances that cause flushing together with hematuria, lumbar pain, and abdominal mass), or a pancreatic tumor (secretion of intestinal vasoactive peptide that also cause chronic diarrhea, hypopotasemia and achloridia) [70, 99, 103].

3.6. Miscelaneous

Hyperthrichosis Lanuginosa Adquisita

Acquired hypertrichosis lanuginosa is a rare but typically paraneoplastic condition characterized by the sudden appearance of fine, unpigmented hair on the face (Figure 18) and then on the trunk, the axillae, and the extremities, with sparing of the palms, soles, and genital area. Accompanying symptoms may include painful glossitis, angular cheilitis, and papillary hypertrophy of the tongue, acanthosis nigricans and diarrea.

Pathogenesis is unclear, with no obvious hormonal dysfunction, but prolongation of the anagen phase of vellus hairs by a tumor-induced serum factor has been hypothesized [16], so there are no other signs of virilization, in women.

It is strongly paraneoplastic, mostly seen in women, and has been reported associated with lung followed by colorectal cancer in men and colorectal, lung, and breast cancer in women. However, the condition has also been described in association with cancers of the ovary, uterus, bladder, pancreas, and kidney, as well as melanoma, lymphoma and leukemia. It can precede or follow the diagnosis of the tumor, and is usually a sign of poor prognosis [55, 66, 104, 105].

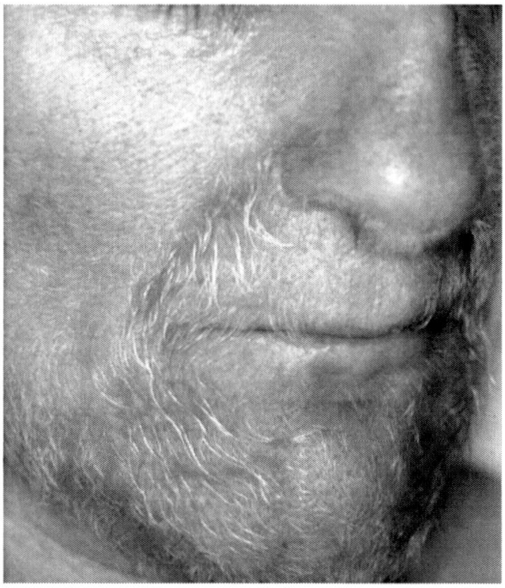

Figure 18. Hyperthrichosis lanuginosa adquisita (courtesy of Dr. J Sánchez Estella): fine and unpigmented hair on the face.

Urticaria and Paraneoplastic Angioedema

Urticaria is characterized by acute onset of pruritic, evanescent and circumscribed areas of erithema and edema secondary to increased vascular permeability. Angioedema is most apparent in distensible tissues, such as lips, eyes, earlobes, and tongue, and also may involve the larynx, extremities, and genitalia.

Urticaria and angioedema are most often associated with allergic reactions, drugs, infections, autoinmune mechanism or may be idiopathic. Rarely, they may be associated with malignancy.

Pathogenetic mechanisms are not known, but an immunological reaction induced by the presence of a malignant tumour has been described [106].

Tabla I. Paraneoplastic syndromes and common malignancies

Dermatomyositis	Ovariy and breast in women Lung and prostate in men
Paraneoplastic pemphigus	Non-Hodgkin lymphoma, chronic lymphocytic leukemia, Castleman's disease, thymoma
Vasculitis	Hairy cell leukemia, chronic myelogenous leukemia, myeloma. Solid tumors: lung and gastrointestinal cancer
	Lung, haematological cancers, breast cancer Non-Hodgkin's lymphoma
Scleroderma	
	Acute myelogenous leukemia, myelodysplastic syndrome
Lupus eritematoso	
Sweet´s syndrome	Acute myelogenous leukemia, myelodysplastic syndrome, myeloma
	Monoclonal gammopathies, multiple myeloma
Pyoderma gangrenosum	
	Lung, esophagus and breast
Subcorneal pustular dermatosis	Glucagonoma
Erythema gyratum repens	Aerodigestive tract and lung
Necrolytic migratory erythema	Hodgkin's lymphoma
Bazex syndrome	Lung, esophagus
Acquired ichthyosis	Gastrointestinal adenocarcinomas (stomach)
Acquired palmoplantar keratoderma	Stomach (Alone: Lung)
Acantosis Nigricans	Gastrointestinal adenocarcinomas
Tripe palms	Cutaneous T-cell lymphoma, Hodgkin lymphoma
	Myeloproliferative disorder: polycythemia vera
Leser-Trélat	Lung, hemathological malignancies
Erythroderma and exfoliative dermatitis	Pheochromocytoma, medullary thyroid cancer, renal carcinoma, pancreatic tumor
Erythromelalgia	Lung, colorectal cancer, and breast
Palmar erithema	Lymphoreticular system malignancies
Facial Redding, swelling and flushing	
Hyperthrichosis lanuginosa adquisita	
Angioedema and paraneoplastic urticaria	

Urticaria is most often reported with lymphoreticular system malignancies, and rarely with lung cancer, ovarian, rectum, bronchus, renal and prostata cancer [106].

The C1-inhibitor angioedema has been associated with chronic lymphocytic leukemia, non- Hodgkin's lymphoma, multiple myeloma, and Waldenström's macroglobulinemia [69].

Screening is recommended in patients with chronic urticaria, especially when the specific therapies are ineffective.

Thoracic radiography, among others laboratoy test (including routine blood examinations, complement C3 and C4, C1 inhibitor, thyroid function test, antithyroid autoantibodies, antinuclear antibodies, rheumatoid factor, serum immunoglobulins level, circulating immune complexes, screening for parasites and yeast, serum electrophoresis, anti-streptolysin O titre, total immunoglobulin E level, and prick-test) are recomendable in the routine study of angioedema to rule out malignant diseases [106, 107].

Table I shows a summary of the main malignancies associated with these classical paraneoplastic syndromes.

3. Other Skin Manifestations of Hormone Secreting Tumors

Cushing´s Syndrome

Cushing's syndrome is characterized by the clinical signs and symptoms resulting from chronic glucocorticoid excess and it can be caused mainly by pituitary hypersecretion of adrenocorticotropic hormone (ACTH, Cushing's disease), ectopic secretion of ACTH by nonpituitary tumors, adrenal hypersecretion of glucocorticoids, or exogenous administration of steroids.

Glucocorticoid excess induces a change in appearance and body habitus: redistribution of the fat to the abdomen, face (moon face), neck, and upper back (buffalo hump) is characteristic, as well as thinning of the skin, easy bruising, development of striae, increased acne, facial hair growth, and scalp hair loss in women. The presence of purple striae most commonly seen on the abdomen and lower flanks is virtually pathognomonic for Cushing's syndrome. Acanthosis nigricans and hyperpigmentation is also seen and is dependent upon the duration and the degree of excess in ACTH secretion [70].

Ectopic ACTH secretion comprises the most cases of paraneoplastic Cushing's syndrome which is induced by neuroendocrine tumors such as small-cell lung carcinoma, carcinoid tumors, medullary carcinomas of the thyroid, pheochromocytoma, and reproductive organ and pancreatic tumors. Weakness, wasting of proximal muscles, emotional disturbances ranging from mood swings to psychosis, edema, hypokalemic alkalosis, and hyperglycemia, as well as a cushingoid features, may develop. Clinical evidence of Cushing's syndrome actually develops in only 1% to 5% of patients with small cell lung cancer, but increased levels of ectopic adrenocorticotropic hormone are detectable in about 50% [16, 55, 66, 70].

Elevated plasma cortisol and corticotropin levels are highly suggestive of a diagnosis of ACTH syndrome. Treatment of choice is resection of the tumor secreting ACTH (pituitary or ectopic) or adrenalectomy if it is localized to the adrenal gland.

Carcinoid Syndrome

Patients with carcinoid syndrome have a carcinoid neuroendocrine tumor that secretes vasoactive substances, such as serotonin, histamine, bradykinin, and prostaglandins, that are responsible for the clinical manifestations of this syndrome. Its presence almost always indicates liver metastasis. Carcinoid tumors confined to the intestinal tract are asymptomatic, because the various mediators are inactivated by the liver as they pass through portal circulation. Hepatic metastases or extraintestinal carcinoids tumors lead to carcinoid syndrome [6].

It is characterized by repeated episodes of flushing, which can progress to severe rosacea, and in some cases even to leonine facies due to metophyma, rhinophyma, and zygophyma. Flushing can become more intense, involving the entire trunk and extremities, and be associated with vasomotor disturbances, such as heat and edema. In more advanced cases, patients may also develop hyperpigmentation, pellagra-like lesions due to tryptophan or niacina depletion (hyperkeratosis, xerosis, scaling, glossitis), pachydermoperiostosis and digital clubbing, scleroderma-like lesions, brown-orange plaques, pruritus, erythema annulare centrifugum, acrocyanosis, and pyoderma gangrenosum. Systemic manifestations include diarrhea, weight loss, cough, dyspnea, and bronchospasms [10, 108, 109].

Carcinoid syndrome should be considered in patients with persistent flushing of the face, neck, and upper aspect of the trunk with associated symptoms of diarrhea, dyspnea, and wheezing.

Diagnosis is confirmed by elevated levels of 5-hydroxyindoleacetic acid in a 24-hour urine test. Chromogranin A is considered to be a preferable marker. Surgical excision, tumor embolization, subcutaneous octreotide, and oral steroids provide therapeutic benefit. In patients with niacin deficiency, treatment focuses on nutritional supplemen- tation and oral nicotinamide [6].

Hyperandrogenism

Hyperandrogenism is defined as androgen excess in females, and it can be caused by ovarian and adrenal tumors secreting androgens. Most commonly is due to polycystic ovary syndrome or it may be idiopathic, with increased sensitivity of the pilosebaceous unit to normal plasma levels of androgens.

Clinical features include: skin thickening, acne, seborrhea, hirsutism and acanthosis nigricans. Abrupt onset suggests the presence of an androgen-producing tumor and is accompanied by hormone changes and other signs of virilization: temporal balding, deeping voice, or clitoromegaly, among others [70].

Elevated testosterona and dehydroepiandrosterone-sulfate levels are highly suggestive of adrenal origin. Elevated androstendiona is seen in polycystic ovarian syndrome. Imaging is performed to localize the tumor.

Mastocytosis

Mastocytosis is a rare disease consists of a group of disorders characterized by a pathologic increase in mast cells in tissues including skin, bone marrow, liver, spleen, and lymph nodes and gastrointestinal tract. Symptoms and signs are typically related to the tissue mast cell burden, to the response of the release of mast cells mediators, or to the presence or absence of an associated non-mast cell hematological disorder.

Different forms of mastocytosis exist which differ by the age of onset (pediatric vs adult), mast cells localization (cutaneous vs systemic), or clinical behavior (indolent vs aggressive). Adult-onset mastocytosis is almost always associated with bone marrow involvement [110].

The most common clinical sign of mastocytosis is the presence of typical skin lesions of urticaria pigmentosa, which appear as fixed, dark red-brown macules or papules. Darier's sign is the local whealing of the urticaria pigmentosa lesion when rubbed or scratched. Other rare forms of cutaneous mastocytosis include mastocytoma, diffuse cutaneous mastocytosis, and telangiectasia macularis eruptiva perstans.

Symptoms typically include pruritus, whealing, flushing, palpitations, and tachycardia Gastrointestinal involvement courses diarrhea and abdominal pain. Anaphylactoid reactions and idiopathic anaphylaxis have been described. They are attributed to the degranulation of mast cells containing substances such as histamine, heparin, cytokines, and tumor necrosis factor. Bone marrow involvement, can lead to anemia and low bone density. Criteria for the diagnosis of systemic mastocytosis have been proposed [111]. Aggressive or systemic forms of this disease can sometimes progress to mast cell leukemia.

Clinical suspicion is based on the patient's history, and diagnosis can be confirmed by biopsy of skin lesions, if present. Serum tryptase levels should also be determined and a bone marrow biopsy performed in adult patients or when signs of a hematologic disorder or aggressive forms, which are commonly associated with flushing [70].

Table II shows the leading malignancies associated with specific endocrine syndromes.

Tabla II. Hormonal disorders and common malignancies

Cushing´s syndrome	Small-cell lung carcinoma, carcinoid tumors, medullary carcinomas of the thyroid, pheochromocytoma, and reproductive organ and pancreatic tumors
Carcinoid syndrome	Hepatic metastases or extraintestinal carcinoids (neuroendocrine) tumors
Hyperandrogenism	Ovarian and adrenal tumors

4. General Cutaneous Manifetstions of Malignancy

Pruritus

Pruritus is a common dermatologic symptom with many possible causes. Patients with advanced malignancy commonly exhibit nonspecific cutaneous signs such as pruritus and xerosis. Patients with severe generalized pruritus may have scratch lesions and excoriated papules, prurigo nodularis and lichen simplex chronicus in accessible areas, namely, the upper third of the back (Figure 19) and the arms and legs [66, 112].

An underlying malignancy is the etiology in 11% of pruritis patients [3]. It has a complex pathogenesis in which T cell-dysregulation and the production of mediators such as histamine and serotonin by certain tumors has been implicated [13, 66].

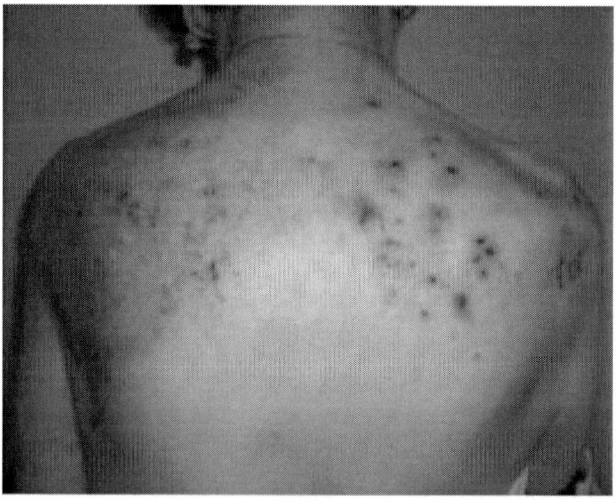

Figure 19. Pruritus: scratch lesions and excoriated papules in the upper third of the back.

Polycythemia vera is the malignancy most commonly associated with pruritus, followed by Hodgkin lymphoma, cutaneous T-cell lymphoma, Sézary syndrome, leukemia, and a variety of solid tumors as breast cancer, gastrointestinal and hepatocellular carcinomas, and carcinoid syndrome [3, 113].

Pruritus may be a significant cause of morbidity in the palliative care stage. Treatable causes such as cholestasis, xerosis, and use of opioids should be identified.

Localized pruritus is very rarely a sign of an underlying malignancy. However, in 40% of patients with meningioma, astrocytoma, and cerebral glioma, pruritus localized to the nares is seen, which is a poor prognostic factor [13, 114]. Recalcitrant intra-nostril pruritus has been associated with fourth-ventricle tumors of the brain [115].

Xerosis

Xerosis is a common sign that can be constitutional and it is also frequently in elderly patients. However, generalized xerosis is attributable to many causes in a patient with an underlying malignancy, including malnutrition, dehydration, and cachexia.

It may occasionally indicate the presence of an underlying malignancy, mainly joined with ichthyosis acquisita and erithroderma [116].

5. Other Skin Signs and Particular Conditions

Skin Induration or Skin Infiltration

Scleredema

Scleredema adultorum of Buschke commonly occurs in association with diabetes mellitus, but it has also been described in lymphomas and myeloma. It starts with nonpitting hardening and swelling of the neck and upper chest and should be clinically distinguished from scleromyxedema and scleroderma. Biopsy shows thickened collagen with mucin in large edematous spaces, but there is no fibroblastic proliferation. It can affect organs other than the skin [66, 117].

Scleromyxedema

Scleromyxedema is the diffuse variant of lichen myxedematosus. The latter consists of millimetric waxy papules that may be present on all over the skin. On the face, it can result in leonine facies (Figure 20) and difficulties with facial expression.

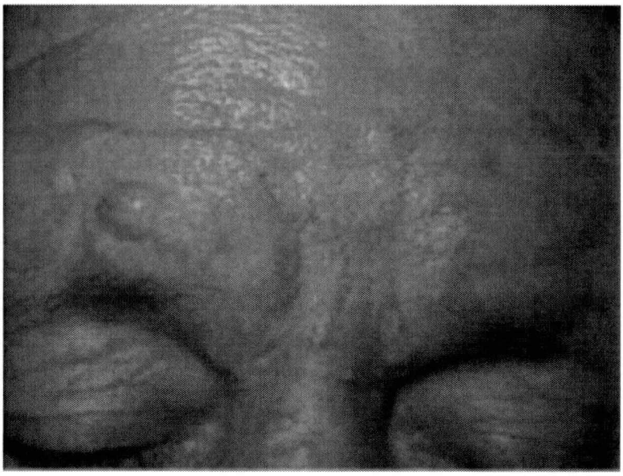

Figure 20. Scleromyxedema: facies leonine.

Systemic manifestations include dysphagia, proximal muscle weakness, peripheral neuropathy, carpal tunnel syndrome, and kidney disorders. Scleromyxedema runs a chronic, progressive course, with skin manifestations preceding systemic involvement [14, 42]. Histology shows a proliferation of fibroblasts, fibrosis, and dermal mucin deposits.

It is associated with monoclonal gammopathy in 80% of cases. Less commonly, it is seen in patients with multiple myeloma, Waldenström macroglobulinemia, Hodgkin and non-Hodgkin lymphoma, and leukemia. It can also indicate POEMS syndrome or thymic carcinoma [118].

Primary Systemic Amyloidosis [27, 117]

Amyloidosis is classified as primary amyloidosis, which includes an idiopathic form and associated with multiple myeloma, or secondary amyloidosis, which is due to chronic inflammatory disease.

Primary systemic amyloidosis is caused by the extracellular accumulation of an insoluble fibrillar protein (immunocyte amyloid) in tissues. Aspiration of subcutaneous abdominal fat is the preferred to obtaining tissue for examination. Furthermore, biopsy of clinically involved skin will yield a diagnosis in almost 100% of patients. The condition can be diagnosed histologically on detection of green birefringence when tissue stained with Congo red is examined under polarized light.

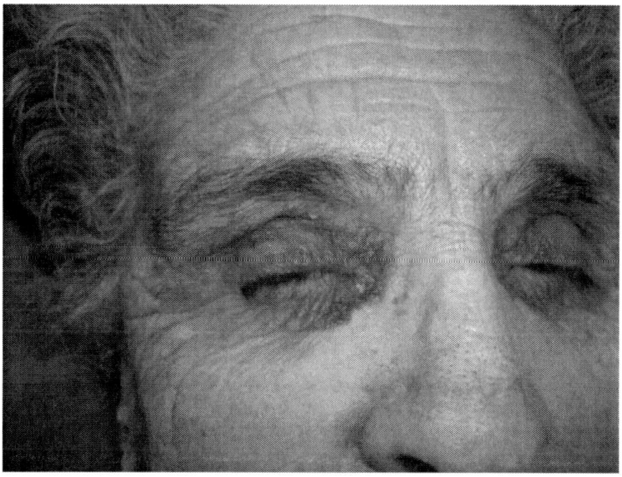

Figure 21. Primary amyloidosis: distinctive purple coloring is marked around the eyes.

The skin is affected in 25% of cases of primary systemic amyloidosis. Patients develop waxy skin and pinch purpura, which refers to the appearance of purpuric lesions following minimal trauma. This purple coloring is marked around the eyes (Figure 21) and on the face and neck. Papules, plaques, blisters, nodules, alopecia, and scleroderma-like manifestations may also appear. Infiltration of the tongue can cause macroglossia. The involvement of other tissues can lead to heart failure, Carpal tunnel syndrome, polyneuropathy, kidney failure, among others.

Between 13% to 26% f patients with primary amyloidosis have or will develop multiple mieloma. Paraneoplastic amyloidosis carries a poor prognosis, with a mean survival of less than 1 year [3].

Acquired Cutis Laxa

Cutis laxa is a elastic fibers disorder resulting in loose, redundant, hypoelastic skin and may be inherited or acquired.

Acquired cutis laxa is presented commonly in adulthood and it is characterized by insidious onset, initially on the face and progresses caudally. Some patients have systemic involvement with emphysema, intestinal diverticula, hernias, and vascular dilatation

It may be associated with inflammatory, infectious or rheumatic conditions and drugs, among others. Myeloma and lymphoma association has also been described [118].

Pachydermoperiostosis/ Hypertrophic Osteoarthropathy

Pachydermoperiostosis is characterized by digital clubbing, hypertrophic osteoarthropathy, and cutaneous manifestations including diffuse, progressive thickening of the skin with seborrhea, acne, folliculitis and dilated pores. Skin presents a furrowed appearance (Figure 22). Others signs include palmoplantar hyperhidrosis and decreased facial and pubic hair. Overall, patients develop coarse and acromegaloid features.

There is a primary form, usually hereditary, which progresses slowly, while other times it is associated with cardiopulmonary disorders. In acquired form, 80% of cases can be a paraneoplastic condition and it is associated with lung cancer, metastases in the lung, nasopharyngeal carcinoma, among others [11, 66, 120, 121].

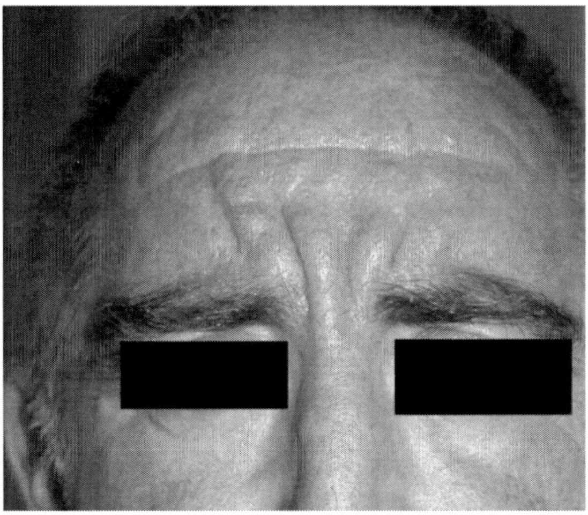

Figure 22. Pachydermoperiostosis: skin thickening and furrowing.

Reticular Erythematous Mucinosis

Reticular erythematous mucinosis has been considered by some authors to be an idio- pathic and primary form of cutaneous mucinosis, and by others as a disorder closely related to cutaneous lupus erythematosus, in particular lupus erythematosus tumidus.

Clinically, erythematous macules and/or papules coalescing into a reticulate pattern on the midline of the back and chest were present in all patients, frequently middle-aged women.

There are sporadically reported associations with malignancies (breast and rectal carcinoma, Hodgkin disease) and with autoimmune disorders, including thyroid disease, diabetes mellitus and ulcerative colitis. Some patients with colon carcinoma and thyroid dysfunctions experienced regression of their lesions after treatment of the associated disorder, althoug it can regress spontaneously [122].

Necrobiotic Xanthogranuloma

Necrobiotic xanthogranuloma is characterized by multiple yellowish plaques and subcutaneous nodules located in the periorbital region and on the head, the neck, the flexures of the extremities, and the trunk. Ulceration and scarring are common. The condition is associated with benign monoclonal gammopathy in 80% of cases. Associated malignancies include lymphoproliferative diseases, myeloma, chronic lymphoid leukemia, and Hodgkin and non-Hodgkin lymphoma [14, 66].

Diffuse Normolipemic Plane Xanthomas

Diffuse normolipemic plane xanthomas are characterized by the presence of yellowish plaques on the eyelids, neck, upper trunk, buttocks and flexures. Histology shows foamy histiocytes in the dermis. Approximately half of all cases are associated with hematological disorders and it often precedes myeloproliferative disorders such as leukemia, paraproteinemia, or lymphoma. On rare occasions, they have been described in the context of cutaneous T cell lymphomas [123, 124].

Other Vascular lesions

Vascular skin manifestations in patients with underlying malignancies are quite nonspecific. They are many and diverse, including telangiectasia, purpura, ischemic lesions, thrombophlebitis, livedo reticularis, and collateral circulation.

Because these manifestations are often benign and have multiple causes, the possibility of an underlying malignancy should be investigated in atypical cases with an unknown etiology. In such cases, a detailed clinical history is required to establish a logical correlation.

Telangiectasias

Clusters of telangiectasias on the anterior surface of the thorax may indicate breast cancer, or reveal the presence of a subcutaneous metastasis. Progressive telangictasias also have been reported in association with carcinoid tumors and hepatic adenocarcinoma. Generalized telangiectasias can indicate the presence of a malignant angioendotheliomatosis (intravascular lymphoma), overlying indurated and painful specific lesions [99].

Telangiectasias can appear on the conjunctivae, eyelids, ears, and cheeks of patients with ataxia-telangiectasia syndrome (Louis-Bar syndrome), which is a hereditary immunodeficiency disorder also characterized by difficulty walking in the second or third year of life. It has been associated with an increased risk of lymphoid tumors [47].

Purpura and Ecchymosis [1, 99]

Nonpalpable purpuric lesions and ecchymosis can sometimes reveal idiopathic thrombocytopenic purpura or thrombocytopenia, commonly seen in multiple myeloma, Waldenström macroglobulinemia, lymphoma, chronic lymphoid leukemia, breast cancer, ovarian cancer, cervical cancer, prostate cancer, and undifferentiated lung cancer. Thrombotic thrombocytopenic purpura is a late sign associated with gastric and breast cancer.

Purpura is also seen in patients with hyperglobulinemia secondary to lymphoma or myeloma. Cryoglobulinemic purpura affects acral sites and occurs in association with Raynaud phenomenon.

Disseminated intravascular coagulation causes purpura fulminans in several malignant hematologic disorders and some solid tumors, such as pancreatic, gastrointestinal, and prostate cancer.

Raynaud´s Syndrome

Raynaud´s syndrome is believed to be the result of vasospams that decrease blood supply causing discoloration of the fingers and toes. First of all, the skin turns pale or white and becomes cold. When the oxygen supply is depleted, the skin color turns blue and finally the blood flow returns and the skin color turns red.

Primary Raynaud's is diagnosed if the symptoms are idiopathic and secondary Raynaud's occurs associated to a wide several conditions: connective tissue disorders obstructive disorders, drugs and malignancy, among others.

Only a few cases of Raynaud's syndrome have been reported with underlying cancers of all types, including lung, stomach, colon, small intestine, pancreas, uterus, ovary, kidney, melanoma, leukemia, and lymphoma [125].

Several unusual features should trigger the clinician's attention, such as a sudden onset, an asymmetrical involvement of the fingers, and a common progression to ischemia, atrophy and necrosis, in men upper 50 years [16].

Cutaneous Ischemia

Cutaneous ischemia may be associated with erithromelagia, Raynaud´s syndrome (Figure 23) and purpura, as it has been mentioned earlier.

Peripheral ischemia may be considerated a paraneoplastic acral vascular syndrome, and has been associated with lymphoma and pancreatic, stomach, small-intestine, ovarian, and renal carcinoma [126]. Patients may develop skin lesions resembling chilblains [127].

Ischemia in patients with cryoglobulinemia is caused by increased blood viscosity and is associated with multiple myeloma, Waldenström macroglobulinemia, and lymphoma. Hyperviscosity also occurs in leukostasis phenomenon seen in acute leukemia or policitemia vera, among others linfoproliferative disorders [71, 99].

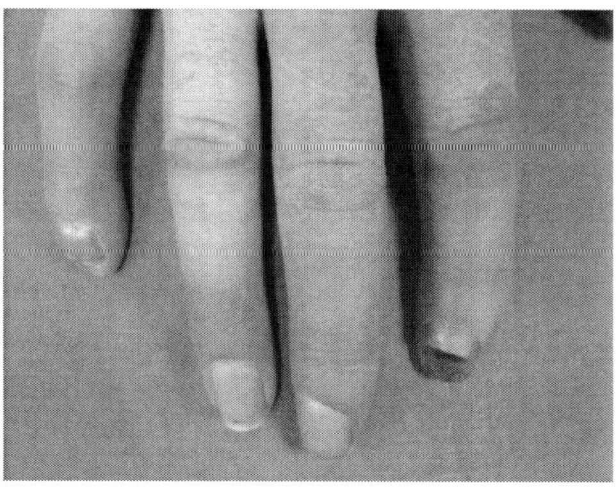

Figure 23. Raynaud´s syndrome: digital ischemia.

Thrombophlebitis

A state of hypercoagulability may occur in the setting of any carcinoma, before or after the diagnosis of neoplasm.

Superficial thrombophlebitis (Figure 24) of lower limbs in isolation is rarely a sign of malignancy. However, spontaneous, recurrent, multiple, superficial, or migratory thrombophlebitis (*Trousseau syndrome*) is paraneoplastic in 50% of patients, and it is has ben described in lymphomas, leukemias, and cancers of the, lung, prostate, stomach, and colon. Actually, pancreatic cancer is considered at major risk for developing Trousseau's syndrome [1].

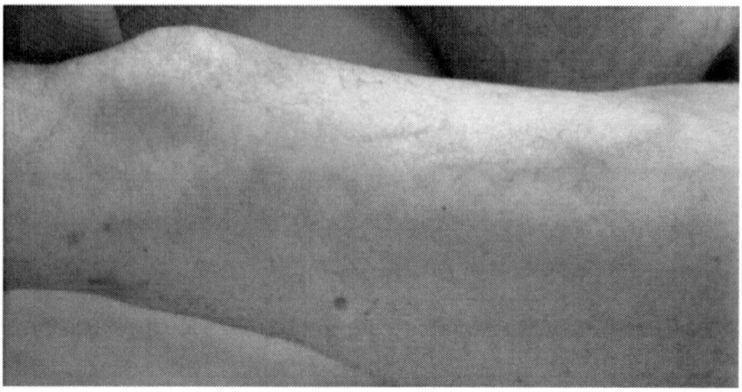

Figure 24. Superficial thrombophlebitis.

Thrombophlebitis of the subcutaneous veins of the anterolateral aspect of the chest and abdomen is known as *Mondor disease*. It is usually the result of trauma, physical activity, inflammatory conditions, breast infections (mastitis, abscesses), or mastoptosis. In several cases it can play a key role in the diagnosis of breast cancer, accordingly mammography is indicated in all patients with Mondor disease [18, 55, 71, 99].

Patients with cancer have a considerably increased prevalence of deep vein thrombosis and thromboembolism is noted in 50% of terminally patients. Underlying malignancy must suspect in patients younger than 50 years, multiple sites affected, and poor response to anticoagulant treatment. Upper extremity involvement is more common than lower extremity, frequently related with Pancoast tumor. The most common tumors detected in this patients are mucin-secreting adenocarcinomas of the gastrointestinal tract, the genitourinary tract, the lung, and the breast [71, 99].

Livedo Reticularis

Livedo reticularis is a common skin finding consisting of a mottled reticulated vascular pattern that appears as a lace-like purplish coloration of the skin (Figure 25). The mains causes are venodilatation and deoxygenation of the blood. Any conditions that cause increased visibility of the venous plexus can give rise to livedo reticularis.

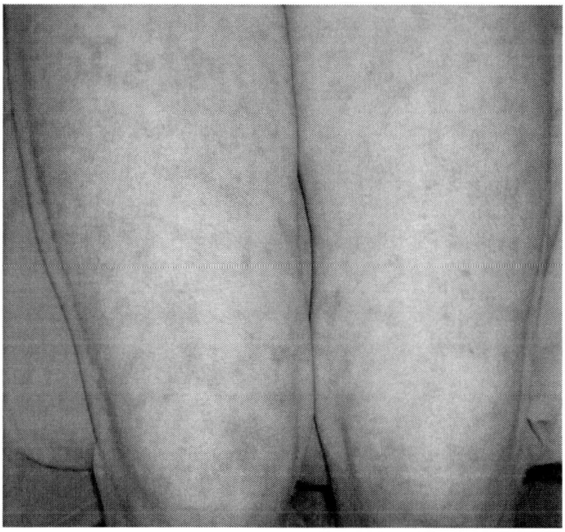

Figure 25. Livedo reticularis: mottled reticulated vascular pattern on the thighs.

Therefore, livedo reticularis can be caused by vasospasm due to cold or mechanical injury, arterial and venous thrombosis, or increased blood viscosity. This explains why patients with malignant conditions, such as multiple myeloma, essential thrombocythemia, and polycythemia may develop livedo reticularis. The condition has also been described in cutaneous T-cell and B-cell lymphoma, angiotropic lymphoma, acute lymphoid leukemia, renal carcinoma, and inflammatory or metastatic breast carcinoma. The cause is vascular obstruction in most of these cases, and the reticular pattern is broken, knowed as livedo racemosa [128, 129].

Superior Vena Cava Syndrome

This syndrome can be caused by extrinsic compression of the superior vena cava by a tumor or by intrinsic thrombosis due to a blood clot. It is characterized by a triad of signs: *a)* swelling of the face, neck, upper trunk, and arms; *b)* facial cyanosis, due to venous stasis; and *c)* collateral circulation in the thoracic and brachial areas. If the syndrome progresses, patients can develop jugular distension, dyspnea, orthopnea, cough, chest pain, and symptoms of cerebral edema (dizziness, nausea, and blurred vision). Classically, facial edema decreases on standing.

Superior vena cava syndrome is caused by a tumor in 85% to 90% of cases. The leading cause is lung cancer, particularly small-cell lung cancer in the right lung. Others common causes are non-Hodgkin lymphoma, germ cell tumors, thymomas, and metastatic tumors mostly breast cancer [130, 131].

Others Erythematosquamous Lesions

Eczema Craquelé, Asteatotic Eczema or Xerotic Eczema

Eczema craquelé occurs when skin becomes abnormally dry, itchy, and cracked. Lower legs tend to be especially affected.

Eczema craquelé has been described in association with lymphomas, gastric adenocarcinoma, glucagonoma, and adenocarcinoma of the pancreas [132].

In patients with inflammatory appearance lesions located on trunk or upper legs, and refractory to topical corticosteroids, it is advisable to examine lymph nodes, check for hepatosplenomegaly, and perform blood tests, chest radiograph, and abdominal ultrasound to rule out the presence of neoplastic disease [133, 134].

Pytiriasis Rotunda

Pityriasis rotunda is a rare disease more common in Japanese, African and Indian individuals characterized by well-delimited circular, scaling lesions, which may be lighter or darker than the surrounding skin, typically found in the trunk. There is no associated inflammation or pruritus. Some authors believe it to be a localized form of acquired ichthyosis.

One third of patients have an underlying disease, including tuberculosis, leprosy, liver and lung diseases, and malnutrition. It is associated with internal malignancies in 6% of cases, most frequently gastric and hepatic carcinomas. Others neoplasms described are hepatocellular carcinoma, cancer of the stomach, esophagus, palate, and prostate, and chronic lymphoid leukemia and multiple myeloma [63, 66, 69].

Erythema Annulare Centrifugum

Erythema annulare centrifugum is an uncommon skin disease consisting of annular and polycyclic, erythematous lesions with scaling on the inner margins of the rims (Figure 26) and borders advance slowly without leave scars.

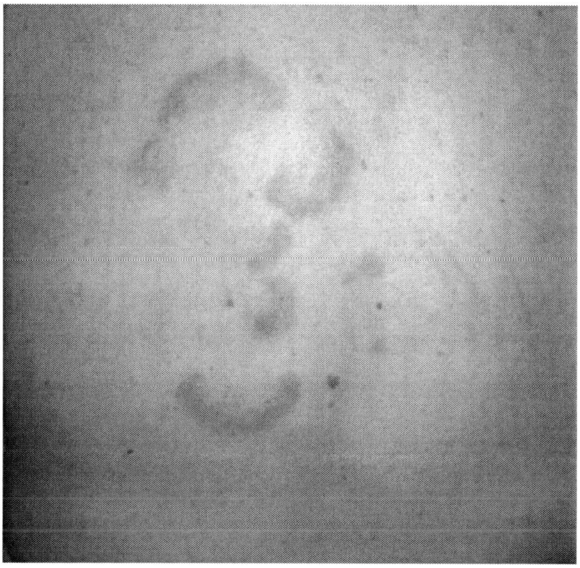

Figure 26. Erythema annulare centrifugum: polycyclic and erythematous lesions with scaling on the inner margins of the rims.

Erythema annulare centrifugum is believed to be a hypersensitivity reaction to a wide variety of antigens, such as those associated with infections, drugs, and endocrine disorders and pregnancy. It is rarely seen in neoplastic disorders, such as lymphomas, leukemias, and malignant histiocytosis [13, 55].

There have also been anecdotal reports of an association with prostate and more frequently with squamous cell laung carcinoma [136].

Others

There have also been anecdotal reports of other erythematosquamous lesions occurring in association with malignant tumors. These lesions include *small plaque parapsoriasis*, described in a liposarcoma[137] and *pityriasis rubra pilaris*, described in Merkel cell carcinoma, cutaneous squamous cell carcinoma, hepatocellular carcinoma, breast carcinoma, lung carcinoma and colon carcinoma [138-140].

Some authors have suggested that *disseminated superficial porokeratosis* might be a paraneoplastic presentation in hematologic malignancies, hepatocellular carcinoma, cholangiocarcinoma, and esophageal and ovarian carcinoma [141-144].

Hyperkeratotic spicules presented as spinous, skin-colored, coalescing papules with keratotic plugs in a generalized distribution has been reported as paraneoplastic phenomenon in myeloma multiple. Keratotic spicules can be either related or not to the hair follicle and they are composed of a columnar precipitation of monoclonal dysprotein in the infundibular epithelium matching the serum monoclonal immunoglobuline type, among keratin [145].

Others Bullous Diseases

Bullous Pemphigoid

Bullous pemphigoid occurs in elderly patients, and the rate of neoplasia not excedes that expected for this age group. However, there have been reports of refractory patients together with cancer [116].

Cicatricial Pemphigoid

Cicatricial pemphigoid has been classified as paraneoplastic in certain cases of antiepiligrin cicatricial pemphigoid [116].

Dermatitis Herpetiforme

Classically, patients with celiac disease and dermatitis herpetiforme, a blistering disease frequently associated with gluten enteropathy, may develop intestinal lymphoma. However, a recent controlled study conducted on the General Practice Research Database in Great Britain did not show a statistically significant increase in risk of malignancy in general nor of non-Hodgkin lymphoma specifically [146].

Linear IgA Bullous Dermatosis

Linear IgA bullous dermatosis has been described in association with lymphoproliferative diseases and renal cell carcinoma [147-149].

Epidermolysis Bullosa Acquisita

Epidermolysis bullosa acquisita is characterized by antibodies to type VII collagen. It may indicate the presence of a lymphoreticular or other tumor [150].

Pemphigus Foliaceus

There has been an anecdotal report of pemphigus foliaceus associated with non-Hodgkin lymphoma that responded to treatment with rituximab [151].

Exudative Multiforme Erithema

Persistent, atypical exudative multiforme erithema has been associated with renal cell carcinoma, gastric adenocarcinoma, and extrahepatic cholangiocarcinoma [152].

Granulomatosus Disorders

Granuloma Annulare

Granuloma annulare is presented as flesh-colored to red papules and small nodules, which appear either as individual lesions or as an annular pattern of confluent lesions. The skin lesions can be localized to a specific area of the body, commonly on dorsum of the hands (Figure 27), or generalized. Perforating and subcutaneous variants of the condition may also occur. A delayed hypersensitivity reaction to an unknown antigen has been implicated in its pathogenesis [58].

Several factors has been associated with granuloma annulare: trauma, insect bites, tuberculin testing, psoralen-UVA therapy and sunburn, viral infection, and drug eruption. Diabetes mellitus and thyroid disease are particularly associated [5].

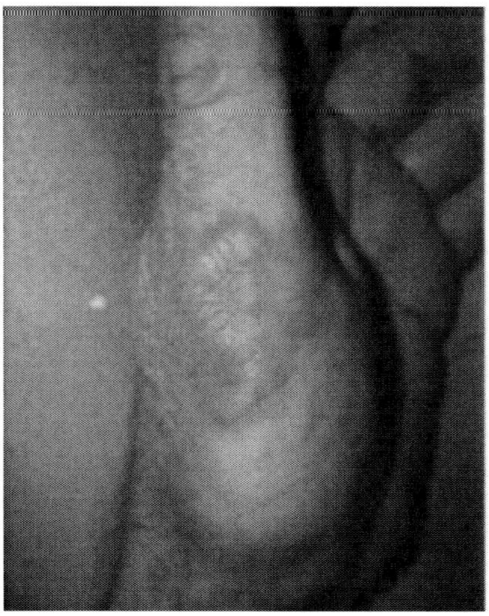

Figure 27. Granulomma annulare: red papules with an annular pattern.

There have also been rare reports of an association with Hodgkin lymphoma and less often with solid tumors [41], such as cancer of the lung, colon, cervix, prostate, stomach, and ovary. In this cases, granuloma annulare presents an atypical clinical pattern, with painful lesions in uncommon locations, as the palms and the soles. It affects older patients, with a peak age of onset of 54 years. The erythematous eruption can precede the detection of an underlying tumor by 18 months or may not appear until up to 7 years later. Additionally, middle-aged patients with persistent generalized granuloma annulare that responds poorly to treatment should undergo screening for an underlying tumor [58, 153].

Sarcoidosis

Sarcoidosis is a multisystem granulomatous disease of unknown origin that can involve lung, lymph nodes, glands and skin, among orhers tissues.

Specific cutaneous lesions of sarcoidosis are associated with chronic disease, and are characterized by noncaseating granulomas in the dermis. They have a wide clinical spectrum including papules, plaques, nodules, lupus pernio, scar induration, ulceration, alopecia, hypopigmentation, lichenoid or psoriasiform lesions, and more rarely, nail dystrophy or ichthyosiform lesions. Nonspecific skin lesions, as erithema nodosum among others, are associated with acute disease and do not reveal granulomatous inflammation in the dermis.

Its association with malignancy is attributed to an immune imbalance. The most common associated malignancies are hematological disorders, but a wide variety of solid tumors have also been reported, most frequently lung cancer or solid tumors in organs known to be affected by sarcoidosis [41, 58].

Unilateral upper limb skin sarcoid reaction after homolateral mastectomy for breast cancer has also been reported [154].

Multicentric Reticulohistiocytosis

Multicentric reticulohistiocytosis is a rare systemic inflammatory granulomatous disease that primarily manifests clinically with severe erosive arthritis and widespread papulonodular skin lesions but can involve multiple other organ systems. Histologic findings include a histiocytic infiltrate with multinucleated giant cells with an eosinophilic cytoplasm and a ground-glass appearance.

Multicentric reticulohistiocytosis starts with skin-colored, pink, or brownish papules measuring between a few millimeters and 2cm in diameter located on the dorsum of the fingers, around the nailfold. They have a characteristic coral-bead appearance. The lesions can subsequently spread to other sites, such as the periorbital region, elbows, knees, feet, and shoulders.

Patients may also develop destructive symmetric arthritis of the hands and knees.

Between 20% and 25% of patients have an associated hematologic malignancy or breast, stomach, ovarian, or cervical cancer [14, 66, 117, 155, 156].

Panniculitis

Erythema Nodosum

Erythema nodosum is presented as red, painful and firm nodules on the extensor surfaces of the legs (Figure 28).

Recalcitrant and persistent lesions has been associated with Hodgkin´s disease. The skin nodules completely regressed with treatment of the malignancy [94].

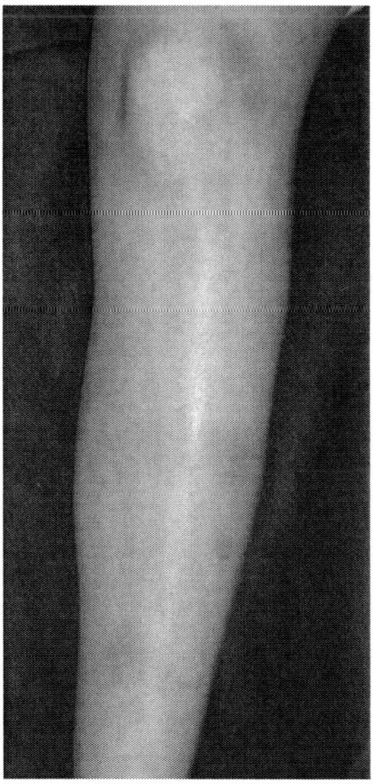

Figure 28. Erythema nodosum: red and firm nodules on the extensor surfaces of the legs.

Furthermore, erythema nodosum may be a nonspecific skin lesion associated to acute sarcoidosis. An association between sarcoidosis and malignancy has been observed in several investigations [41].

Necrotizing Panniculitis or Subcutaneous Fat Necrosis

Necrotizing panniculitis is also known as pancreatic panniculitis because it occurs in pancreatic disorders. It is caused by the excessive production of pancreatic lipase, an enzyme that induces fat necrosis.

It is clinically characterized by the presence of painful erythematous plaques or nodules on the buttocks and pretibial regions. Less often, trunk and the upper limbs may also be affected. The lesions frequently ulcerate, acquiring an abscess-like appearance, and discharge a brownish substance resulting from the liquefaction of subcutaneous fat. Other symptoms like fever, arthralgia, and eosinophilia, are also occasionally observed. The latter is quite specific of this condition.

Patients with necrotizing panniculitis should be evaluated for the presence of acinar cell carcinoma of the pancreas, among others pancreatic disorders [157].

Pigmentary Disordes

Diffuse Hyperpigmentation

Sometimes, hyperpigmentation may be a nonspecific cutaneous manifestation of leukemia and Hodgkin and non-Hodgkin lymphoma or less frequently, mycosis fungoides. Its pathogenesis is believed to be associated with the secretion of factors stimulating the production of melanin by mast cells, fibroblasts, keratinocytes, endothelial cells, and lymphoid tumor cells [25, 158].

Hyperpigmentation may be present in hormone-secreting tumors like acromegaly and Cushing Syndrome, as mentioned earlier. The hyperpigmentation in latter case is diffuse, similar to that seen in Addison disease, and more intense in exposed areas (face, neck, back of hands), areas affected by trauma or subject to slight pressure, and mucous membranes. The cause is unclear, but the pigmentary changes have been linked to the production of the polypeptidelipotropin, which is capable of inducing the production of MSHs, which in turn, stimulate the production of melanocytes in the skin [5, 70].

Diffuse hyperpigmentation is also a feature of hemochromatosis (bronze diabetes), which manifests with hyperpigmentation in advanced states, diabetes mellitus, and hepatic cirrhosis, being a risk factor for liver câncer [5].

Late-stage metastatic melanoma is not often associated with diffuse melanosis, which is characterized by a blue-gray color and believed to be caused by tumor lysis [5].

Cronkhite-Canada Syndrome

Cronkhite-Canada syndrome is a rare, nonhereditary polyposis syndrome that is characterized by diffuse gastrointestinal polyposis and ectodermic cutaneous findings. Despite its similarities to Peutz-Jeghers syndrome, Cronkhite-Canada syndrome does not have a genetic component.

The most common presenting symptoms are diarrhea, weight loss, nausea, vomiting, hypogeusia, and anorexia. The cutaneous manifestations of the disease possibly result from malabsorption and malnutrition and include nail dystrophy, alopecia, and diffuse hyperpigmented lentiginous macules, ranging from a few millimeters in size to 10cm, located on the palms, arms, neck, and scalp [159].

14% of patients develop gastrointestinal carcinoma [6, 55].

Pigmented Macules and Papules

Eruptive melanotic macules and papules in the perianal and genital regions have been reported in association with esophageal and lung adenocarcinoma The pigmented lesions were histologically characterized by a lentiginous melanocytic proliferation of large and heavily pigmented melanocytes associated with hyperpigmentation of adjacent keratinocytes [158].

Numerous associations with eruptive nevi have been described as following chemotherapy for hematological malignancies, after bullous eruptions such as bullous erythema multiforme, epidermolysis bullosa, and toxic epidermal necrolysis and in immunosuppresed patients treated with azathioprine and biological agents, as well as in the renal transplant population and those with HIV. Eruptive nevi on the forearmas and thighs have also been described as paraneoplastic phenomenon in prostatic adenocarcinoma [160].

Acral eruptive lentigines on palms and soles have been described associated with bowel lymphoma, breast carcinoma and stomach adenocarcinoma. Authors described a new paraneoplastic condition because of the closely relationship with tumor and skin lesions [161].

Hyperhidrosis and Anhidrosis [162, 163]

Hyperhidrosis has multiple causes and on rare occasions can indicate the presence of an underlying tumor.

Generalized Hyperhidrosis

Generalized hyperhidrosis is observed in pheochromocytoma, carcinoid tumors, Hodgkin lymphoma (night sweating), and tumors of the cerebral cortex.

Localized Craniofacial Hyperhidrosis

Localized craniofacial hyperhidrosis occurs in situations of minimum stress.

Frey syndrome, also known as gustatory sweating, is triggered by the ingestion of certain foods and is characterized by sweating on a single cheek toquether with salivation. This results from damage to the parasympathetic fibers in the auriculotemporal nerve that may oaccurs in parotid disorders, including neoplasia.

Segmental Hyperhidrosis

Segmental hyperhidrosis is caused by intrathoracic neoplasms that alter the trunk of the sympathetic nerve (lymphomas, mesotheliomas, Pancoast tumor, contralateral lung cancer, or superior mediastinal neurinoma [131]). This condition is also known as *Harlequin syndrome* and is characterized by asymmetric flushing and unilateral sweating induced by heat and exercise. It can also be idiopathic.

Anhidrosis

Anhidrosis occurs in neurogenic tumors that affect the central nervous system at the level of the hypothalamus or the spinal cord. It can also occur in association with segmental hyperhidrosis [116].

Nails Changes

Digital Clubbing

Digital clubbing is defined as broadening and thickening of the distal phalanges of the fingers or toes, due to an accentuation in the convexity of the nails (Figure 29).

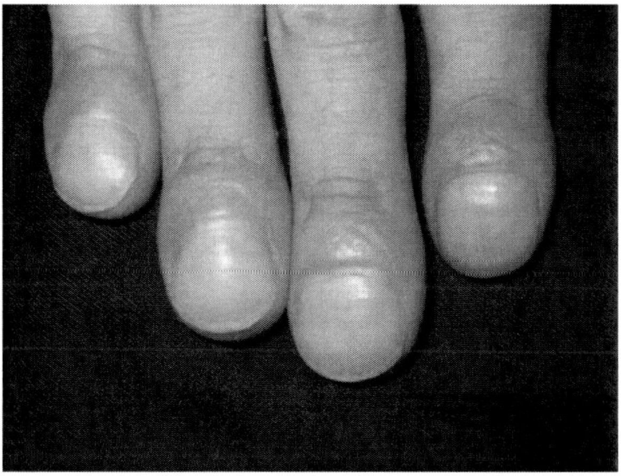

Figure 29. Digital clubbing.

It is seen in chronic heart and lung disorders resulting in low blood oxygen, and in up to 29% of patients with lung cancer, particularly in women [16]. Digital clubbing may also be associated wiht thyroid disorders [164].

Hypertrophic osteoarthropathy is characterized by a symmetrical painful arthropathy involving of the ankles, wrists, and knees, and periostitis of distal long bones of the limbs. It may also be observed in less than 5% of patients [16].

Yellow Nail Syndrome

Yellow nail syndrome is characterized by thick, overcurved yellow-greenish nails with loss of cuticle and occasionally onycholysis (Figure 30). Nail growth cessation is not uncommon. Etiology is unknown, although hypoplasia of the lymphatic system plays an important role. There have also been occasional reports of the syndrome affecting members of the same family. The changes can occur alone or together with a systemic disorder. It is advisable to rule out respiratory diseases, primary lymphedema, autoimmune diseases such as rheumatoid arthritis, and malignant tumors such as breast cancer and lymphomas [165].

Skin Cancers

Paget´s Disease

Paget´s disease is a rare intraepithelial adenocarcinoma with a high rate of recurrence and invasiveness.

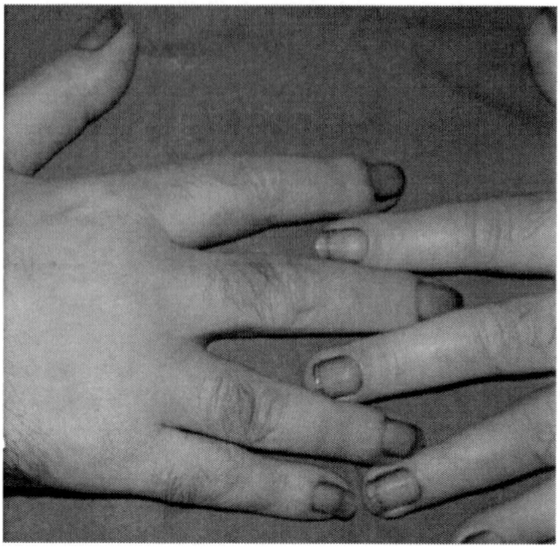

Figure 30. Yellow nail syndrome is characterized by thick, overcurved yellow-greenish nails with loss of cuticle.

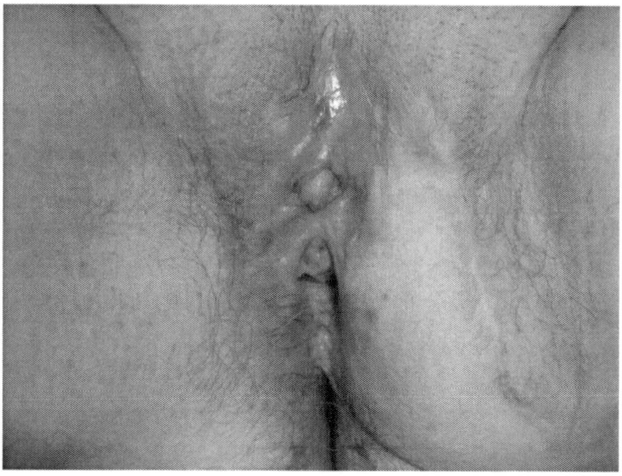

Figure 31. Vulvar Paget´s disease: erythematous plaque refractory to treatment, in vulvar area.

The initial presentation of Paget´s disease of the breast is an eczematous lesion, similar to contact dermatitis, in the skin of the breast at the areola and/or nipple and is refractory to usual topical treatments. It is frequent among women, especially those in their 50s and 60s. The significance of the disease lies in its association with underlying malignancy as well as its inherent ability to invade the dermis and metastasise. Most cases are associated with an in situ or underlying invasive breast neoplasia [166].

Vulvar Paget´s disease (Figure 31) is the most common site of extramammary Paget´s disease. The disease is frequently associated with the underlying invasive skin adnexal carcinoma or representing the migration of underlying internal malignancy, especially anorectal and genitourinary cancer, but the coexisting with primary breast cancer is rare [167].

Perianal Paget disease associated with underlying anorectal carcinoma carries a poor prognosis. Long term follow-up for 5 years is recommended. This includes an annual physical examination, proctosigmoidoscopy, and random biopsy specimens of surgically resected margins and unexcised perianal skin. A colonoscopy should be performed every 2 to 3 years [6].

Kaposi Sarcoma

Classic Kaposi's sarcoma is a a solitary or multifocal lymphatic tumor likely associated with human herpes virus 8 infection. Tumor lesions are characterized by slow progression of purple macules or patches on the lower extremities (Figure 32). This lesions could acquire nodular characteristics when the disease progresses. Associated lymphedema, especially of the feet, is common. Dissemination to to oral cavity, lymph nodes, or internal organs may occur in advanced forms.

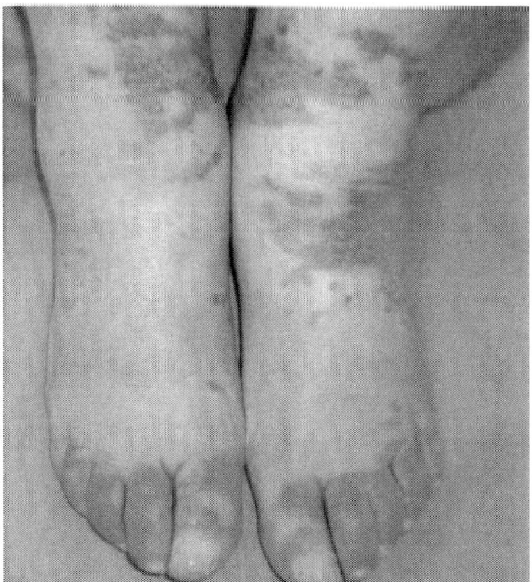

Figure 32. Classic Kaposi's sarcoma: purple macules, patches and nodules on the lower extremities. Note associated lymphedema, especially of the feet.

Classic Kaposi's sarcoma is associated with other primary malignancies, often of the reticuloendothelial system, that may precede, coincide with or follow the occurrence of itself [168].

Dermatofibrosarcoma Protuberans

Dermatofibrosarcoma protuberans begins as a small pearl to brownis plaque with a cicatricial appearance (Figure 33) usually found on the trunk but can also be found on the arms, legs, head and neck. It is a slow growing tumor, and it acquire nodular characteristics when the disease progresses.

Tabla III. Skin changes in particular conditions and common malignancies

Scleredema Scleromyxedema Primary Systemic Amyloidosis Acquired cutis laxa Pachydermoperiostosis/ Hypertrophic Osteoarthropathy Reticular erythematous mucinosis Necrobiotic xanthogranuloma Diffuse normolipemic plane xanthomas Telangiectasias Purpura and Ecchymosis Raynaud´s syndrome Cutaneous Ischemia Trousseau syndrome Mondor disease Deep vein thrombosis Livedo reticularis Superior vena cava syndrome Pityriasis rotunda Erythema annulare centrifugum Granuloma annulare Sarcoidosis Multicentric reticulohistiocytosis Erythema nodosum Necrotizing panniculitis Diffuse hyperpigmentation Cronkhite-Canada syndrome Eruptive melanotic macules and	Lymphomas and myeloma Monoclonal gammopathy, myeloma Myeloma Myeloma and lymphoma Lung cancer, metastases in the lung, nasopharyngeal carcinoma breast and colorectal carcinoma, Hodgkin disease Monoclonal gammopathy and hemathological malignancies Leukemia, paraproteinemia, lymphoma Carcinoid tumors and hepatic adenocarcinoma, intravascular lymphoma Hematologic disorders Hematologic disorders among several solid tumors Lymphoma and pancreatic, stomach, small- intestine, ovarian, and renal carcinoma Pancreatic cancer, lymphomas, leukemias Breast cancer Gastrointestinal tract; Upper extremity: Pancoast tumor Myeloproliferative disorders

papules Eruptive nevi Acral eruptive lentigines on palms and soles Digital clubbing/ Hypertrophic osteoarthropathy Yellow nail syndrome Paget´s disease Extramammary Paget´s disease Classic Kaposi's sarcoma Dermatofibrosarcoma protuberans	Lung cancer, non-Hodgkin lymphoma, thymomas Gastric and hepatic carcinomas Lymphomas, leukemias, and malignant histiocytosis Hodgkin lymphoma Hematological disorders, lung cancer Hematologic malignancy, and breast, stomach, ovarian, cervical cancer Hodgkin´s disease acinar cell carcinoma of the pancreas hormone-secreting tumors, metastatic melanoma, hemochromatosis (liver cancer) Gastrointestinal carcinoma Esophageal and lung adenocarcinoma Prostatic adenocarcinoma Bowel lymphoma, breast carcinoma and stomach adenocarcinoma Lung cancer Breast cancer and lymphomas Breast neoplasia Anorectal and genitourinary cancer Other primary malignancies of the reticuloendothelial system Melanoma, breast cancer, and soft tissue cancer

Dermatofibrosarcoma protuberans is a skin cancer that can be locally destructive, with high rates of recurrence after surgical excision. Metastasis to lymph nodes are uncommon. More than 90% of DFSP lesions contain a t(17;22) translocation that creates a fused platelet-derived growth factor PDGF β-collagen type1 alpha1 gene that constitutively produces collagen [169].

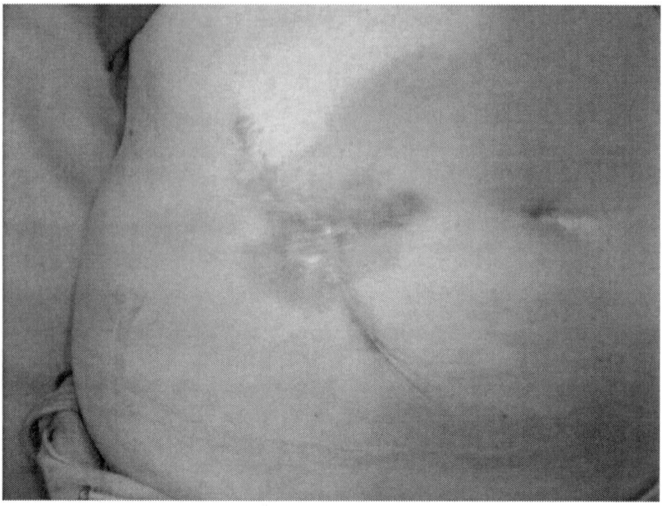

Figure 33. Recidivant dermatofibrosarcoma protuberans: pearl-browned plaque over prior scar.

Patients with Dermatofibrosarcoma protuberans are at greater risk than the general population for several subsequent primary malignancy. This increased risk is possibly the result of common genetic and environmental mechanisms. PDGFβ has been implicated in melanoma, breast cancer, and soft tissue cancer [170].

Table III shows the main neoplasms associated with certain characteristic cutaneous signs and others that only in specific situations do it.

6. Cutaneous Features of Familial Cancer

6.1. Neurocutaneous Syndromes

Neurofibromatosis

Neurofibromatosis type 1 (NF1) is an autosomal dominantly inherited neurocutaneous disorder due to mutations in NF1 gene on 17q11.2.

Diagnosis is made by the presence of at least two major criteria: 6 or more café-au-lait macules (Figure 34) 5 mm or greater size in prepubertal patients or 15 mm or greater in size in post-pubertal patients, axillary of inguinal freckling, two or more cutaneous neurofibromas or one plexiform neurofibroma, optic glioma, characteristic bony abnormalities (such as sphenoid wing dysplasia, thinning of long bone cortex), two or more Lisch nodules, or a first-degree relative with NF1.

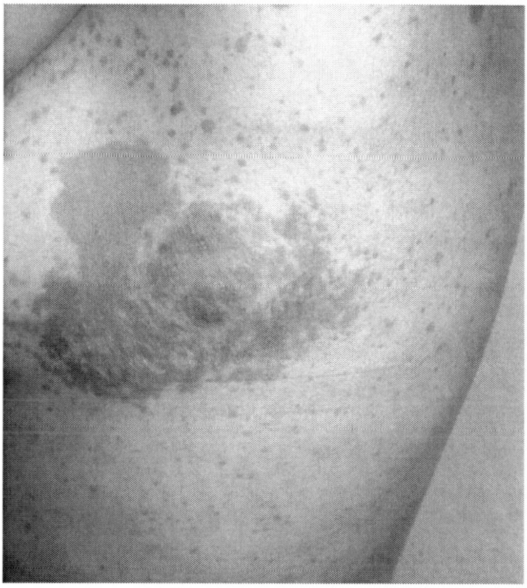

Figure 34. Neurofibromatosis: multiple café-au-lait macules involving left side of the trunk.

Other reported cutaneous findings associated with NF1 are: juvenile xanthogranuloma, glomus tumor, blue-red macules, and pseudoatrophic macules [171].

Neurofibromatosis can be complicated by the malignant transformation of plexiform neurofibromas. As the disease evolves, patients can develop certain malignancies, such as Wilms tumor, rhabdomyosarcoma, retinoblastoma, melanoma, intestinal leiomyosarcoma, medulloblastoma, and leukemia. Pheochromocytomas are benign in 90% of cases. Neurofibromatosis has been linked to Lynch syndrome in patients with homozygous mutations of DNA mismatch repair genes [6], and to familial gynecologic and breast malignancies [13, 55]. Genetic studies have shown that a common haplotype involving the NF1 and breast cancer (BRCA)-1 loci, both located on chromosome 17 [13].

Individuals with NF1 are recommended to undergo annual clinical reviews, including measurement of blood pressure. Symptomatic cutaneous neurofibromas may be surgically excised [13].

Tuberous Sclerosis

Tuberous sclerosis is an autosomal dominant neurocutaneous disorder due to a heterozygous mutation in one of two separate genes, TSC1 gene on chromosome 9q34 or TSC2 gene on chromosome 16p13. The main clinical findings in TSC are cutaneous lesions, epilepsy, and mental retardation.

Cutaneous features occur in more than 90% of patients, including hypomelanotic macules, facial angiofibromas (Figure 35), shagreen patches, fibrous facial plaques, and ungual fibroma (Figure 36). Oral signs include gingival fibromas and dental pits.

Non-cutaneous abnormalities involve the brain (cortical tubers, subependymal glial nodules, subependymal giant-cell astrocytomas, seizures, mental retardation, and behavioural disorders), kidney (angiomyolipomas, cysts, renal tumours), and heart (rhabdomyomas and arrhythmias) [171].

Cardiac rhabdomyomas are the most common neoplasm in Tuberous Sclerosis. Kidney involvement is the most frequent cause of death usually caused by angiomyolipomas. Renal carcinoma (2–3%) may also arise in these patients, usually in childhood. Hystopathology is heterogeneous, including clear-cell, oncocytomas, papillary, and chromophobe tumours [171, 172].

Diagnostic evaluation of this conditon include cranial magnetic resonance imaging, ECG, echocardiogram, and renal ultrasound at diagnosis and every 1–3 years.

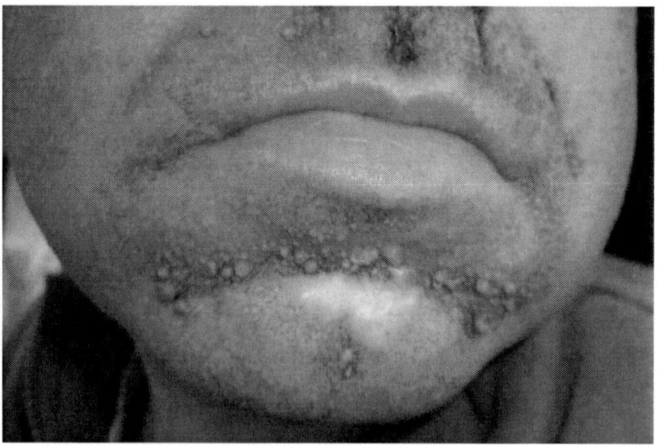

Figure 35. Tuberous sclerosis: facial angiofibromas.

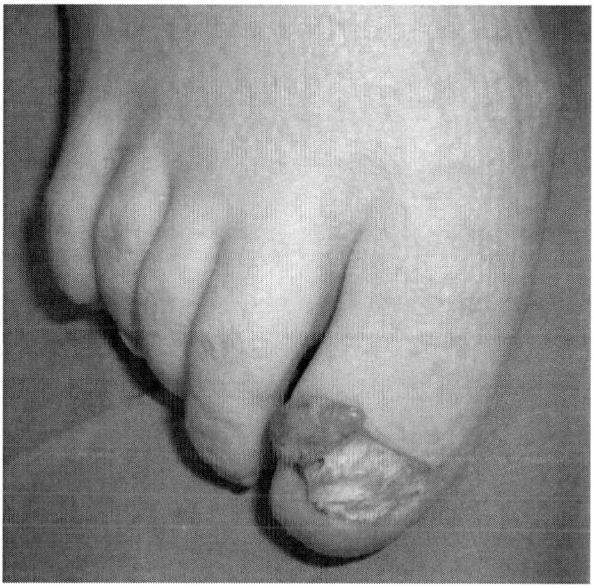

Figure 36. Tuberous sclerosis: ungual fibroma.

6.2. Syndromes That Predispose to Colorectal Cancer

Hereditary Non-Poliposis Colorectal Cancer (Lynch Syndrome)

Hereditary non-polyposis colorectal cancer is a familial cancer syndrome or Lynch syndrome, with onset in young people, which results from mutations in one of the mismatch repair genes. Cellular loss of expression of *MLH1, MSH2, MSH6,* or *PMS2* results in the accumulation of undetected and unrepaired DNA mismatches, and consequently, increased tumour formation [171].

Lynch syndrome is associated with colon cancer and also has an increased risk of developing endometrial, urologic, small bowel, ovarian, hepatobiliary, and brain cancers [6].

Muir-Torre Syndrome

Muir-Torre syndrome is a phenotypic subset of Lynch syndrome. The vast majority of cutaneous findings associated with Lynch syndrome are found in this variant.

The suggested diagnostic criteria for Muir-Torre syndrome is the finding of a sebaceous adenoma epithelioma, carcinoma, or keratoacanthoma and any visceral malignancy. Alternatively, the development of multiple keratoacanthomas in combination with multiple visceral malignancies and a family history of Muir-Torre syndrome [172].

Sebaceous adenomas are presented as yellow papules or nodules predominantly on the face. Malignant transformation results in sebaceous carcinoma, commonly found on the eyelids as yellow nodules with a propensity toward ulceration.

Up to 42% of patients with a sebaceous neoplasm will have an associated visceral malignancy. When there is a single tumor located on the head or neck, it is not usually indicative of malignancy[55]. Tumors can arise anywhere within the urogenital or digestive tract. Cancer of the proximal colon is the most frequent tumor associated. Surveillance includes colonoscopy beginning at 25 years of age and repeated every 2 to 3 years [6, 172]. Others tumours associated include endometrial, ovarian, stomach, small intestine, hepatobiliary, upper urinary tract, brain, and skin cancer [172].

Familial Adenomatous Polyposis

Familial adenomatous polyposis is an autosomal dominant cancer syndrome, due to heterozygous mutations in APC on chromosome 5q21-22.23.

Gardner Syndrome

Gardner syndrome is a phenotypic variant of the familial adenomatous polyposis syndrome characterized by numerous gastrointestinal adenomatous polyps with multiple mucocutaneous findings and others extraintestinal features involving eye, bone, and thyroid.

Cutaneous manifestations include epidermoid cysts, fibromas, leiomyomas, trichoepitheliomas, neurofibromas, lipomas, and desmoid tumors as well as dental abnormalities including osteomas, odontomas, and supernumerary or unerupted teeth. Epidermoid cysts are usually multiple, typically manifesting on the face or extremities, and frequently predate the appearance of intestinal polyps. Desmoid tumors are located intraabdominally, within the abdominal wall, and extraabdominally often in the shoulder girdle, chest wall, and inguinal regions These tumours occur at the site of trauma and surgery, and are rapidly proliferating masses of fibrous tissue with a locally aggressive manner. A skin examination may reveal a nontender, well-circumscribed, firm, flesh-colored tumor. Lipomas and pilomatricomas can precede the development of polyps [6, 55, 171].

Congenital hypertrophy of retinal pigmented epithelium can be an early sign in this patients. It is considered a phenotypic marker for FAP [6].

Patients with Gardner syndrome are predisposed to duodenal, thyroid, brain (medulloblastomas), adrenal, and liver cancers in addition to colorectal cancer. The latter is preceded by hundreds or thousands of colonic polyps; if these polyps are left untreated, cancer is invariable after the second decade. Annual colon screening should begin at 10 to 15 years [13]. Upper gastrointestinal endoscopy is recommended every 1 to 3 years beginning at 25 to 30 years of age along with an annual thyroid examination [6].

Hamartomatous Polyposis Syndrome

Peutz-Jeghers Syndrome

Peutz-Jeghers syndrome is a dominantly inherited cancer predisposition syndrome due to heterozygous mutations in STK11 gene on chromosome 19p13.3. It si characterized by hyperpigmentation of mucosa and digits, small bowel hamartomatous polyps an increased risk of visceral malignancy.

The pigmentation is macular dark brown or dark blue, most commonly on the border of the lips and the oral mucosa, and on the nostrils, eyes, and perianal area, digits and volar aspects of the hands and feet. The skin pigmentation begins in childhood and usually fades in adolescence and adulthood, however oral-buccal mucosal pigmentation is usually permanent. Macules that often precede GI symptoms, making early dermatologic diagnosis essential [6, 171].

Hamartomatous polyps occur in the small intestine, stomach, and large bowel. Mucosa pigmentation may also be seen on the bowel at proctoscopy or colonoscopy.

These patients have a higher risk of pancreatic, breast, gastrointestinal, uterux, cervical, ovarian, testicular and lung cancer than the general population [47, 171].

Colonoscopy being initiated during the late teenage years. Annual transvaginal ultrasound, endoscopic ultrasound for evaluation of pancreatic malignancy, computed tomographic scans of the abdomen, and assays for CA-125 biomarkers are also recommended [6]. Men should have regular testicular exams [172].

Syndromes That Predispose to Renal Cancer

Birt-Hogg-Dube Syndrome

Birt-Hogg-Dube syndrome is a variable autosomal dominant renal cancer predisposition condition due to a heterozygous mutation in FLCN gene which encodes folliculin it is preferentially expressed in the skin, kidney, and lung [173].

Skin lesiosns include fibrofolliculomas, trichodiscomas, and acrochordons (skin tags). Fibrofolliculomas and trichodiscomas are characteristic benign hair-follicle hamartomas, which present as many small asymptomatic skin-coloured papules on the face, neck, scalp, and upper trunk, usually in the third decade of life.

Pulmonary features include spontaneous pneumothorax and lung cysts [173].

The renal neoplasms associated with Birt-Hogg-Dube are of varying histological type and can be unilateral, bilateral, solitary, or multifocalThe most frequent renal tumours are chromophobe renal-cell carcinomas and hybrid chromophobe- oncocytomas [171].

Some authors suggest using renal ultrasound and/or abdominal CT on diagnosis and then every 3 or 5 years [173].

Reed Syndrome

Reed Syndrome or hereditary leiomyomatosis renal-cell carcinoma is an autosomal dominantly inherited cancer predisposition syndrome due to a heterozygous mutation in the fumarate hydratase gene on chromosome 1q42 [171].

These patiens have an inherited predisposition to the development of cutaneous leiomyomas, uterine leiomyomas and papillary renal-cell carcinoma

Cutaneous leiomyomas appears as ill-defined, flesh-coloured papules or well-circumscribed, reddish-purple nodules on the face, back (Figure 37), and extensor surfaces of extremities. Characteristically, painful is precipitated by cold and trauma.

Renal cell carcinoma is present in only 20% of those with the gene mutation at a younger age than sporadic patients, and the tumors are associated with aggressive metastatic disease with poor prognosis. A few cases of leiomyosarcoma have also been described [171, 173].

6.3. Syndromes with Endocrine Neoplasia

MEN 1

Multiple endocrine neoplasia type 1 is an autosomal dominant syndrome due to heterozygous MEN1 mutations on 11q13, which results in a genetic predisposition to tumours of the pituitary gland, pancreas, and parathyroid glands, and to peptic ulcer disease.

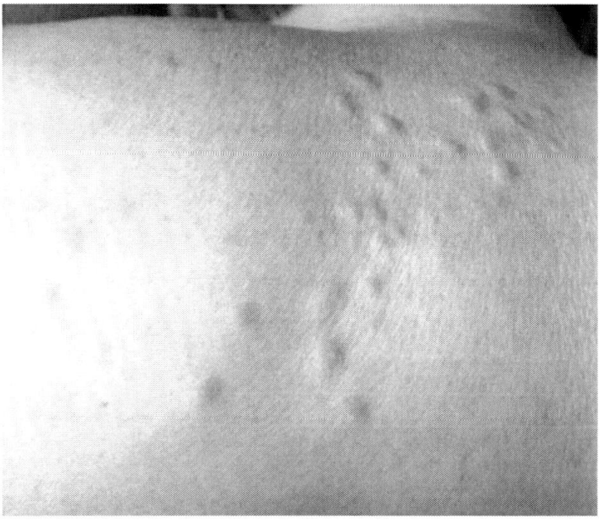

Figure 37. Segmentary cutaneous leiomyomas on the back.

The coexistence of multiple angiofibromas and collagenomas is a sensitive diagnostic indicator of MEN1. Other skin signs include subcutaneous lipoma, café au lait macules, confetti-like hyperpigmented macules, and many gingival polyps [171].

MEN 2A

MEN2A is a dominantly inherited condition due to a heterozygous mutation in the RET proto-oncogene on 10q11.2, and is characterised by a predisposition to medullary thyroid cancer pheochromocytoma, and primary parathyroid hyperplasia [171].

Frequent association between MEN 2A and cutaneous lichen amyloidosis has been described, with dry and scaly skin area with substantial pruritus, mainly in the inter- scapular region [174].

MEN 2B

MEN2B a phenotypic subset of the MEN2 syndrome characterized by pheochromocytoma without hyperparathyroidism, medullary thyroid carcinoma, mucosal and cutaneous neuromas, and marfanoid habitus [172].

These patients has characteristic phenotypic features, including mentioned marfanoid body habitus, coarse facial features, and developmental delay [171].

Mucosal and cutaneous neuromas present as 2–7 mm, yellowish-white, sessile, painless nodule of the lips, anterior tongue and buccal mucosa [172].

PTEN Hamartoma Tumour Syndrome

PTEN hamartoma tumour syndrome includes Cowden syndrome, Bannayan-Riley-Ruvalcaba syndrome Proteus syndrome, and Proteus-like syndrome, where a heterozygous mutation is identified in the phosphate and tensin gene (PTEN) on 10q23.31.6 [171].

Cowden Syndrome

Cowden syndrome is the most common phosphatase and tensin homolog hamartomatous tumor syndrome that is characterized by multiple hamartomas with cutaneous and gastrointestinal manifestations predominating and an increased risk for malignancy.

Diagnostic criteria include pathognomonic mucocutaneous signs, which include multiple trichilemmomas, oral papillomatosis and facial papules, and acral keratoses [6, 171].

Trichilemmomas, a benign hamartomas of the outer sheath of hair follicles, are flesh-colored smooth papules, ranging from 1- to 5 mm in size and are present predominantly on the face, head, and neck, close to the hairline. Papillomatous papules are benign mucocutaneous lesions usually seen on the face, oral mucosa, and acral surfaces. They produce a cobblestone appearance on the buccal and gingival mucosa. Keratosis punctata may be seen on the palms and sides and soles of the feet.

Lipomas are seen in 30% of the patients and cafè au lait spots in 9% of patients with CS [6].

Affected individuals are highly susceptible to malignancies: breast, colon, and thyroid cancers are most commonly associated. Others neoplasias including, ovarian cancer, cervical cancer, meningioma, and transitional-cell carcinoma of the bladder [6, 171].

Bannayan-Riley-Ruvalcaba Syndrome

Bannayan-Riley-Ruvalcaba syndrome is characterized by hamartomatous gastrointestinal polyps, macrocephaly, hemangiomas, and developmental delay.

Hyperpigmented macules involving the glans penis or vulva are the most specific cutaneous finding. Less common lesions include facial verrucous papules, lipomas, acanthosis nigricans, and vascular malformations Facial lesions, histologically, show the characteristics of verruca vulgaris or trichilemmomas, suggesting an overlap with Cowden Syndrome [6].

Any patient with a PTEN mutation, regardless of the phenotypic expression, has an elevated risk of malignancy. A multidisciplinary approach is imperative in these patients.

Carney Complex

Carney complex, also known as LAMB (lentigines, atrial myxomas, blue naevus) syndrome or NAME (naevus, atrial myxoma, endocrinopathy) syndrome, is an autosomal dominantly inherited condition due to heterozygous mutations in the PRKAR1A chromosome 17q23-24.

This syndrome affects endocrine glands as the adrenal cortex, the pituitary and the thyroid, including primary pigmented nodular adrenocortical disease an adrenocorticotropin hormone ACTH-independent cause of Cushing's syndrome, growth hormone -secreting and prolactin-secreting pituitary adenomas, thyroid adenomas or carcinomas, and ovarian lesions (cysts and cancinomas) [167]. It is associated with many other nonendocrine tumors, including cardiac myxomas, testicular tumors, melanotic schwannoma, breast myxomatosis, and abnormal pigmentation (lentiginosis) or myxomas of the skin [176].

The typical spotty brown or black pigmentation is centrofacial, eyelid, inner or outer canthal signs, or mucosal lentigines. Nevi including blue nevi, ephilides, and café au lait macules, can occur, along with profuse pigmentation and hypopigmentation. Cutaneous and subcutaneous myxomas occur in about half of affected individuals, usually in young adulthood. The most common sites for these myxomas are eyelids, nipples, and ears [171].

6.4. Others Cutaneous Genodermatosis and Skin Disorders with Internal Malignancies

Naevoid Basal-Cell Carcinoma Syndrome

Naevoid basal-cell carcinoma syndrome, also known Gorlin syndrome, is a clinically variable condition due to an autosomal dominantly inherited mutation in PTCH gene on 9q22 [171].

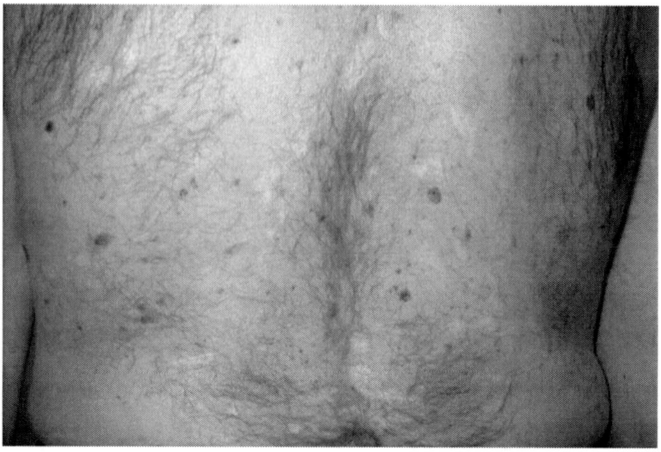

Figure 38. Gorlin Syndrome: multiple basal cell carcinomas on the back.

Gorlin Syndrome consists on multiple basal cell carcinomas (Figure 38), palmoplantar pits (Figure 39), jaw cysts, falx calcification, macrocephaly, cleft lip or palate, frontal bossing, coarse face, and moderate or severe hypertelorism, among others bone abnormalities.

Patients affected may also develop other malignancies such as medulloblastomas, oligodendrogliomas, ovarian fibrosarcoma, and Hodgkin and non-Hodgkin lymphoma [13].

Melanoma/Pancreatic Cancer Syndrome

Melanoma/pancreatic cancer syndrome is caused by an autosomal dominant germline mutation in the CDKN2A gene on chromosome 9p21.

It has been known as familial atypical multiple mole-melanoma syndrome, dysplastic nevus syndrome, atypical mole syndrome, and B-K mole syndrome. Later pancreatic carcinoma and possibly other tumors were found to be associated with this syndrome as well.

The clinical diagnostic criteria for familial atypical multiple mole-melanoma syndrome syndrome has been suggested as: (1) one of more cutaneous malignant melanoma in a family member (2); presence of atypical nevus or multiple atypical nevi at least 5 mm in diameter resembling early cutaneous malignant melanoma; and (3) patient with multiple nevi, usually more than 50.

Affected patients with familial atypical multiple mole-melanoma syndrome have been reported to have a 50% chance of developing cutaneous malignant melanoma. The risk of pancreatic cancer in individuals with

CDKN2A mutations has been estimated at 17% and it presents with symptoms including jaundice, pruritus, and weight loss [172].

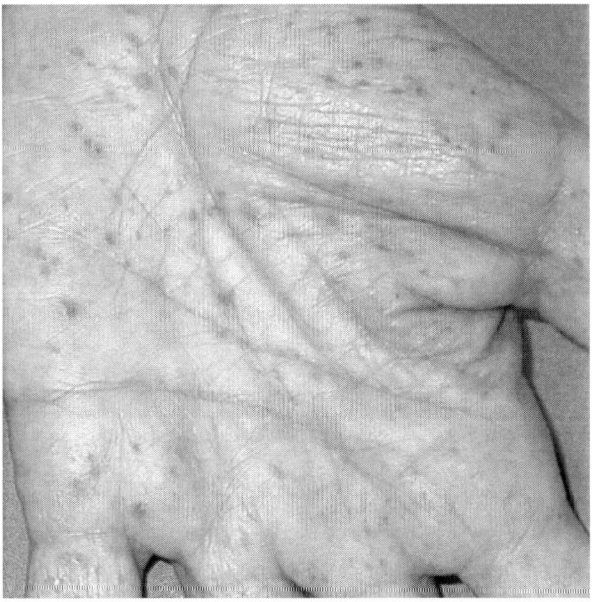

Figure 39. Gorlin Syndrome: palmar pits.

Disorders with Photosensitivity

Bloom Syndrome

BS is an autosomal recessive disorder with an abnormal BLM protein caused by a mutation in the RecQ2 DNA helicase family on chromosome 15.

Cutaneous findings include skin photosensitivity with redding of the face and telangiectasia, atrophy and scarred lesions on malar regions, nose, ears and hands. Also is often the appearance of spots café au latte dispersed in 50% of patients.

Associated malignancies include non-Hodgkin's lymphoma, leukemia, lymphosarcoma, Willms tumour, gastrointestinal adeocarcinoma and skin cancer [55, 172].

Rothmund–Thomson Syndrome

Rothmund–Thomson syndrome is an autosomal recessive disorder with a mutation in the RecQ4 DNA helicase family on chromosome 8, leading to genomic instability as a result of a sensitivity to oxidative stress and defective DNA repair mechanisms [172].

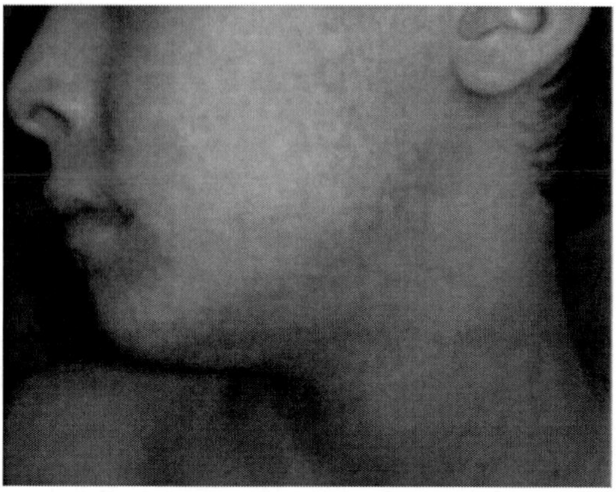

Figure 40. Rothmund-Thomsom syndrome: poikiloderma, erythema and telangiectasia on the face.

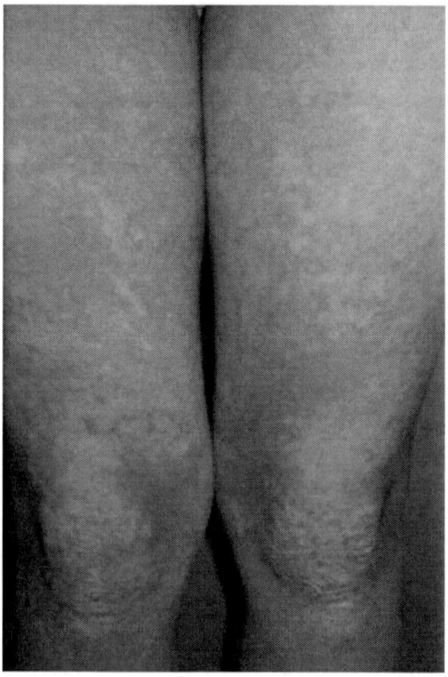

Figure 41. Rothmund-Thomsom syndrome: poikiloderma, erythema and telangiectasia on extensor surface of the extremities. Note hyperkeratotic plaques on the knees.

Photosensitivity and poikiloderma are noted at an early age beginning with the appearance of striated erythema and telangiectasia on the face (Figure 40) and ears, which then progresses to involve the buttocks and extensor surface of the extremities (Figure 41). Early aging, ungual changes, and alopecia have been described. Non-skin manifestations include cataracts, and skeletal or dental abnormalities.

On rare occasions, patients can also develop osteosarcoma, fibrosarcoma, gastric carcinoma, and cutaneous squamous cell carcinoma [55].

Xeroderma Pigmentosa

XP is an autosomal recessive disorder consisting of seven complementation groups, A to G, involving defects in the function of nucleotide excision repair.

Patients with xeroderma pigmentosa have a severe cellular sensitivity to ultraviolet light, which predisposes them to cutaneous malignancy at an early age, poikiloderma, premature cutaneous aging, neurologic, and ophthalmologic problems, and in some variants an increased risk for internal malignancy, developmental disorders and neurodegenerative problems.

Patientes have been reported to develop fibrosarcoma, angiosarcoma, astrocytoma, medulloblastoma, glioblastoma, malignant schwannoma, conjunctival and eyelid epitheli mas, and leukemia [172].

Dyskeratosis Congenita

Dyskeratosis congenita is a multisystemic X-linked recessive disorder characterized by the triad of nail changes, reticulated hyperpigmentation, and leukoplakia of any of the mucous membranes, although the oral mucosa is the most frequently affected.

Nail changes occur early on in the disease. The nails are initially fragile and uneven. They remain small and can even be absent or barely noticeable. The changes first affect the fingernails and then the toenails.

Patients with dyskeratosis congenita have a high risk of aplastic anemia, myelodysplastic syndrome, leukemia, and solid tumors. Leukoplakia is associated with a higher incidence of squamous cell carcinoma of the mouth, rectum, cervix, vagina, esophagus, and skin [177].

Acknowledgments

Both authors have contributed equally in the proposing of this manuscript.
Authors declare not to have any conflict of interest.
Authors declare not to have received any kind of external funding.
Attached Copyright Transfer Form signed by the authors
Permission request form has not been required.

Conclusion

The dermatologist is in a unique position to impact the clinical course of patients with internal malignancies, as many of them may be associated with skin disorders.

Early recognition of these cutaneous signs can help enter these patients in to appropriate screening and treatment programs that will improve the diagnosis and patient outcome.

Cutaneous lesions may also be useful for monitoring the activity and response to treatment of malignant disease.

References

[1] Buggiani G, Krysenka A, Grazzini M, Vaskù V, Hercogová J, Lotti T. Paraneoplastic vasculitis and paraneoplastic vascular syndromes. *Dermatol. Ther.* 2010;23:597-605.

[2] Curth HO. Cancer associated with acanthosis nigricans. *Arch. Surg.* 1943;47:517-52.

[3] Steele HA, George BJ. Mucocutaneous paraneoplastic syndromes associated with hematologic malignancies. *Oncology* (Williston Park). 2011 Oct;25(11):1076-83.

[4] Brenner S, Tamir E, Maharshak N, Shapira J. Cutaneous manifestations of internal malignancies. *Clin. Dermatol.* 2001; 19: 290-7.

[5] M. Yuste-Chaves, P. Unamuno-Pérez. Cutaneous Alerts in Systemic Malignancy: Part I. *Actas Dermosifiliogr.* 2013;104(4):285-298.

[6] Shah KR, Boland CR, Patel M, Thrash B, Menter A. Cutaneous manifestations of gastrointestinal disease: part I. *J. Am. Acad. Dermatol.* 2013 Feb;68(2):189.e1-21; quiz 210.

[7] Nishigori K, Yamamoto T, Yokozeki H. Vesiculo-bullous dermatomyositis: report of three cases. *Dermatol. Online J.* 2009;15:6.
[8] Martorell-Calatayud A, Serra Guillén C, Ciudad-Blanco C, San Martín O. Skin necrosis as a predictive factor for neoplasia in dermatomyositis. *Actas Dermosifiliogr.* 2010;101:455-6.
[9] Vílchez F, Camacho E, Alcaraz I, López N, Herrera E. Dermatomyositis and livedoid vasculopathy as the initial manifestation of a tumor. *Actas Dermosifiliogr.* 2011;102:155-7.
[10] Choi YS, Ryu KH, Kwon GY, Jeon SS, Choi HY, Lee HM. Ureteral cancer associated with dermatomyositis. *Int. J. Urol.* 2006;13:442-4.
[11] Toro C, Rinaldo A, Silver CE, Politi M, Ferlito A. Paraneoplastic syndromes in patients with nasopharyngeal cancer. *Auris Nasus Larynx.* 2009;36:513-20.
[12] Yosipovitch G, Tan A, LoSicco K, Manabat CG, Kannagra A, Carroll C, et al., A comparative study of clinical characteristics, work-up, treatment, and association to malignancy in dermatomyositis between two tertiary skin centers in the USA and Singapore. *Int. J. Dermatol.* 2013; 52(7): 813–19.
[13] Kleyn CE, Lai-Cheong JE, Bell HK. Cutaneous manifestations of internal malignancy: diagnosis and management. *Am. J. Clin. Dermatol.* 2006;7:71-84.
[14] Chung VQ, Sci M, Moschella SL, Zembowicz A, Liu V. Clinical and pathologic findings of paraneoplastic dermatoses. *J. Am. Acad. Dermatol.* 2006;54:745-62.
[15] Scheinfeld N. A review of the cutaneous paraneoplastic associ- ations and metastatic presentations of ovarian carcinoma. *Clin. Exp. Dermatol.* 2008;33:10-5.
[16] Thomas I, Robert A. Schwartz Cutaneous paraneoplastic syndromes: uncommon presentations. *Clin. Dermatol.* 2005; 23(6): 593–600.
[17] Bielsa I. Nuevos autoanticuerpos en la dermatomiositis. *Actas Dermosifiliogr.* 2009;100:182-9
[18] Braverman IM. Skin manifestations of internal malignancy. *Clin. Geriatr Med.* 2002;18:1-19.
[19] András C, Ponyi A, Constantin T, Csiki Z, Szekanecz E, Szodoray P, et al., Dermatomyositis and polymyositis associated with malignancy: a 21-year retrospective study. *J. Rheumatol.* 2008;35:438-44.
[20] Anhalt GJ, Kim SC, Stanley JR, Korman NJ, Jabs DA, Kory M, et al., Paraneoplastic pemphigus: An autoimmune mucocutaneous disease associated with neoplasia. *N. Engl. J. Med.* 1990;323:1729 – 1735.

[21] Billet SE, Grando SA, Pittelkow MR. Paraneoplastic autoimmune multiorgan syndrome: Review of the literature and support for a cytotoxic role in pathogenesis. *Autoimmunity* 2006; 39(7): 617–630.
[22] Cummins DL, Mimouni D, Tzu J, Owens N, Anhalt GJ, Meyerle JH. Lichenoid paraneoplastic pemphigus in the absence of detectable antibodies. *J. Am. Acad. Dermatol.* 2007;56:153-9.
[23] Yokokura H, Demitsu T, Kakurai M, Umemoto N, Azuma R, Yamada T, et al., Paraneoplastic pemphigus mimicking erosive mucosal lichen planus associated with primary hepatocellular carcinoma. *J. Dermatol.* 2006;33:842-5
[24] Kaplan I, Hodak E, Ackerman L, Mimouni D, Anhalt GJ, Calderon S. Neoplasms associated with paraneoplastic pemphigus: A review with emphasis on non-hematologic malignancy and oral mucosal manifestations. *Oral. Oncol.* 2004;40:553 – 562.
[25] De Saint Paul G, Busam B, Bayle P, Lamant L, Bazex J. Cutaneous T-cell lymphoma, cutaneous hyperpigmentation and paraneoplastic pemphigus (French). *Ann. Dermatol. Venereol.* 2002;129 (6-7):896–900.
[26] Sánchez NB, Canedo IF, García-Patos PE, Unamuno P, Benito AV, Martín A. Paraneoplastic vasculitis associated with multiple myeloma. *J. Eur. Acad. Dermatol.* 2004;18:731-5.
[27] Solans-Laqué R, Bosch-Gil JA, Pérez-Bocanegra C, Selva- O'Callaghan A, Simeón-Aznar CP, Vilardell-Tarres M. Paraneoplastic vasculitis in patients with solid tumors: report of 15 cases. *J. Rheumatol.* 2008;35:294-304.
[28] Wilson D, McCluggage WG, Wright GD. Urticarial vasculitis: a paraneoplastic presentation of B-cell non-Hodgkin's lymphoma. *Rheumatology.* 2002;41:476-7.
[29] Ducarme G, Rey D, Bryckaert PE, Reguiai Z, Bernard P, Staerman F. Paraneoplastic urticarial vasculitis and renal carcinoma. *Prog. Urol.* 2003;13:495-7.
[30] Wong M, Grossman J, Hahn BH, La Cava A. Cutaneous vasculi- tis in breast cancer treated with chemotherapy. *Clin. Immunol.* 2008;129:3-9.
[31] Hutson TE, Hoffman GS. Temporal concurrence of vasculitis and cancer: a report of 12 cases. *Arthritis Care Res.* 2000;13:417-23. 74.
[32] Simon Z, Tarr T, Tóth L, Szucs G, Illés A. Cutaneous vasculitis as an initiating paraneoplastic symptom in Hodgkin lymphoma. *Rheumatol. Int.* 2008;28:719-23.75.

[33] Podjasek JO, Wetter DA, Pittelkow MR, Wada DA. Cutaneous small-vessel vasculitis associated with solid organ malignancies: The Mayo Clinic experience, 1996 to 2009. *J. Am. Acad. Dermatol.* 2012;66:55-65.

[34] Bonifazi M, Tramacere I, Pomponio G, Gabrielli B, Avvedimento EV, La Vecchia C, et al. Systemic sclerosis (scleroderma) and cancer risk: systematic review and meta-analysis of observational studies. *Rheumatology* (Oxford) 2013;52:143-54.

[35] Reyes CM, Rudinskaya A, Kloss R, Girardi M, Lazova R. Scleroderma-like illness as a presenting feature of multiple myeloma and amyloidosis. *J. Clin. Rheumatol.* 2008;14:161-5.

[36] Szekanecz E, Szamosi S, Gergely L, Keszthelyi P, Szekanecz Z, Szucs G. Incidence of lymphoma in systemic sclerosis: a retrospective analysis of 218 Hungarian patients with systemic sclerosis. *Clin. Rheumatol.* 2008;27:1163-6.

[37] Vettori S, Staibano S, Mascolo M, Ilardi G, Valentini G. Non-Hodgkin's lymphoma in systemic sclerosis: case and literature review. *Clin. Rheumatol.* 2010;29:1-6.

[38] Hounkpati A, Marie I, Paillotin D, Muir JF, Cuvelier A. Paraneoplastic sclerodermiform syndrome. *Rev. Mal. Respir.* 2010;27:251-6.

[39] Sakauchi F, Mori M, Ishikawa O, Endo H. The association of systemic sclerosis with malignant neoplasms. *Nihon Rinsho Meneki Gakkai Kaishi* 2004; 27(6): 402-6.

[40] Vallés L, Arrue I, González M, Polo I, Guerra A, Vanaclocha F. Esclerodermia sistémica y cáncer de mama. *Med. Cutan Iber Lat. Am.* 2009;37(6):258-261.

[41] Cohen PR Granuloma annulare, relapsing polychondritis, sarcoidosis, and systemic lupus erythematosus: conditions whose dermatologic manifestations may occur as hematologic malignancy- associated mucocutaneous paraneoplastic syndromes. *Int. J. Dermatol.* 2006; 45(1):70–80.

[42] Sánchez-Cano D, Callejas-Rubio JL, Vilanova-Mateu A, Gómez-Morales M, Ortego-Centeno N. Intravascular lymphoma in a patient with systemic lupus erythematosus: a case report. *Lupus.* 2007;16:525-8.

[43] Dawn G, Wainwright NJ. Association between subacute cutaneous lupus erythematosus and epidermoid carcinoma of the lung: a paraneoplastic phenomenon? *Clin. Exp. Dermatol.* 2002;27:717-8.

[44] Chaudhry SI, Murphy LA, White IR. Subacute cutaneous lupus erythematosus: a paraneoplastic dermatosis? *Clin. Exp. Dermatol.* 2005;30:655-8.

[45] Gantzer A, Regnier S, Cosnes A, Ortonne N, Wolkenstein P, Bagot M, et al., Subacute cutaneous lupus erythematosus and cancer: two cases and literature review. *Ann. Dermatol. Venereol.* 2011;138:409-17.

[46] Bernatsky S, Ramsey-Golman R, Labrecque J, Joseph L, Boivin JF, Petri M, et al., Cancer risk in systemic lupus: An updated international multi-centre cohort study. *J. Autoimmun* 2013;42:130-5.

[47] Evans KG, Heymann WR. Paraneoplastic subacute cutaneous lupus erythematosus: an underrecognized entity. *Cutis.* 2013 Jan;91(1):25-9.

[48] Mellemkjaer L, Andersen V, Linet MS, et al., Non- Hodgkin's lymphoma and other cancers among a cohort of patients with SLE. *Arthritis Rheum* 1977; 40: 761–768.

[49] DiCataldo A, Villari L, Milone P, et al., Thymic carcinoma, systemic lupus eythematosus, and hypertrophic pulmonary osteoarthropathy in an 11-year-old boy: a novel association. *Pediatr Hematol. Oncol.* 2000; 17: 701– 706.

[50] Loche F, Schwarze HP, Durieu C, et al., A case of systemic lupus erythematosus associated with cancer of the lung: a paraneoplastic association? [Letter]. *Br. J. Dermatol.* 2000; 143: 210 –211.

[51] Imaoka K, Kaneko S, Harada Y, Ota M, Furumura M, Morita E. Neutrophilic dermatosis of the palms. *J. Dermatol.* 2012;39(11):949-51.

[52] Cohen PR. Sweet's syndrome: a comprehensive review of an acute febrile neutrophilic dermatosis. *Orphanet J. Rare Dis.* 2007; 2: 34.

[53] Hospach T, von den Driesch P, Dannecker GE. Acute febrile neutrophilic dermatosis (Sweet's syndrome) in childhood and adolescence: two new patients and review of the literature on associated diseases. *Eur. J. Pediatr.* 2009;168:1-9.

[54] Yuste M, González-Morán A, Narváiz J, Cermeño F, Velasco R. Síndrome de Sweet asociado a adenocarcinoma gástrico. *Actas Dermosifilogr.* 1989;80:205-8.

[55] Thiers BH, Sahn RE, Callen JP. Cutaneous manifestations of internal malignancy. *CA Cancer J. Clin.*. 2009;59:73-98.

[56] Talsania N, Harwood CA, Piras D, Cerio R. Paraneoplastic Acan- thosis Nigricans: The importance of exhaustive and repeated malignancy screening. *Dermatol. Online J.* 2010;15:16-8.

[57] Cohen RP. Neutrophilic Dermatoses A Review of Current Treatment Options. *Am. J. Clin. Dermatol.* 2009; 10 (5): 301-312.

[58] Alexandrescu DT, Riordan NH, Ichim TE, Kauffman CL, Kabigting F, Dutton CT, et al., On the missing link between inflammation and cancer. *Dermatol. Online J.* 2011;17:10.

[59] Eubanks LE, McBurney E, Reed R. Erythema gyratum repens. Am. J. Med Sci 2001; 321: 459-81. Kawakami T, Saito R. Erythema gyratum repens unassociated with underlying malignancy. *J. Dermatol.* 1995; 22: 587-9.

[60] Lomholt H, Thestrup-Pedersen K. Paraneoplastic skin manifestations of lung cancer. *Acta Derm. Venereol.* 2000;80:200-2. 37.

[61] Ameen M, Chopra S, Darvay A, Acland K, Chu C. Erytema gyratum repens and acquired ichtyosis associated with transitional cell carcinoma of the kidney. *Clin. Exp. Dermatol.* 2001;26:510-2.

[62] Kaminsky A. Eritemas figurados. *Actas Dermosifilogr.* 2009;100 Suppl. 2:88-109.

[63] Silva JA, Mesquita Kde C, Igreja AC, Lucas IC, Freitas AF, Oliveira SM, Costa IM, Campbell IT. Paraneoplastic cutaneous manifestations: concepts and updates. *An Bras Dermatol.* 2013 Jan-Feb;88(1):9-22.

[64] Endo Y, Fujisawa A, Tanioka M, Miyachi Y. Erythema gyratum repens preceding the onset of rheumatoid arthritis. *Eur. J. Dermatol.* 2013 Jun 1;23(3):399-400.

[65] Campbell L, Freedman JR, O'Donoghue M, Chevalier M, Dy LC, Tharp MD Erythema gyratum repens without associated malignancy. *J. Am. Acad. Dermatol.* 2011 Jul;65(1):e22-3.

[66] Pipkin CA, Lio PA. Cutaneous manifestations of internal malignancies: an overview. *Dermatol Clin.* 2008;26(1):1-15,vii.

[67] De La Torre Lugo EM, Sánchez JL. Erythema gyratum repens. *J. Am. Acad. Dermatol.* 2011;64:89-90.

[68] Technau K, Renkl A, Norgauer J, Ziemer M. Necrolytic migratory erythema with myelodysplastic syndrome without glucagonoma. *Eur. J. Dermatol.* 2005;15:110-2.

[69] Abreu Velez AM, Howard MS. Diagnosis and treatment of cutaneous paraneoplastic disorders. *Dermatol. Ther.* 2010;23:662-75.

[70] Jabbour SA. Skin manifestations of hormone-secreting tumors. *Dermatol Ther.* 2010;23:643-50.

[71] Boyce S, Harper J. Paraneoplastic dermatoses. *Dermatol. Clin.* 2002;20:523-32.

[72] Bazex A, Salvador R, Dupre´ A, Christol B. Syndrome paraneoplasique a type d'hyperkeratose des extremits; Guerison apres le traitement de le´ pithe´ lioma larynge´. *Bull Soc. Fr. Dermatol. Syphiligr* 1965;72:182.

[73] Gougerot H, Grupper C. Dermatose erythemato-squameuse avec hyperke´ratose palmoplantaire, porectasies digitales et cancer de la langue latent. *Paris Med.* 1922;43:234 - 7.

[74] González-Morán A, Román C, Galván C, Yuste M, Pascual JA, Revestido R. Acroqueratosis paraneoplásica de Bazex asoci-ada a Carcinoma epidermoide oculto. *Actas Dermosifilogr.* 1993;841:63.

[75] Santos-Silva AR, Correa MB, Vargas PA, Almeida OP, Lopes MA. Bazex syndrome (acrokeratosis paraneoplastica) diagnosed in a patient with oral persistent ulcerations. *Head Neck Pathol.* 2010;4:312-7.

[76] Yuste M, González-Morán A, Galván C, Santiago M, Aramendi T. Acroqueratosis paraneoplásica de Bazex asociada a adenocarcinoma de próstata. *Actas Dermosifilogr.* 1991;82:577-80.

[77] Sator PG, Breier F, Gschnait F. Acrokeratosis paraneoplastica (Bazex's syndrome): Association with liposarcoma. *J. Am. Acad. Dermatol.* 2006;55:1103-5.

[78] Moore RL, Devere TS. Epidermal manifestations of internal malignancy. *Dermatol. Clin.* 2008;26:17-29.

[79] Ennibi K, Rabhi M, Al Bouzidi A, Bahrouch L, Boudlal M, Zinebi A, et al., Acquired ichthyosis revealing an Hodgkin's disease. *Rev. Med. Interne.* 2008;29:418-20.

[80] Berrady R, Baybay H, Khammar Z, Lahlou M, Lamchachti L, Gallouj S, et al., Acquired ichthyosis and haematological malig- nancies: five cases. *Ann. Dermatol. Venereol.* 2012;139:9-14.

[81] Ulla JL, García-Doval I, Posada C, Soto S, Alvárez C, Ledo L, et al., Plantar keratoderma as a presenting sign of pancreatic adenocarcinoma. *J. Clin. Ultrasound.* 2008;36:108-9.

[82] El Bakkal A, Idrissi R, Meziane M, Mikou O, Sekal M, Belghiti H, et al., Tripe palms and a hypertrophic osteoarthropathy syndrome revealing a neuroendocrine carcinoma of the lung. *Ann. Dermatol. Venereol.* 2011;138:668-72.

[83] Kebria MM, Belinson J, Kim R, Mekhail TM. Malignant acanthosis nigricans, tripe palms and the sign of Leser-Trélat, a hint to the diagnosis of early stage ovarian cancer: A case report and review of the literature. *Gynecol. Oncol.* 2006;101:353-5.

[84] Janniger EJ, Schwartz RA. Florid cutaneous papillomatosis. *J. Surg. Oncol.* 2010;102:709-12.

[85] Singhi MK, Gupta LK, Bansal M, Jain V, Kachhawa D. Florid cutaneous papillomatosis with adenocarcinoma of stomach in a 35 year old male. *Indian J. Dermatol. Venereol. Leprol.* 2005;71:195-6.

[86] Csete B, Moezzi M, Lengyel ZS, Hodosi B, Zombai E, Battyani Z. Florid Cutaneous papillomatosis leading to social exclusion. *Br. J. Dermatol.* 2005;153:664-99.

[87] Zustovich F, Lombardi G, Cartei G. Paraneoplastic diffuse cutaneous papillomatosis. *J. Eur. Acad. Dermatol. Venereol.* 2009;23:220-1.

[88] Cohen PR, Grossman ME, Almeida L, Kurzrok R. Tripe palms and malignancy. *J. Clin. Oncol.* 1989;7:669-78.

[89] Breathnach SM, Wells GC. Acanthosis palmaris: tripe palms. A distinctive pattern of palmar keratoderma frequently associ- ated with internal malignancy. *Clin. Exp. Dermatol* 1980;5:181-9.

[90] Cruz M, Mota A, Baudrier T, Azevedo F..- Tripe palms revealing renal cell carcinoma. *Int. J. Dermatol.* 2013, 52, 1019–32.

[91] Bursztejn AC, Doumat-Batch F, Granel-Brocard F, Perrin A, CunyJF, Barbaud A, et al., Sézary syndrome and Leser- Trélat sign: a chance association? *Ann. Dermatol. Venereol.* 2008;135:287-90.

[92] Rampen HJ, Schwengle LE. The sign of LesereTrèlat: does it exist? *J. Am. Acad. Dermatol* 1989;21:50-5.

[93] Schwartzberg JB, Ricotti Jr CA, Ballard CJ, Nouri K. Eruptive dermatosis papulosa nigra as a possible sign of internal malig- nancy. *Int. J. Dermatol.* 2007;46:186-7.

[94] Rubenstein M, Duvic M. Cutaneous manifestations of Hodgkin's disease. *Int. J. Dermatol.* 2006;45:251-6.

[95] Andriamanantena D, Boye T, Gervaise A, Vieu C, Splingard B, Dot JM, et al., An unusual paraneoplastic manifestation in lung cancer: eosinophilic erythroderma. *Rev. Pneumol. Clin.* 2009;65:32-5.

[96] Scrivener Y, Jeandidier N, Asch PH, et al., Erythroderma induced by hypercalcitonemia: two cases. *Ann. Dermatol. Venereol.* 2002;129: 221-4. Cohen PR. Cutaneous paraneoplastic syndromes. *Am. Fam. Physician.* 1994;50:1273-82.

[97] Rothe MJ, Bialy TL, Grant-Kels JM. Erythroderma. Dermatol Clin 2000;18:405 - 415 Cohen PR, Kurzrock R. Mucocutaneous paraneo-plastic syndromes. *Sem. Oncol.* 1997;24:334-59.

[98] Berlin AL, Pehr K. Coexistence of erythromelalgia and Raynaud's phenomenon. *J. Am. Acad. Dermatol* 2004;50:456-60.

[99] El Tal AK, Tannous Z. Cutaneous vascular disorders associated with internal malignancy. *Dermatol. Clin.* 2008;26:45-57.

[100] Cohen PR, Kurzrock R. Mucocutaneous paraneo- plastic syndromes. *Sem. Oncol.* 1997;24:334-59.

[101] Noble JP, Boisnic S, Branchet-Gumila MC, Poisson M. Palmar erythema: cutaneous marker of neoplasms. *Dermatology.* 2002; 204:209-13.

[102] Metcalfe DD. Differential diagnosis of the patient with unexplained flushing/anaphylaxis. *Allergy Asthma Proc*. 2000;21:21-4.

[103] Batalla Cebey A y De la Torre Fraga C. Signos guıía / diagnóstico diferencial. Rubor facial transitorio. Metodología diagnóstica y tratamiento. *Piel* 2012; 27(7):390-400.

[104] Sánchez-Estella J, Yuste M, Santos JC, Alonso MT. Hipertrico- sis lanuginosa adquirida paraneoplásica. *Actas Dermosifilogr*. 2005; 96:459-61.

[105] Vulink AJ, ten Bokkel Huinink D. Acquired hypertrichosis lanug- inosa: a rare cutaneous paraneoplastic syndrome. *J. Clin. Oncol.* 2007; 20:1625-6.

[106] Adone Baroni A, Faccenda F, Teresa R, Piccolo V. *Figurate Paraneoplastic Urticaria and Prostate Cancer Ann. Dermatol.* Vol. 24, No. 3, 2012.

[107] Rodrguez Trabado A, Riesco Miranda JA, Porcel Carreño S, Rodríguez Martín E, Fletes Peral C, Jiménez Timón S, et al., Angioedema as a single manifestation of carcinoid syndrome in a bronchial carcinoid tumor. *Allergol Immunopathol.* (Madr) 2004 Jul-Aug;32(4):235-7.

[108] Bell HK, Poston GJ, Vora J, Wilson NJE. Cutaneous manifes- tations of the malignant carcinoid syndrome. *Br. J. Dermatol.* 2005;152:71-5.

[109] Bofek A, Rachowska R, Krajewska J, Paliczka-Cieslik E, Fil- ipowska B, Jarzab J. Carcinoid syndrome with angioedema and urticaria. *Arch. Dermatol.* 2008;144:691-2.

[110] Escribano L, Akin C, Castells M, Orfao A, Metcalfe DD. Mastocytosis: current concepts in diagnosis and treatment *Ann. Hematol.* (2002) 81:677–690.

[111] Valent P, Horny H-P, Escribano L, Longley-BJ J, Li CL, Schwartz LB, et al., Diagnostic criteria and classification of mastocytosis: a consensus proposal. *Leuk Res.* 2001;25:603–625.

[112] Dalle S, Merle P, Gouillat C, Thomas L. Hepatocellular carci- noma revealed by prurigo. *Ann. Dermatol. Venereol*. 2006;133: 243-5.

[113] Ahern K, Gilmore ES, Poligone B. Pruritus in cutaneous T-cell lymphoma: A review. *J. Am. Acad. Dermatol.* 2012;67:760-8.

[114] Silvestris N, Chetta G, Sasso N, et al., Mucocutaneous paraneoplastic syndromes (MCPS). A clinical-pathologic review. *J. Exp. Clin. Cancer Res.* 1998;17:453-64.

[115] Sadollah Shamsadini, Majid Varesvazirian, and Ayeh Shamsadini. Urticaria and lip fasciculation may be prodromal signs of brain malignancy. *Dermatology Online Journal* 2006 12 (3): 23.

[116] M. Yuste Chaves, P. Unamuno Pérez. Cutaneous Manifestations of Systemic Malignancies: Part 2 *Actas Dermosifiliogr.* 2013;104(7):543-553.

[117] Bayer-Garner IB, Smoller BR. The spectrum of cutaneous disease in multiple myeloma. *J. Am. Acad. Dermatol.* 2003;48:497-507.

[118] Chan JC, Trendell-Smith NJ, Yeung CK. Scleromyxedema: a cutaneous paraneoplastic syndrome associated with thymic carcinoma. *J. Clin. Oncol.* 2012;30:27-9.

[119] Berk DR, Bentley DD, Bayliss SJ, Lind A, Urban Zlt. Cutis laxa: A review. *J. Am. Acad. Dermatol.* 2012 May 66 (5):842.

[120] Santos JC, Yuste M, Martínez O, Alonso MT, Sánchez J. Paquidermatoperiostosis (Síndrome de Touraine-Solente- Golé). Descripción de un caso. *Actas Dermosifilogr.* 2007;98: 116-20.

[121] Ikeda F, Okada H, Mizuno M, Kawamoto H, Okano N, Okazaki H, et al., Pachydermoperiostosis associated with juvenile polyps of the stomach and gastric adenocarcinoma. *J. Gastroenterol.* 2004;39:370-4.

[122] Rongioletti F, Merlo V, Riva S, Cozzani E, Cinotti E, Ghigliotti G, Parodi A, Kanitakis J. Reticular erythematous mucinosis: a review of patients' characteristics, associated conditions, therapy and outcome in 25 cases. *Br. J. Dermatol.* 2013 Dec;169(6):1207-11.

[123] García-Arpa M, Rodríguez-Vázquez M, Vera E, Romero G, González-García J, Cortina P. Normolipemic plane xanthomas and mycosis fungoides *Actas Dermosifiliogr.* 2005 Jun;96(5):307-10.

[124] Koçak M, Keleş H, Yakaryilmaz F, Bozdoğan O, Güliter Diffuse plane xanthomatosis in a patient with Budd-Chiari syndrome and monoclonal gammopathy. *Indian J. Dermatol.* 2009;54(4):369-71.

[125] Wong A, Hon Yoon K. Paraneoplastic Raynaud phenomenon and idiopathic thrombocytopenia. *Am. J. Clin. Oncol.* 2003;26:26 - 9.

[126] Poszepczynska-Guigné E, Viguier M, Chosidow O, Orcel B, Emmerich J, Dubertret L. Paraneoplastic acral vascular syn- drome: epidemiologic features, clinical manifestations, and disease sequelae. *J. Am. Acad. Dermatol.* 2002;47:47-52.

[127] Yuste M, Galván C, Román C, González-Morán A, Gil S, Aramendi T. Perniosis como manifestación inicial de leucemia mielomonocítica crónica. *Actas Dermosifilogr.* 1993; 841:63.

[128] Gibbs MB, English JC, Zirwas MJ. Livedo reticularis: An update. *J. Am. Acad. Dermatol.* 2005;52:1009-19.

[129] Gambichler T, Baier P, Altmeyer P. Generalized livedo reticularis as the first sign of metastatic breast carcinoma. *Clin. Exp. Dermatol.* 2009 Mar;34(2):253-4.

[130] Jansen T, Romiti R, Messer G, Stucker M, Altmeyer P. Supe- rior vena cava syndrome presenting as persistent erythematous oedema of the face. *Clin. Exp. Dermatol.* 2000;25:198-200.

[131] Yuste M, Santos JC, Sánchez-Estella J, Alonso MT. Edema facial en síndrome de vena cava superior: descripción de dos casos. *Med. Cutan Iber Lat Am.* 2004;32:254-8.

[132] Kraigher O, actas S. Eczema craquelé with purpura: a sign of internal malignancy or malabsorption syndrome? *Cutis.* 2009;83:75-6.

[133] Sparsa A, Boulinguez S, Liozon E, Roux C, Peyrot I, Doffoel- Hantz V, et al., Predictive clinical features of eczema craquelé associated with internal malignancy. *Dermatology.* 2007;215: 28-35.

[134] Pierard GE, Quatresooz P. What do you mean by eczema craquelé? *Dermatology.* 2007;215:3-4.

[135] Matzkin H, Braf Z. Paraneoplastic syndromes associated with prostatic carcinoma. *J. Urol.* 1987;138:1129-33.

[136] Atalay AA, Abuaf OK, Dogan B. Squamous cell lung carcinoma presenting with erythema annulare centrifugum. *Acta Dermatovenereol Croat* 2013 May;21(1):52-8.

[137] Tartaglia F, Blasi S, Sgueglia M, Polichetti P, Tromba L, Berni A. Retroperitoneal liposarcoma associated with small plaque parapsoriasis. *World J. Surg. Oncol.* 2007;5:76.

[138] Kurzydlo AM, Gillespie R. Paraneoplastic pityriasis rubra pilaris in association with bronchogenic carcinoma. *Australas J. Dermatol.* 2004;45:130-2.

[139] Vitiello M, Miteva M, Romanelli P, Castaneda J, Garces-Milanes D, Kirsner R, Kerdel FA. Pityriasis rubra pilaris: Was it the first manifestation of colon cancer in a patient with pre-existing psoriasis?. *J. Am. Acad. Dermatol* 2013, february :43-44.

[140] CB Garretson, ML Machan, J Krejci-Manwaring, Daniel Aires, V Tonkovic-Capin. Adenocarcinoma of the lung associated with pityriasis rubra pilaris. *Dermatology Online Journal* 2011, November 17 (11): 14.

[141] Cannavó SP, Borgia F, Adamo B, Guarneri B. Simultaneous development and parallel course of disseminated superficial porokeratosis and ovarian cancer: Coincidental association or true paraneoplastic syndrome? *J. Am. Acad. Dermatol.* 2008;58:657-.

[142] Schena D, Papagrigoraki A, Frigo A, Girolomoni G. Eruptive disseminated porokeratosis associated with internal malignancies: a case report. *Cutis*. 2010;85:156-9.

[143] Torres T, Velho GC, Selores M. Disseminated superficial poroker- atosis in a patient with cholangiocarcinoma: a paraneoplastic manifestation? *An Bras. Dermatol*. 2010;85:229-31.

[144] Lee WJ, Kim CH, Park GH, Won CH, Chang SE, Lee MW, et al., Disseminated superficial porokeratosis in a patient with esophageal cancer. *J. Dermatol*. 2010;37:747-8.

[145] Vivas AC, Chimento SM, Herschthal J, Spock C, Alonso-Llamazares J. Disseminated keratotic spicules: A rare manifestation in multiple myeloma and successful response to lenalidomide. *J. Am. Acad. Dermatol* 2013; 68 (6) June:179-80.

[146] Thrash B, Patel M, Shah KR, Boland CR, Menter A. Cutaneous manifestations of gastrointestinal disease. Part II. *J. Am. Acad. Dermatol*. 2013;68:211.e1-33.

[147] Van Der Waal RIF, Van de Scheur MR, Pas HH, Jonkman MF, Van Groeningen CJ, Nieboer C, et al., Linear IgA bullous der- matosis in a patient with renal cell carcinoma. *Br. J. Dermatol*. 2001;144:870-3.

[148] Benoit Corven C, Khalaf A, Courville L, Sibert L, Gobet F, Joly P. Renal chromophobe cell carcinoma and paraneoplastic linear IgA bullous dermatosis. *J. Urol*. 2003;169:270-1.

[149] Gantzer A, Bouaziz JD, Valeyrie-Allanore L, Ingen-Housz-Oro S, Ortonne N, Bagot M. Acute linear IgA bullous dermatosis with circulating IgA monoclonal antibody associated with Hodgkin's disease. *Ann. Dermatol. Venereol*. 2010;137:819-20.

[150] Etienne A, Ruffieux P, Didierjean L, Saurat JH. Epydermolyse bulleuse acquise et cancer du col utérin metastatique. *Ann. Dermatol. Venereol*. 1998;125:321-3.

[151] Prodanovic EM, Korman NJ. A case of non-Hodgkin's lymphoma-associated pemphigus foliaceus and use of rituximab for treatment. *J. Dermatol. Treat*. 2008;19:1-3.

[152] Tzovaras V, Liberopoulos EN, Zioga A, Pavlidis N, Elisaf M. Persistent erythema multiforme in a patient with extrahepatic cholangiocarcinoma. *Oncology*. 2007;73:127-9.

[153] Chiu ML, Tang MB. Generalized granuloma annulare associa- ted with gastrointestinal stromal tumour: case.

[154] Badri T, Kerkeni N, Marrak H, Khelifa E, Benmously-Mlika R, Mokhtar I, Fenniche S. Unilateral upper limb skin sarcoid reaction after

homolateral mastectomy for breast cancer. *Int. J. Dermatol.* 2013;52:124–125.

[155] Kishikawa T, Miyashita T, Fujiwara E, Shimomura O, Yasuhi I, Niino D, et al., Multicentric reticulohistiocytosis associated with ovarian cancer. *Mod. Rheumatol.* 2007;17:422-5.

[156] Nicol C, Quereux G, Renaut JJ, Renac F, Dreno B. Paraneoplas- tic multicentric reticulohistiocytosis. Ann. Dermatol. Venereol. 2011;138:405-8. Bayer-Garner IB, Smoller BR. The spectrum of cutaneous disease in multiple myeloma. *J. Am. Acad. Dermatol.* 2003;48:497-507.

[157] Lakhani A, Maas L. Necrotizing panniculitis: a skin condition associated with acinar cell carcinoma of the pancreas. *South Med. J.* 2008;101:554-5.

[158] Busam KJ, Sachs DL, Coit DG, Halpern A, Hwu WJ. Eruptive melanotic macules and papules associated with adenocarcinoma. *J. Cutan Pathol.* 2003;30:463-9.

[159] Dourmishev LA, Draganov PV. Paraneoplastic dermatological manifestation of gastrointestinal malignancies. *World J. Gas- troenterol.* 2009;15:4372-9.

[160] Collette McCourt, Cliona Feighery, Gemma McIntyre, Maureen Walsh, and Susannah Hoey. Eruptive nevi in prostate cancer: is this a paraneoplastic phenomenon? *International Journal of Dermatology* 2013, 52, 212–13.

[161] Ronni Wolf, Edith Orion, Batya Davidovici. Acral lentigines, a new paraneoplastic syndrome. *Int. J. Dermatol.* 2008;47: 168-70.

[162] Díez-Caballero N, Blanco G, Fournier D, Hernando F, Jarabo JR, López E. Alternativas actuales en el tratamiento de la hiperhidrosis. Dermatología-Información y avances. 2006 (mayo):4-11.

[163] Callejas MA, Grimalt R. Hiperhidrosis. Visión actual. *Clin. Dermatol.* 2009;9:8-19.

[164] Fatourechi V, Ahmed DD, Schwartz KM. Thyroid acropachy: report of 40 patients treated at a single institution in a 26-year period. *J. Clin. Endocrinol. Metab.* 2002 Dec;87(12):5435-41.

[165] Ginarte M, Monteagudo B, Toribio J. Yellow nail syndrome and lung lymphoma. *Clin. Exp. Dermatol.* 2004;29:432-3.

[166] Marques-Costa JC, Cuzzi T, Carneiro S, Parish LC, Ramos-e-Silva M. Paget's disease of the breast. *Skinmed.* 2012 May-Jun;10(3):160-5; quiz 165.

[167] Aroonroch R, Visetsiri Y, Wongwaisayawan S, Charakorn C, Kanchanapanjapol S, Rochanawutanon M. J Coexisting vulvar Paget's disease and mucinous carcinoma of the breast: a case report and review of the literature. *Med. Assoc. Thai*. 2012 Jun;95(6):847-52.
[168] Errihani H, Berrada N, Raissouni S, Rais F, Mrabti H, Rais G. Classic Kaposi's sarcoma in Morocco: Clinico - epidemiological study at the National Institute Of Oncology. *BMC Dermatology* 2011, 11:15.
[169] McArthur GA, Demetri GD, van Oosterom A, Heinrich MC, Debiec-Rychter M, Corless CL, et al., Molecular and clinical analysis of locally advanced dermatofibrosarcoma protuber- ans treated with imatinib: imatinib target exploration consor- tium study B2225. *J. Clin. Oncol.* 2005;23:866-73.
[170] Kurlander DE, Martires KJ, Chen Y, Barnholtz-Sloan JS, Bordeaux, JS. Risk of subsequent primary malignancies after dermatofibrosarcoma protuberans diagnosis: A national study. *J. Am. Acad. Dermatol.* 2013 Mayo;68:790-6.
[171] Winship IM, Dudding TE. Lessons from the skin—cutaneous features of familial cáncer. *Lancet Oncol.* 2008; 9: 462–72.
[172] Reyes MA, Bisent DB. Inhereted syndromes. *Dermatology Therapy*. Vol 23,2010,606-642.
[173] V. López, E. Jordá, C. Monteagudo. Actualización en el síndrome Birt-Hogg-Dubé. *Actas Dermosifiliogr*. 2012;103:198-206.
[174] Verga U, Fugazzola L, Cambiaghi S, et al., Frequent association between MEN 2A and cutaneous lichen amyloidosis. *Clin. Endocrinol.* 2003; 59: 156–61.
[175] Courcoutsakis NA, Tatsi C, Patronas NJ, Lee CC, Prassopoulos PK, Stratakis CA. The complex of myxomas, spotty skin pigmentation and endocrine overactivity (Carney complex): imaging findings with clinical and pathological correlation. *Insights Imaging*. 2013 Feb;4(1):119-33.
[176] Espiard S, Bertherat J. Carney complex. *Front Horm. Res.* 2013; 41:50-62.
[177] Walne AJ, Dokal I. Advances in the understanding of dyskeratosis congenita. *Br. J. Haematol.* 2009;145:164-72.

In: Paraneoplastic Syndromes
Editor: Lora H. Winter
ISBN: 978-1-63117-878-8

Chapter III

Paraneoplastic Syndromes in Patients with Malignancies of the Genitourinary Tract

Emilio Sacco*, M.D., Ph.D. and Riccardo Bientinesi, M.D.
Urology Department, "Agostino Gemelli" Academic Hospital, Catholic University Medical School, Rome, Italy

Abstract

Paraneoplastic syndromes may represent a major clinical problem also in patients with malignancies of the genitourinary tract. In this context, some paraneoplastic syndromes are of particular interest because of their clinically relevant incidence, such as endocrine paraneoplastic syndromes caused by inappropriate release of hormonal peptides, syndromes caused by inappropriate release of biologic amines, syndromes caused by inappropriate release of growth factors and renal cell carcinoma-related syndromes. The neuroendocrine differentiation of the tumour is often associated with paraneoplastic syndromes, especially endocrine syndromes.

Although with a low incidence, neurological paraneoplastic syndromes have been also reported in the published literature in

* Email: emilio.sacco@gmail.com.

association with genitourinary tumours. However, neurological syndromes are of clinical relevance because they may dominate the clinical picture in some patients and the diagnosis is often difficult due to the high index of suspicion needed to be recognized.

Renal cell carcinoma is the most frequent urological malignancy involved in paraneoplastic syndromes of urological interest. Prostate cancer is the second urological tumour associated with these syndromes. Bladder and testicular cancers, on the other hand, are less commonly associated with paraneoplastic manifestations.

Important technical advances in diagnostic tools have sensibly improved our ability to detect the primary tumours.

Generally, the radical therapy of the underlying cancer represent the most effective treatment strategy, although specific therapeutic options are available in particular clinical situations.

Endocrine Paraneoplastic Syndromes Caused by Inappropriate Release of Hormonal Peptides

The endocrine paraneoplastic syndromes are related to the aberrant hormonal production by tumors [1-3]. These syndromes can be classified broadly into several different types. The first is the production of a hormonal substance by a cell type that normally produces the hormone. Some examples include parathyroid hormone production by a parathyroid cancer, production of calcitonin by medullary thyroid carcinoma, and serotonin by carcinoid tumours. The second type is the "ectopic" production of a hormone by a cell type that does not normally produce the hormonal substance or produces it normally at very low levels. In some cases, the cell may have produced the hormonal product at an earlier stage in its development. An example of this is parathyroid hormone-related peptide (PTHrP) production by a squamous cell carcinoma. A second type of "ectopic" hormone production occurs in a hormone-producing cell whose machinery has been co-opted to produce another hormone. Many neuroendocrine tumours, for example, produce ACTH. Production of peptides by neuroendocrine tumours represents the most common "ectopic" hormone syndromes [2, 3]. Neuroendocrine cells are dispersed throughout nearly all organs, prevalently lungs, gastrointestinal tract, pancreas, thyroid gland, adrenal medulla, breast, prostate, and skin. These cells are most commonly derived from neural crest and produce biogenic amines and polypeptide hormones. The nature of tumour-produced hormones seems to be essentially the same of that of native hormones, although many tumours can produce precursors or hormone fragments with less biological activity. The production of multiple hormones by a tumour is not uncommon [1-4].

Paraneoplastic Hypercalcemia

Hypercalcemia is a serious and frequent complication of most malignancies, occurring in 10% to 20% of patients with cancer [5, 6]. The incidence of hypercalcemia is low at the initial presentation of cancer (1%–5%) but increases dramatically in patients with advanced disease and generally associated prognosis is poor. In fact, the median duration of survival for patients with malignancy-associated hypercalcemia is only 2–6 months from the onset of hypercalcemia [7, 8].

Alterations of calcium regulation in patients with hypercalcemia of malignancy can be divided into three general categories [2]. First, most common are humoral factors secreted in a paracrine or endocrine fashion (humoral hypercalcemia of malignancy, HHM). Second, in patients with substantial tumour burden metastatic to bone, the local effects of tumour can directly facilitate bone dissolution and calcium mobilization (local osteolysis). Third, less commonly, absorptive hypercalcemia results from excess vitamin D activation by the neoplasm. The cellular basis for the former two mechanisms includes changes in the activity and balance at the level of the bone-remodelling unit.

Up to 80% of hypercalcemias are due to HHM [6-9]. HHM is often associated with metastatic breast cancer (48%), lung cancer (22%), renal cell carcinoma (RCC) (15%) and ovarian cancer (5%) [10].

Often HHM is due to ectopic production of PTHrP, a paracrine and/or autocrine factor produced in almost every cell type in the body at some point, whether in childhood or adult life, with involvement of cellular growth regulation and differentiation [11].

Tumours that commonly produce ectopic PTHrP include squamous cell carcinomas of the lung, cervix, and oesophagus; certain lymphomas; RCC; and adenocarcinoma of the breast, prostate, and ovary [12, 13]. HMM is the most common paraneoplastic syndrome in patients affected by RCC, interesting between 13% and 20% of patients [14], and is occasionally reported in patients affected by bladder cancer [15].

Pathophysiology is related to the expression by osteoblasts of a cell surface receptor for parathyroid hormone (PTH) and parathyroid hormone–

related hormone (PTHrP), which is called PTH1R [16]. Both PTH and PTHrP stimulate PTH1R, which, in turn, increases osteoblast activity and RANKL signalling to the osteoclast. In sum, PTH/PTHrP signalling results in an increased bone turnover with a greater increase in bone reabsorption than formation, resulting in a net efflux of calcium and hypercalcemia from the bone microenvironment.

Given that the malignancy is usually advanced by the time hypercalcemia develops, a thorough history and physical examination can often lead to the correct diagnosis with limited laboratory evaluation. Clinical signs often are represented by itching, asthenia, anorexia, polydipsia and dehydration; organ-related signs, in particular renal signs, are: polyuria, lithiasis and renal failure; gastro-intestinal: nausea, vomiting, stipsis, paralytic ileus; cardiologic: bradicardya, arrhythmias; neurological: drowsiness, mental confusion, hyporeflexia. Measurement of intact PTH through an immunoradiometric or immunochemoluminescent assay will confirm a PTH-independent process. In this case, the PTH levels will be suppressed (often <20 pg/ml) and should prompt further testing to distinguish among the multiple possible causes in patients with malignancy. This would include measurement of PTHrP, 1,25-$(OH)_2D$ levels, serum and urine protein electrophoresis, assessment of serum free light chains, and possibly imaging studies (such as a skeletal survey). Patients presenting with acute and symptomatic hypercalcemia require prompt therapy that rapidly reduces the serum calcium level, restores the GFR, and leads to longer-term normalization of the serum calcium level. Patients with hypercalcemia are usually volume depleted. Furthermore, patients will present with poor fluid intake and may have had nausea and vomiting that further worsen the volume depletion. The decrease in GFR leads to impaired calcium clearance; thus, restoration of extracellular fluid volume and of GFR is a key goal of therapy.

When the tumour treatment is oncologically effective, a complete resolution of the hypercalcemic syndromes is usually achieved. Otherwise or before radical tumor treatment, there are two different therapeutic approaches for treating cancer-related hypercalcemia: to increase the urinary excretion of calcium, or to inhibit osteoclastic bone resorption, RANK ligand or the action of PTHrP. The first step of management of hypercalcemia should be to assess the hydration state; saline infusion is currently the standard of treatment, depending upon the severity of dehydration. However, if employed alone, volume expansion is ineffective in restoring normocalcemia because rehydration does not interfere with osteoclastic function. Association of diuretics (saline-induced diuresis) is recommended; this association enhances calcium excretion only after normovolemia has been reached.

Bisphosphonates represent at present the drugs of choice for treating patients with paraneoplastic hypercalcemia. They inhibit osteoclasts, induce apoptosis in these cells and bind to bone, blocking osteoclastic resorption and osteolysis [17]. Calcitonin, gallium nitrate, and corticosteroids can serve as adjunctive therapies. Denosumab, a fully human monoclonal antibody that binds to RANKL and inhibits osteoclast maturation, activation, and function, is an attractive therapeutic option for refractory cases of hypercalcemia; in phase III studies, Denosumab was shown to prevent skeletal-related events or HCM in patients with advanced malignancies involving bone [18-20]. In these trials, patients with breast cancer had a 52% lower incidence of HCM with denosumab than with zoledronic acid. However, more data are required before this therapy can be recommended [21]. In Patients with acute renal failure, haemodialysis should be considered [22].

Paraneoplastic Hypercortisolism

Different states of inappropriate neoplastic hormonogenesis can cause an overproduction of gluco- and/or mineralo-corticoids from the adrenal gland leading to paraneoplastic hypercortisolism (PNHC). Generally, these conditions can be divided into ectopic production of corticotropin-releasing hormone, or ectopic production of pro-opiomelanocortin, a polypeptidic precursor ACTH, which can directly stimulate and induce hyperplasia of the adrenal cortex [2, 3]. Both these situations result, finally, in production and release of cortisol from the adrenal glands. Approximately 5% to 10% of cases of Cushing syndrome (the clinical syndrome associated to the hypercortisolism) are paraneoplastic.

Neuroendocrine lung tumours (small cell lung cancer and bronchial carcinoids) are accountable of 50-60% of these paraneoplastic cases; other paraneoplastic Cushing cases are due to carcinoids, prostate cancer, RCC and small cell carcinoma (SCC) of prostate and bladder [2, 23, 24].

In contrast to other endocrine and metabolic paraneoplastic syndromes, patients often present with symptoms of paraneoplastic Cushing syndrome before a cancer diagnosis is made. Similarly, relapse of paraneoplastic Cushing syndrome may herald tumour recurrence [25].

Clinically, patients with PNHC may present clear signs and symptoms of Cushing's syndrome: rapid weight gain with central obesity (weight gain with centripetal fat distribution is more common in nonparaneoplastic than in paraneoplastic Cushing syndrome, because of the cachectic effects of the underlying neoplasm), a round face, excess sweating, telangiectasia, red striae, proximal muscle weakness, osteoporosis, hyperpigmentation and lipodystrophy, persistent hypertension, insulin resistance and various psychological disturbances. Muscle weakness is due to marked hypokalaemia and may be the first manifestation of the syndrome; sometimes, as reported in rare cases in association with bladder cancer, that symptom can be the main symptom in the clinical picture [26].

Laboratory findings include a baseline serum cortisol level greater than 29 μg/dL, a urinary free cortisol level greater than 47 μg/24 h, and a midnight adrenocorticotropic hormone level greater than 100 ng/L. Failure to respond to high-dose dexamethasone suppression distinguishes ectopic (paraneoplastic) Cushing syndrome from a pituitary source. For the high-dose dexamethasone suppression test, 2 mg of dexamethasone is given orally every 6 hours for 72 hours, and levels of urine 17-hydroxycorticosteroid are measured at 9 am and midnight of days 2 and 3 of the test. The suppression test is considered positive if 17-hydroxycorticosteroid levels are reduced by 50% or more. Imaging studies, including computed tomography (CT), magnetic resonance imaging, and somatostatin receptor scintigraphy (octreotide scan), are then used to locate the primary tumour.

Aside from the radical treatment of the underlying tumour, the goal of pharmacological therapy for paraneoplastic Cushing syndrome is the inhibition of steroid production. Usually, most common drugs include ketoconazole, mitotane, metyrapone, and aminoglutethimide. Despite associated nausea and hepatotoxicity, ketoconazole is usually the best tolerated of these agents. Antihypertensive agents and diuretics, with careful monitoring of serum potassium, may also be used to control symptoms. Less commonly used options include octreotide, which blocks the release of adrenocorticotropic hormone, and etomidate, which inhibits aspects of steroid synthesis and has been used to decrease serum cortisol levels in patients who are unable to take oral medications. Mifepristone, which binds competitively to the glucocorticoid receptor, has recently been shown to improve clinical and biochemical parameters of Cushing syndrome, although it is not currently approved by the US Food and Drug Administration for this indication. When medical therapy is not successful, bilateral adrenalectomy may be considered [27, 28].

Paraneoplastic Inappropriate ADH Production

The syndrome of inappropriate antidiuretic hormone secretion (SIADH), which is characterized by hypo-osmotic, dilutional hyponatremia, is found in 1-2% of patients with cancer [2, 3]. SCC of the lung accounts for most of these cases, with approximately 10% to 45% of all patients with this cancer developing SIADH. The syndrome has also been reported in association with SCC of genitourinary organs and in some cases of poorly or undifferentiated prostate cancer [29-32].

Paraneoplastic SIADH arises from tumor cell production of antidiuretic hormone (ADH, also known as arginine vasopressin or vasopressin) and atrial natriuretic peptide. ADH is normally produced by neurons in the hypothalamus when the plasma osmolality falls below 275 mOsm/kg or when baroceptors detect a hypovolemic state. Antidiuretic hormone leads to increased free-water reabsorption in distal convoluted renal tubules [33].

The fundamental problem in SIADH is the failure to maximally suppress vasopressin secretion. ADH excess results in water retention and volume expansion, leading to weight gain and natriuresis. Serum osmolality falls below the reference range. Hyponatremia does not develop unless the patient is ingesting or receiving some source of free water. The natriuresis, which occurs in SIADH despite hyponatremia and further contributes to hyponatremia, is produced by a decrease in proximal tubular sodium reabsorption secondary to the expansion of the extracellular fluid volume. Hypervolemia initially suppresses the renin-angiotensin-aldosterone system during the water retention phase, but later levels of renin and aldosterone rise again, perhaps in response to hyponatremia. The main mediator of the natriuresis in SIADH is probably the atrial natriuretic peptide (ANP), which may suppress proximal tubular reabsorption of sodium in response to expanded ECF volume. Sodium balance is maintained in SIADH, and the sodium output equals the intake. Clinical manifestations of SIADH are largely related to the cellular swelling and cerebral oedema due to hyponatremia.

Most patients with SIADH are asymptomatic if the serum osmolality remains above 240 mOsm/kg, and the diagnosis is only made by routine biochemical exams. The clinical manifestations of SIADH are those of water intoxication and are usually related to the degree of the hyponatremia and to the rate at which hyponatremia develops. Symptoms are more likely to develop in elderly patients and young children, and usually include anorexia, nausea and vomiting, lethargy, apathy, agitation, disorientation, irritability, muscle cramps or weakness. On laboratory exams, classic SIADH usually presents with hyponatremia (serum sodium<135 mM), low serum osmolarity (<280 mosm/kg), persistent urinary sodium excretion with urine less than maximally dilute. Additional diagnostic criteria include absence of clinical evidence of volume depletion, normal skin turgor and blood pressure, correction of hyponatremia by fluid restriction, absence of other causes of hyponatremia such as hypovolemia, renal disease, liver and cardiac failure, adrenal and pituitary insufficiency, hypothyroidism, psychogenic polydypsia and medications to be considered. Plasmatic ADH is typically elevated, but its determination is not crucial for the diagnosis of SIADH [34].

Most patients affected by SIADH develops hyponatremia in many weeks or months, so a rational therapy is to correct hyponatremia gradually, except when convulsions or mental status alteration is present. Initial management includes fluid restriction or intravenous hypertonic saline depending on severity. The best therapy for paraneoplastic SIADH is treatment of the underlying tumor, which, if successful, can normalize the sodium level in a matter of weeks. Pharmacologic treatments of SIADH include demeclocycline and vasopressin receptor antagonists. Demeclocycline (150-300 mg, 4-4 times per day) interferes with the renal response to ADH and does not require simultaneous fluid restriction to achieve its effect, which in every case are noted after 1-2 weeks of therapy. In recent years, vasopressin receptor antagonists (e.g., conivaptan, tolvaptan) have become available for the treatment of hyponatremia. These agents, which block arginine vasopressin binding to receptors in the renal collecting ducts, result in the excretion of free water [35, 36].

Syndromes Caused by Inappropriate Release of Biologic Amines

The inappropriate secretion of neuroendocrine substances, like serotonin (5-hydroxytryptamine), kallikrein, bradykinin or histamine, is a tipical manifestation of neuroendocrine tumors, wich can affect genitourinary organs, in particular the prostate [2]. Malignant carcinoid syndrome is the constellation of symptoms typically exhibited by patients with metastases from carcinoid tumors, which usually secrete excessive amounts of serotonin. Carcinoid tumors arise from neuroendocrine cells, which are widespread in the human body, especially in the organs derived from the primitive intestine. Malignant carcinoid syndrome occurs in less than 10% of patients with a carcinoid tumor. Typically, 90% of cases of carcinoid tumors originate from the distal ileum or appendix (the embryologic midgut) and represent 90% of appendiceal tumors [37].

Tumors arising from the foregut and hindgut are considered atypical; however, tumors can originate from any cell of the amine precursor uptake and decarboxylation system and, therefore, produce several intestinal hormones. Most of these tumors produce 5-hydroxytryptamine, which, in physiological conditions, is taken up and stored in the platelets while the excesses are inactivated from the liver and lung and transformed into 5-hydroxyindoleacetic acid (5-HIAA). In order of frequency, carcinoids may occur in the appendix (35%), ileum (28%), rectum (13%), and bronchi (13%). Incidence is less than 1% in the pancreas, gallbladder, liver, larynx, testes and ovaries; however, these tumours have been described to affect kidney, urinary bladder, urethra and prostate [38].

Physiologically, serotonin causes vasodilation and determines increased blood clotting, stimulating platelet aggregation (diffuse intravascular coagulation [DIC]); however, serotonin is converted to 5-HIAA in the body. In many cases, carcinoid tumours often cause no symptoms. In advanced cases, when the tumour has spread, the increased release of hormonal substances can cause a diverse set of symptoms. These may include:

Facial flushing, redness, and sudden rush of warmth in the face
Diarrhoea
Dyspnoea
Tachycardia
Wheezing
Sudden hypotension
Fatigue
Dizziness

The Carcinoid Syndrome, due to the presence of a functioning carcinoid tumor, is easily diagnosed when all the features of the syndrome are present or even when 1 or 2 of the main symptoms are present and the Carcinoid Syndrome is thought of. The biggest impediment to making the diagnosis is not thinking of the Carcinoid Syndrome, or even considering it because of its rarity. Once considered, the diagnosis usually can be confirmed quickly and painlessly by doing a urine 5-HIAA test. This stands for 5-hydroxy indole acetic acid, which is the main breakdown (waste) product of Serotonin. Its quantitative measurement in the urine which an individual excretes in a 24 hour period tells how much Serotonin is being made in the body during that time. In the presence of Carcinoid Syndrome the amount of 5-HIAA is usually distinctly increased above normal. Certain foods and medicines must be avoided for a day or two before, and on the day of the urine collection, since they can cause false test results. These are: bananas, pineapple and its juice, red plums, avocado, walnuts and other nuts, kiwi fruit, tomatoes, various cough medicines muscle relaxing medicines, acetaminophen (Tylenol), caffeine, fluorouracil, iodine solutions (Lugol's solution), phenacetin, MOA inhibitors (certain antidepressant drugs), isoniazid, and phenothiazine drugs (Compazine, Thorazine). Sometimes urine 5-HIAA is not increased but other carcinoid "markers" in the blood can be measured and will be increased. These are chromogranin A (CgA) and serotonin. Blood tryptophan may be decreased below normal values. The measurement of CgA is considered "the gold standard" of chemical tests for confirming the diagnosis of carcinoid and neuroendocrine tumours and following their course. A universally approved (though costly) way of finding carcinoid tumours, as well as other neuroendocrine tumours, is the OctreoScan (or somatostatin receptor scintigraphy). It is successful in 85% of carcinoids and consists of a harmless injection of a minute dose of a short duration radioactive isotope which is specifically attracted to, and concentrated in, carcinoid tumor tissue (and any other neuroendocrine tumor) where it lights up when a radiation scan is taken over the entire body. The ^{11}C-labeled 5-hydroxy-L-tryptophan (5-HTP) was developed for positron emission tomography (PET) imaging of neuroendocrine tumors. The ^{11}C-5-HTP-PET is based on the metabolic capacity of amine-precursor uptake decarboxylation (APUD) tumours cells, such as those of carcinoids, to accumulate and decarboxylate 5-HTP, precursors of serotonin [39].

The usefulness of these nuclear medicine diagnostic tools is limited in the diagnosis of neuroendocrine tumors of genitourinary tract due to the high radioactivity of urine. Interestingly, the premedication of patients with Carbidopa orally before PET examination, in order to block the aromatic amino acid decarboxylase enzyme, decreased the decarboxylation rate of ^{11}C-5-http, leading to a higher tumor uptake and a considerably lower urinary radioactivity concentration [39].

Carcinoid tumours vary greatly in their size, location, symptoms and growth. Therefore the treatment in each case should be individualized to what is best for each particular patient. Surgery, with complete removal of all of the tumor tissue, is the first and best treatment when it is possible, and if detected early can result in a complete and permanent cure. Chemotherapy for carcinoid given by intravenous injection or by mouth has been in use for over 20 years. There are many drugs available. Individual drugs used alone have been disappointing but a number of combinations of these drugs have been beneficial. Somatostatin analogue (octreotide/lanreotide and vapreotide) injections not only usually squelch the symptoms of Carcinoid Syndrome but are now believed to sometimes inhibit or even reverse growth of the tumours. This has become the mainstay of treatment for most carcinoid tumors, with or without the Carcinoid Syndrome. Additional drug treatments include serotonin and histamine antagonists (e.g., cyproheptadine) and blockers of serotonin synthesis (e.g., parachlorophenylalanine).

Syndromes Caused by Inappropriate Release of Growth Factors

Non-Islet-Cell Tumor Hypoglycemia

Non-islet-cell tumor hypoglycaemia (NICTH) is a rare condition, usually caused by tumor cell production of IGF-2, IGF-2 precursors ('big IGF-2') or insulin. NICTH often presents as recurrent or constant hypoglycaemic episodes with glucose levels as low as 20 mg/dL (0.0555mmol/L) and typically affects elderly patients with advanced cancer [40]. Soft tissue sarcomas, in particular retroperitoneal sarcomas (adrenal and renal) have been associated with NICTH in several reports [41]. The optimal initial approach to NICTH is to treat (if possible, resect) the underlying tumor. When such an approach is not feasible, the goal of medical therapy is to maintain adequate blood glucose levels. For recurrent or chronic hypoglycaemic episodes, longer-term management includes corticosteroids, growth hormone, diazoxide, octreotide, or glucagon.

Acanthosis Nigricans

Acanthosis nigricans is characterized by eruption of many, symmetric, velvety hyperkeratotic lesions with brownish hyperpigmentation, predominantly in the axilla and neck regions. Other regions frequently involved are flexures, skin folds, bend of the elbow, nipples, navel and anogenital regions. Most cases of acanthosis nigricans occur in persons with insulin resistance or other nonmalignant endocrine disorders. The occurrence of acanthosis nigricans in adult is almost in up to 90% of cases associated with cancers. The syndrome is proposed to be due to the inappropriate production of TGF-alpha, EGF and a MSH-like peptide by undifferentiated malignancies. Most often involved tumors are carcinomas (gastric especially), sarcomas and haematological proliferations. Although rarely, acanthosis nigricans has been reported also in urological cancers, such as RCC, urothelial cancer and prostate cancer, and its presence seems to be related to a bad prognosis [42, 43]. Symptomatic treatment, such as topical corticosteroids, seems to have minimal benefit, but successful treatment of the underlying malignancy may result in improvement and occasionally resolution of the condition [44].

Paraneoplastic Leukocytosis

Paraneoplastic leukocytosis is a common condition in cancers and has been described in urological malignancies, such as RCC, urotheliomas and penile cancer, alone or in association with other PNSs [45-49].

Paraneoplastic eosinophilia represents a subset of secondary eosinophilia that is due to tumor production of interleukins acting as eosinophil growth factors (IL-3, IL-5 and GM-CSF). Patients with paraneoplastic and other forms of secondary eosinophilia may have elevated serum levels of IL-3, IL-5, and GM-CSF, as well as elevated IL-2, an eosinophil chemoattractant. Other causes of secondary eosinophilia include allergic reactions, parasitic infections, and collagen vascular diseases. Paraneoplastic eosinophilia is usually asymptomatic, but in some cases wheezing and dyspnoea may be present; these symptoms usually respond to corticosteroid therapy [50]. After successful cancer treatment, return of eosinophilia may herald tumour recurrence. Several studies have shown that paraneoplastic eosinophilia is a poor prognostic sign and indicates metastatic and extensive disease [51].

Paraneoplastic granulocytosis occurs in approximately 15% of patients with solid tumours. In patients with cancer, several factors may contribute to leukocytosis. In a recent series of greater than 750 cancer patients with white blood cell counts exceeding 40×10^9/L, the following aetiologies were identified: hematopoietic growth factors (69%), infection (15%), paraneoplastic (10%), glucocorticoids or vasopressors (5%), and newly diagnosed leukaemia (1%) [52]. The tumor production of colony-stimulating factor (G-CSF) can promote the development of mature neutrophils from hematopoietic progenitor cells. Paraneoplastic granulocytosis does not require specific therapy.

Fasciitis-Panniculitis Syndromes

The fasciitis-panniculitis syndromes (FPS) are a group of disorders characterized by induration of the skin due to chronic inflammation and fibrosis of the subcutaneous septa, muscular fascia and subjacent muscle [53]. Clinically, FPS are characterized by swelling and induration of the skin of the upper or lower extremities and sometimes of the trunk or neck. The indurated segments present large, circumferential sleeve-like or round to elongated patchy lesions. Chronic inflammation and fibrosis occur in the subcutaneous fat tissue and deep fascia. These signs can be important clues to an underlying malignancy, although the incidence of cancer in patients with FPS is rather small and a meticulous search for occult cancer does not seem cost-effective. Occurrence of FPS has been rarely reported in patients with prostate cancer [54, 55].

Neurological PNS

Neurological PNS (NPNS) affect 6% of all patients with cancer. NPNS sporadically reported in patients with urological tumors are summarized in table 1 [2]. Generally, neurologic PNS are immune-mediated and are due to the production, from the tumor cells, of neuronal antigens that are recognized as foreign by dendritic cells of the immune system. Neuronal antigens are normally shielded in immune privileged sites within the central nervous system. The generation of neuronal antibodies to these antigens by plasma cells results in immune-mediated neuronal damage.

Peripheral neuropathy is the most common NPNS and is usually a distal sensorimotor polyneuropathy that produces mild motor weakness, sensory loss and absent distal reflexes. Subacute sensory neuropathy is a more specific but rare peripheral neuropathy. Between urological malignancies, peripheral neuropathy is usually associated with small cell carcinomas of the prostate and of the bladder [56, 57].

Limbic encephalitis clinically presents with personality disturbance, memory loss (short-term and long-term) with preserved cognitive function, sleep disturbance, irritability, seizures, hallucinations and bizarre behaviour. MRI or PET demonstrates lesions in the medial temporal lobes. It is a paraneoplastic syndrome seldom seen in prostate cancer and testicular neoplasms [58, 59]. The syndrome is characterized by progressive amnesia and psychiatric disturbances resulting from an inflammatory reaction probably related to an immune response to the neuronal proteins expressed by tumours. Frequently, this disorder is accompanied by subacute sensory neuronopathy (SSN) due to involvement of the dorsal root ganglia. Anti-Hu antibodies may be detected in both of these conditions. Symptoms consist of irritability, depression, seizures, severe memory deficit, and dementia. These symptoms are due to dysfunction of the limbic system (hippocampus, amygdala, hypothalamus, and insular and cingulate cortex), which is the area of the nervous system where most of the pathological changes that characterize the syndrome occur. Brain-stem encephalitis and abnormalities in other areas of the nervous system are frequent, but they may be clinically silent. Clinically, Ma-2 antibodies have been correlated with symptoms associated with limbic, diencephalic, or brainstem encephalopathy. Neurological symptoms preceded the tumor diagnosis in the majority of patients. Identification of the tumor is particularly important in Ma-2associated paraneoplastic syndrome as the neurologic complications responds to treatment of the tumor in over one third of the patients. The most common malignancy associated with Ma-2 antibody is testicular cancer. This correlation and subsequent diagnosis are very important, as this is a highly curable tumour, even in the presence of metastatic disease. Cranial magnetic resonance imaging may show increased signal intensity in the limbic cortex. Genitourinary examinations are sometimes inadequate. Testicular ultrasonography is recommended if no tumor is detected on the chest and abdominal computed tomography scan. The outcome of the treatment of the underlying cancer on the paraneoplastic syndrome is variable [60-62].

Table 1. Neurological paraneoplastic syndrome (NPNS) reported in urological malignancies

Syndrome	Clinical Features	Associated urological cancers	Antibodies	Ref.
Pheripheral neuropathy	The most common NPNS. It is usually a distal sensorimotor polyneuropathy that produces mild motor weakness, sensory loss, and absent distal reflexes. Subacute sensory neuropathy is a more specific but rare peripheral neuropathy. Dorsal root ganglia degeneration and progressive sensory loss with ataxia but little motor weakness develop.	SCC of prostate and bladder	Anti-Hu autoantibody can be found in the serum of some patients	[56,57]
Limbic encephalitis	Characterized by rapid development of irritability, depression, sleep disturbances, seizures, hallucinations, and short-term memory loss. Approximately 80% of patients with limbic encephalitis have MRI T2 hyperintensities involving medial temporal lobes. PET studies may show radionuclide uptake in the temporal lobes, even when the MRI is normal. Approximately 30% of patients respond to treatment of the tumor, usually a testicular cancer, and to immunotherapy.	Testicular cancer, SCC of prostate, RCC. Testicular cancer can be confined to the testis and may be found in a microscopic stage.	Anti-Ma2-associated encephalitis is associated with testicular cancer. Some patients (usually with SCC) have anti-Hu in the serum and CSF.	[58-62]
Paraneoplastic cerebellar degeneration	Paraneoplastic cerebellar degeneration is a heterogeneous group of disorders characterized by the subacute onset in cancer patients of a cerebellar syndrome: progressive bilateral leg and arm ataxia, dysarthria, vertigo, diplopia, nystagmus, ophthalmoplegia, dementia with or without brain stem signs, extensor plantar signs, with prominent dysarthria and arm involvement. The disease usually progresses	BCa and PCa	Anti-Yo, a circulating autoantibody binding to cytoplasmatic protein antigens of Purkinje cells, and anti-Hu are found in the serum	[63]

Table 1. (Continued)

Syndrome	Clinical Features	Associated urological cancers	Antibodies	Ref.
	over weeks to months, often causing profound disability. Cerebellar degeneration may precede the discovery of the cancer (usually SCC or breast and gynecologic tumors) by weeks to years. MRI or CT may show cerebellar atrophy.		and/or CSF of some patients.	
Opsoclonus-myoclonus-ataxia syndrome	Opsoclonus (spontaneous chaotic eye movements) is usually associated with cerebellar ataxia and myoclonus of the trunk and extremities. Usually accompanying childhood neuroblastoma, in adults the most frequent causes are idiopathic (50%) and paraneoplastic (20%). This cerebellar syndrome has been reported in patients with lung, breast and gynecologic tumors.	RCC, adenocarcinoma and urothelioma of bladder	The autoantibody anti-Ri may be present in the serum and CSF directly resulting in the damage to the neurons causing the symptomatology.	[64]
Lambert-Eaton myasthenic syndrome	Lambert-Eaton myasthenic syndrome is an immunemediated, myasthenia-like disorder of neuromuscular and autonomic transmission with weakness usually affecting the limbs and sparing ocular and bulbar muscles. It results from impaired release of acetylcholine from nerve terminals. The diagnosis is confirmed by serum test for autoantibodies and by finding an incremental response to repetitive nerve stimulation. The syndrome can precede, occur with, or develop after the diagnosis of cancer. It occurs most commonly in men with intrathoracic tumors such as lymphomas, thymomas or (70% of cases) pulmonary SCC.	PCa, prostatic SCC, BCa. The association of the syndrome with PCa can be a marker of neuroendocrine differentiation and hormonal independency.	An IgG autoantibody (anti-VGCC) leading to presynaptic voltage-gated calcium channel loss is involved (a serum test for anti-VGCC is commercially available).	[65]

Syndrome	Clinical Features	Associated urological cancers	Antibodies	Ref.
Myositis	Polymyositis and dermatomyositis are idiopathic inflammatory myopathy characterized by asthenia, pain, progressive hypertrophy of proximal muscles and dermatologic manifestations such as violet-colored rashes of the face and hands. There are some evidences of the autoimmune basis of paraneoplastic polymyositis and dermatomyositis such as the presence of a lymphoplasma cellular infiltrate of the muscular interstices.	Most urological tumors		[110-112]
Paraneoplastic encephalomyelitis	Paraneoplastic encephalomyelitis (PEM) is pathologically characterized by neuronal loss and inflammatory infiltrates in particular areas of the nervous system. The location and severity of the neuronal loss predicts the clinical symptoms of the patient that may be confined to one area of the nervous system or, more frequently, involve over time, multiple areas.		Hu-Ab	[66-68]

Modified from Sacco et al. [2], with permission.

Paraneoplastic cerebellar degeneration is another neurological manifestation of urological cancers, in particular associated with prostate and bladder cancer, and can vary in its presentation. Patients often present with ataxia, vertigo, dysarthria, and ocular symptoms, such as diplopia, nystagmus and ophthalmoplegia. Paraneoplastic cerebellar syndrome can occur in conjunction with LEMs, and has been linked to production of the autoantibodies anti-Hu and anti-Yo. Paraneoplastic cerebellar degeneration usually presents many years before the detection of the tumor and is associated with profound disability. Cerebellar atrophy results in ataxia, vertigo, dysarthria, nystagmus, truncal weakness, ophthalmoplegia and therefore, immobility, respiratory dysfunction and severely reduced function. Reported cases in prostate cancer have demonstrated variable response to treatment of the underlying malignancy and further symptomatic deterioration that led to death [63].

Opsoclonus has been associated with infections, trauma, toxins, and numerous neoplasms such as small cell lung carcinoma, thyroid carcinoma, breast carcinoma, and other gynaecologic tumors. In the paediatric population, 2% of children with neuroblastoma have opsoclonus. In adults, opsoclonus/myoclonus is a rare symptom in patients with tumors. It is characterized by rapid, involuntary, multivectorial (horizontal and vertical), unpredictable, conjugate fast eye movements without intersaccadic intervals; cerebellar ataxia. Although opsoclonus and ataxia are not life threatening, they can cause significant disability. The overall prognosis of adult patients with opsoclonus and an associated malignancy appears to depend on the nature of the malignancy and its prognosis [64].

Lambert-Eaton myasthenic syndrome (LEMs) is caused by a sensorial and motor peripheral neuropathy due to immune-mediated neuronal damage; in particular, autoantibodies against voltage-gated calcium channels (VGCCs) affect the release of acetylcholine from the presynaptic terminal of the neuromuscular junction. Patients often present with increasing weakness of proximal muscles, with the ocular and bulbar muscles spared. Symptoms improve with stimulation of the proximal muscles by the brain through normal electrical impulse or with electromyography. This is particular to LEMs, and thus electromyography is used diagnostically [65].

Paraneoplastic encephalomyelitis (PEM), one of the most frequent remote effects of cancer, is pathologically characterized by neuronal loss and inflammatory infiltrates in particular areas of the nervous system [66]. The location and severity of the neuronal loss predicts the clinical symptoms of the patient that may be confined to one area of the nervous system or, more frequently, involve over time, multiple areas. At present, early diagnosis and treatment of the tumor gives the best chance of being able to stabilize the disease. The outcome of patients with PEM depends on the evolution of the neurologic syndrome and the possibility of curing the tumor, although the prognosis of PEM remains poor in terms of survival and neurological disability; in fact, many patients with PEM die from progression of the neurologic disorder rather than the tumor. In patients with PEM and Hu-Ab, complete response of the tumor to therapy is the best predictor to arrest the evolution of the neurologic dysfunction. Immunotherapy does not modify the clinical course of PEM [67], but its use is not detrimental to the tumor evolution. Treatment of the underlying tumor cannot represent the only approach to the management of the neurologic paraneoplastic syndrome despite its beneficial effect. Many patients deteriorate in the months preceding the discovery of the tumor and PEM sometimes develops during treatment of the tumor, and sometimes PEM progresses even when a complete response of the tumor was achieved [68]. Severe neurological symptoms, such as cerebellar dysfunction, truncal ataxia, chaotic eye movements, seizures, hallucinations, and ocular and bulbar muscle dysfunction, often persist despite treatment of the underlying malignancy or plasmapheresis.

Renal Cell Carcinoma-related Syndromes

Renal cell carcinoma (RCC) is the third most common genitourinary malignancy in general population. The incidence of RCC is increasing in the United States, and it is slightly higher among African Americans than the Caucasian population. In 2011, there were approximately 60,920 new cases of kidney cancer reported in the United States (37,120 males and 23,800 females), which resulted in about 13,120 deaths (8,270 males and 4,850 females) [69]. RCC incidence rates has increased steadily between 1975 and 1995, by 2.3% annually among Caucasian men, 3.1% among Caucasian women, 3.9% among African-American men, and 4.3% among African-American women [70]. Since then, the annual incidence rate has steadily increased by 2.6% (National Cancer Institute [NCI], 2011). A likely cause for the increase in the incidence of RCC is the widespread use of abdominal imaging in the last 15 to 20 years. The historical classic triad of flank pain, haematuria, and abdominal mass is seen less and less frequently because many patients are being diagnosed incidentally. Symptoms, if present, may be the result of local tumor growth, haemorrhage, metastatic disease, or paraneoplastic syndromes [71].

High-quality computed tomography (CT) scan with administration of intravenous contrast remains the radiologic modality for choice to work up a renal mass. Magnetic resonance imaging (MRI) may be useful in the setting of locally advanced disease, venous involvement, renal insufficiency, or allergy to IV contrast. Colour flow Doppler imaging may be useful in detecting renal vein/vena cava involvement. Metastatic evaluation includes CT of the abdomen and pelvis, chest X-ray, and liver function tests. If chest x-ray is abnormal, then a CT of the chest is warranted. Bone scan should be ordered if there is an elevation of alkaline phosphatase and/or bone pain.

The treatment options for RCC are surgery, radiation therapy (palliative), targeted therapy (bevacizumab, sumitinib, sorafenib, everolimus, temsirolimus), biological therapy (immunotherapy), and combinations of these [72]. Surgical resection can be curative in patients who present with localized RCC. Unfortunately, most RCCs are asymptomatic for most of their natural history. Therefore, sometimes the diagnosis is made when the disease has progressed locally to the extent where it cannot be resected or has already metastasized. Historically, radical nephrectomy (removal of kidney, ipsilateral adrenal gland, and Gerota's fascia) was advocated for the surgical treatment of RCC. Nephron-sparing surgery was indicated for those with a solitary kidney, those at risk for inheritable forms of RCC (such as VHL), or patients with baseline or at risk for renal insufficiency (such as with diabetes mellitus). However, the current trend is to consider nephron-sparing surgical procedures when the lesion is amenable. For patients with Stage I or Stage II disease, surgery is usually curative. For Stage IV disease, surgery may be considered in carefully selected patients. Cytoreductive nephrectomy can be considered for palliation of local symptoms before initiating systemic immunotherapy.

Table 2. Paraneoplastic syndromes in renal cell carcinoma

Endocrine	Non-endocrine
Hypercalcemia	Amyloidosis
Hypertension	Anemia
Polycythemia	Neuromyopathies
Stauffer's Syndrome	Coagulopathy
Cushing Sindrome	Vasculopathy
Alterations in glucose metabolism	Dermopathies

RCC is unique among the genitourinary malignancies because close to one third of affected patients show signs and symptoms of a PNS [2]. It is estimated that from 10% to 40% of patients affected by RCC will develop a PNS and, although more than 50% of RCC cases today are diagnosed incidentally, approximately 20% of patients diagnosed with RCC present with paraneoplastic symptoms at diagnosis. The most common RCC-related paraneoplastic syndromes are reported in table 2. They are classically divided into endocrine PNS and non-endocrine PNS. The endocrine group is less common and occurs in patients with hormonal manifestations secondary to neoplasm. The non-endocrine group consists of patients with a variety of systemic manifestations of the neoplastic disease [73].

Among patients with RCC, hypercalcemia is the most common PNS, affecting between 13%–20% of patients. Among patients with hypercalcemia and RCC, approximately 75% have high-stage lesions. Neither the presence nor degree of hypercalcemia, however, has been shown to have a significant correlation with tumor grade or overall survival. Mechanisms and pathophysiology of hypercalcemia, such as symptoms, have been yet discussed in this chapter. It has BEEN recently studied the correlation between PTHrP, erythropoietin (EPO), and vascular endothelial growth factor (VEGF) expression in clear cell renal cell carcinoma (ccRCC) and it has been seen that PTHrP and EPO are related to VEGF expression and to the progression of RCC [74, 75]. This syndrome is similar to that of primary hyperparathyroidism except that patients with RCC may present decreased renal and intestinal calcium absorption in addition to decreased 1,25-vitamin D synthesis. Moreover, transforming growth factor (TGF) α and β, osteoclast activating factor (OAF), interleukin 1 (IL-1), and tumor necrosis factor (TNF) are also believed to exacerbate the non-metastatic hypercalcemia seen in RCC patients. Volume repletion can be accomplished with normal saline and total serum calcium can be reduced with loop diuretic administration. Moreover, bisphosphonates are effective for long-term management of hypercalcemia. Some studies showed that administration of nonsteroidal anti-inflammatory drugs, such as indomethacin, could lower the serum calcium concentration when serum prostaglandin levels are elevated. Despite these palliative measures, nephrectomy is the most effective way to treat the nonmetastatic hypercalcemia seen with RCC.

Another common paraneoplastic syndrome found in patients with RCC is hypertension. Whereas the incidence of hypertension among age-matched controls is close to 20%, almost 40% of those with RCC experience hypertension. Hypertension is typically associated with low-grade tumours of clear-cell histology. Several studies have failed to demonstrate a clear relationship between the presence of hypertension in patients with RCC and prognosis. Potential mechanisms of hypertension in these patients include increased renin secretion, ureteral or parenchymal compression, presence of an arteriovenous fistula, and polycythaemia. Although hypertension is not a prognostic indicator, some studies have investigated the use of renin as a potential tumor marker, showing that serum renin levels do not strictly correlate with the degree of hypertension; however, renin levels drop after nephrectomy [76]. Therefore, treatment for hypertension caused by RCC is nephrectomy. This is highlighted by the fact that 85% of those with hypertension secondary to RCC are normotensive following tumour resection.

Constitutional symptoms, such as fever, anaemia, weight loss, and fatigue, can be the first symptoms of RCC in up to one third of cases. Fever is present in 20–30% of patients with RCC and is the only symptom in approximately 2% of patients. These symptoms in RCC patients are mediated by cytokines such as TNF-β, IL-6, IL-1, interferons and prostaglandins. Anaemia is observed in about 20% of patients affected by RCC. Poor nutritional status and the presence of a chronic disease are two main reasons for the anaemia that, however, has been also related to tumor production of iron-binding protein, such as ferritin and lactoferrin. Cachexia, defined as hypoalbuminaemia, weight loss, anorexia or malaise, is associated with lower overall survival [77]. Once non-neoplastic causes of constitutional symptoms in patients with RCC have been ruled out, nephrectomy is the most effective treatment.

Polycythaemia has been reported in 1–8% of RCC cases. In these patients has been noted an elevated red blood cell concentrations, which is believed to be mediated by erythropoietin (EPO), a glycoprotein produced by peritubular renal interstitial cells that induces differentiation of erythrocyte colony-forming units in the bone marrow. An inappropriate and often clinically silent EPO production occurs in up to 66% of RCC cases making this neoplasm the leading cause of ectopic EPO production. The aberrant EPO production occurs in the tumor cells themselves, but perineoplastic cells may also contribute to total EPO levels secondary to local tumor compression and resultant tissue hypoxia. Recent studies showed that expression of EPO in RCC is adversely associated with overall survival [78]. The majority of clear cell RCC displays a strong activation of the transcription factor regulating EPO, the Hypoxia-inducible Factor (HIF). Therefore, it is unclear why only a small minority of patients develop polycythaemia. In patients with organ-confined disease, EPO levels fall to normal following nephrectomy, whereas they remain elevated in those with metastatic disease. Similarly, EPO levels frequently rise with tumor recurrence when the primary lesion was associated with elevated EPO levels

In 1961, Stauffer described abnormal liver function tests, hepato-splenomegaly, histologic changes consistent with non-specific hepatitis with lymphocytic infiltration and elevation of liver enzymes in patients suffering from RCC; these abnormalities were reversible after nephrectomy (Stauffer's syndrome). Hepatic dysfunction, in absence of liver metastases, occurs in 10 to 15% of patients with RCC and is related to the production of cytokines from the tumor, including interleukin-6. It has been postulated that tumour-secreted hepatotoxins could cause hepatocyte injury with activation of the immune system that is mediated by the local recruitment of T cells and the production of antibodies against liver antigens [79]. Clinically, patients may present with hepatosplenomegaly, fever and weight loss and generally they have an unfavourable prognosis [80, 81].

Many other non-endocrine paraneoplastic syndromes have been described in RCC. Some of these are extremely rare and their association with RCC is not well defined. Nonetheless, diseases such as amyloidosis have been found with a recognized incidence in conjunction with RCC and have been studied in some detail [82].

Amyloidosis is a disease associated with the pathological production and deposition of fibril proteins between cells in a variety of tissues and organs in a wide variety of clinical settings. The condition is present in 3–8% of patients affected by RCC. In those patients, the amyloid protein, that is AA protein, is the same of the form seen in the chronic systemic disease of amyloidosis. Of note is that AA protein is thought to be a derivative of the acute phase reactant SAA, a protein that may be elevated in cases of RCC regardless of amyloid status. The mechanism of amyloid production in RCC is not well understood but may involve prolonged stimulation of the immune system by growth of the malignancy or tumor necrosis. Symptoms of amyloidosis depend on the entity of the deposits and the particular organs affected. Initial complaints include weakness, weight loss, and syncope. Eventually, clinical findings are related to the specific organ systems affected, such as the cardiac, renal, and gastrointestinal systems. Elevated serum SAA in patients with RCC seems to be related to a lower survival rate [83, 84].

Neuromyopathies have been described in cases of non-metastatic RCC. Degrees of severity vary from nonspecific myalgias to bilateral phrenic nerve paralysis. A case of amyotrophic lateral sclerosis in a patient with RCC that resolved after nephrectomy has also been reported. There is evidence to suggest that some RCCs may secrete a substance that may mediate such neuromyopathies. The neuropathies associated with RCC may be either sensory or motor. Unfortunately, the low frequency with which these syndromes occur along with RCC precludes prognostic value and a meaningful study of their mechanisms. [85, 86]

Abnormalities in glucose metabolism have also been described in RCC. There are several case reports of hyperglycaemia and hypoglycaemia that have resolved after nephrectomy for RCC. This finding has led to research into possible factors that may be either secreted or stimulated by the tumor, showing that hormones such as insulin and glucagon could be secreted by tumor [87].

Many other syndromes such as light chain nephropathy and various vasculities, coagulopathies, neutrophilia have been described in patients with RCC. Similarly, abnormalities involving prostaglandins, fibroblast growth factors, and α-fetoprotein have also been reported. Although these phenomena are not commonly seen in patients with RCC, their associations may provide some insight into the pathogenesis of this cancer.

Prostate Cancer-related Syndromes

Prostate cancer is the most common non-cutaneous cancer in men in the United States [88]. It is estimated that 1 in 6 white men and 1 in 5 African American men will be diagnosed with prostate cancer in their lifetime, with the likelihood increasing with age. Most prostate cancers (95%) are adenocarcinomas, while approximately 4% of cases of prostate cancer have transitional cell morphology and are thought to arise from the urothelial lining of the prostatic urethra. Only few cases of prostate cancer have neuroendocrine differentiation and are believed to arise from the neuroendocrine stem cells normally present in the prostate or from aberrant differentiation programs during cell transformation. Squamous cell carcinomas constitute less than 1% of all prostate carcinomas. In many cases, prostate carcinomas with squamous differentiation arise after radiation or hormone treatment. About 70% of prostate cancer cases arise in the peripheral zone, 15-20% arise in the central zone, and 10-15% arise in the transitional zone [88].

Currently, screening in asymptomatic men identifies most cases of prostate cancer. Diagnosis in most cases is based on abnormalities in a screening prostate-specific antigen (PSA) level or findings on digital rectal examination (DRE). In addition, prostate cancer can be an incidental pathologic finding when tissue is removed during transurethral resection to manage symptoms due to benign prostatic hyperplasia. Advanced prostate cancer results from any combination of lymphatic, haematogenous, or contiguous local spread. Skeletal manifestations are especially common, because prostate cancer has a strong predilection for metastasizing to bone.

Prostate cancer is the second most common urological malignancy to be associated with PNS after RCC. Paraneoplastic syndromes associated with prostate cancer include endocrine manifestations, neurological entities, dermatological conditions, and other syndromes. In over 70% of cases, the PNS arises at the initial clinical manifestation of prostate cancer, while in just under 20% the syndrome was an initial sign of disease progression to the castrate-resistant state. The vast majority of cases is related to advanced metastatic cancer. Generally, serum PSA tends to be high and histology reveals moderately to poorly differentiated adenocarcinoma, frequently with neuroendocrine features, or small cell carcinoma (SCC) of the prostate. Given that most cases involve metastatic disease, treatment is generally androgen deprivation therapy (ADT). The syndromes generally resolve upon institution of treatment for the underlying prostate cancer, but some syndromes require specific therapies.

Endocrine Syndromes

Less than 2% of patients with prostatic carcinoma are reported to have associated hypercalcemia [89]. Given the predilection of prostate cancer for osseous metastases, the mechanisms of calcium control are likely to be complex. Notably, patients affected by PCa with neuroendocrine pattern and expression of PTHrP frequently show normal calcaemia or even hypocalcaemia due to the so-called 'bone hunger syndrome', a well-recognized metabolic derangement of metastatic PCa patients. This syndrome is characterized by calcium entrapment in bone as a consequence of excessive osteoblastic activity leading to hyperparathyroidism in response to calcium demand; PTH elevation stimulates osteoclasts at sites distant from those involved by the tumor [90]. Furthermore, PTHrP in PCa patients may be cleaved and inactivated by the PSA [90]. The net effect is low or normal ionized calcium values with hypophosphatemia and raised PTH levels. Symptoms of asthenia, nausea, constipation and lethargy are associated with hypercalcemia, but severe cases might present with confusion and possible coma. Almost all reported cases have metastatic disease with poor treatment response and rapid disease progression.

SIADH is frequently observed in patients with tumors that exhibit neuroendocrine differentiation, such as SCC of the bronchus. SIADH has also been reported in patients with poorly differentiated malignancies of the pancreas, duodenum, adrenal glands and stomach. Although rare, SIADH arising from prostatic adenocarcinoma is well-documented in the literature, with more than ten cases reported [31, 32, 91].

Paraneoplastic Cushing's syndrome is most commonly associated with SCC of the lung, but has been reported in association with carcinoid tumors, medullary thyroid carcinoma, pheochromocytomas, pancreatic islet cell tumors, prostate adenocarcinoma [24] and SCC of other organs. In the setting of prostatic malignancy, paraneoplastic Cushing's syndrome is notable for the unique management challenge it poses and the particularly poor prognosis it carries; it is associated with rapidly progressive castrate-resistant prostate cancer owing to *de novo* SCC or neuroendocrine differentiation occurring within an adenocarcinoma. Androgen production occurs through hyperadrenalism despite maximal androgen blockade because ADT acts at the level of the pituitary gland and cannot prevent adrenal stimulation by ACTH-like peptides [27]. Testosterone levels are therefore likely to remain in the normal range despite castration. Ketaconazole, an adrenal steroid synthesis inhibitor, can reduce cortisol levels and is preferable in prostate cancer with paraneoplastic Cushing's syndrome, but hypercortisolism remains difficult to control. This has prompted some advocacy for bilateral adrenalectomy before therapy for prostate cancer in these patients. Another attractive alternative first-line therapeutic option is abiraterone, a CYP17a1 inhibitor, which is a more effective inhibitor of adrenal androgen production than ketoconazole and is currently being evaluated in clinical trials for castrate-resistant prostate cancer [27].

Haematological Syndromes

The spectrum of haematological disorders associated with prostatic malignancy ranges from acute bleeding diathesis to thrombosis and embolic events. Disseminated intravascular coagulation (DIC), however, is the most commonly observed disorder in patients with prostate cancer. DIC can be chronic or acute and is characterized by the increased production of fibrin, increased fibrinolysis and unchecked coagulation throughout the systemic circulation. Thrombin activation can cause microthrombosis at the small-vessel to mid-vessel level, while consumption of coagulation factors and aggressive fibrinolysis can cause acute bleeding. In either instance the prognosis is poor and patients often have aggressive or progressive DIC [92]. The mechanisms by which malignancies cause paraneoplastic DIC is unclear. However, platelet tissue factor and a cysteine proteinase, which are procoagulant mediators, are expressed on prostate tumor cells and might be responsible for triggering the coagulation cascade by activating factor X and, in the case of the latter, without the need for factor VII. It has been reported that needle biopsy of the prostate can initiate the release of tumor procoagulant substances into the systemic circulation, and in one case ADT was instituted before histological confirmation of prostate cancer in order to avoid significant bleeding after biopsy. Less-common haematological paraneoplastic disorders associated with prostate cancer include thrombotic thrombocytopenia (TTP), primary fibrinolysis, sterile thrombotic endocarditis and thrombosis. TTP can cause microangiopathic haemolytic anaemia, neurological dysfunction, renal failure and fever [93, 94].

Other PNS Associated with Prostate Cancer

Most reported cases of paraneoplastic neurological syndromes associated with prostate cancer are caused by adenocarcinoma, although paraneoplastic encephalitis is usually associated with SCC. Treatment is generally of the underlying malignancy. In some cases plasmapheresis might be required to treat the neurological syndrome. Peripheral neuropathy is thought to be the commonest paraneoplastic neurological syndrome associated with prostate cancer, but still appears to be very rare. Other NPNS associated with prostate cancer, but very rare, are paraneoplastic cerebellar degeneration, that has demonstrated a variable response to treatment of the primary malignancy and a further symptomatic deterioration that often lead to death [63], limbic encephalitis and LEMs [65].

Several paraneoplastic dermatological conditions have been reported in association with prostate cancer, but they are mostly single cases. Dermatomyositis appears to be more frequently reported, and has a strong association with malignancy in general, in particular related to lung, gastrointestinal tract, breast, pancreas, kidney and lymphoreticular system cancers.

Reports of paraneoplastic fevers secondary to prostate cancer are rare in the literature; other symptoms common with prostate adenocarcinoma-related systemic inflammatory syndrome (described by Mauri and colleagues) include night sweats, weight loss and fatigue. Back pain is also common, but is more likely to be the result of bone metastases than inflammatory mediators.

Other PNSs associated with prostate carcinoma that have been reported include liver dysfunction, idiopathic cholestatic jaundice, carcinoma-associated retinopathy and osteomalacia. For some syndromes, such as idiopathic cholestatic jaundice, the mechanism remains completely elusive and there does not exist a mediator or marker for the firm diagnosis of the paraneoplastic syndrome. In others, study of the paraneoplastic phenomenon across different cancers has allowed the pathogenesis to be elucidated, such as in retinopathy, where circulating antibodies to retinal antigens have been studied. Despite the difference in mechanisms, most paraneoplastic syndromes appear to resolve upon treatment of the underlying prostate cancer [95, 96].

Transitional Cell Carcinoma-Related Syndromes

The most common type of urothelial tumor diagnosed is transitional (urothelial) cell carcinoma (TCC); it represents more than 90% of bladder cancers. TCC can arise anywhere in the urinary tract, including the renal pelvis, ureter, bladder, and urethra, but it is usually found in the urinary bladder. The American Cancer Society predicted that 72,570 new cases of bladder cancer will be diagnosed in the United States in 2014 and that 15,210 people will die of the disease. The incidence of bladder cancer increases with age, with the median age at diagnosis being 65 years; bladder cancer is rarely diagnosed before age 40 years. [97]. Bladder cancer is about 3 times more common in men than in women. Over the past 2 decades, however, the rate of bladder cancer has been stable in men but has increased in women by 0.2% annually. Up to 80% of bladder cancer cases are associated with environmental exposure. Tobacco use is by far the most common cause of bladder cancer in the United States and is increasing in importance in some developing countries. Smoking duration and intensity are directly related to increased risk [98]. Approximately 80-90% of patients with bladder cancer present with monosymptomatic gross haematuria. All patients with this classic presentation should be considered to have bladder cancer until proof to the contrary is found. Irritative bladder symptoms such as dysuria, urgency or frequency of urination occur in 20-30% of patients with bladder cancer. Therefore, patients presenting with unexplained or refractory irritative symptoms should be considered for cystoscopy and urine cytology, especially if they smoke or have other risk factor.

The gold standard to diagnose bladder cancer is cystoscopy; once diagnosed, any patient should undergo imaging studies of urinary tract. CT-scan with contrast administration or MRI are recommended. The WHO histological classification from 1973 differentiates 3 groups of bladder cancer, such as well (G1), moderately (G2), and poorly differentiated (G3) bladder cancer. TCC can be single or multifocal. 1.7%–5% of the patients have synchronous upper tract TCC, while metachronous recurrence can also develop several years after the initial diagnosis.

TCC associated with PNS is a rare entity with few cases being described in the literature and most of these are high grade and aggressive in nature.

Cutaneous manifestations of TCC of the bladder are extremely rare. Inclusion body myositis in association with dermatomyiositis, seborrheic keratosis and prurigo nodularis have been reported as paraneoplastic cutaneous manifestations in patients affected by TCC of the bladder. Inclusion body myositis (IBM) is a unique category of inflammatory myopathy. It is characterized histologically by the presence of muscle fibres with rimmed vacuoles and abnormal intracellular accumulations of proteins [99]. Clinically, IBM manifests by slowly progressive weakness and wasting of both distal and proximal muscles, most apparent in the muscles of the arms and legs. This weakness tends to progress over weeks to months, with variable involvement of the pharynx, upper oesophagus, or respiratory muscles. A number of autoantibodies are associated with DM and have prognostic implications, such as anti-Jo-1, anti-Mi-2 or anti-p155, which is associated with a greater frequency of malignancy [100]. Prurigo nodularis is a skin disease characterised by itchy nodules, that are either stable or increasing in number and which usually appear on the arms or legs, usually bilaterally symmetric, and in some cases is associated with cancer. It has rarely been described in association with TCC of the bladder. Patients often present with multiple excoriated lesions caused by scratching. Prurigo nodularis is a benign condition and does not increase mortality; however, severe morbidity can occur in untreated and even in some treated persons who are affected. Topical, oral, and intralesional corticosteroids have all been used in prurigo nodularis in attempts to decrease inflammation and sense of itching and to soften and smooth out firm nodules. The improvement with corticosteroids is variable, and corticosteroids are sometimes not helpful [101].

Paraneoplastic hypercalcemia due to ectopic production of PTHrP has been also described in association with TCC, although this association is a very rare condition. The presence of paraneoplastic hypercalcemia in patients with TCC is usually associated to a poor prognosis [15, 102].

Neurological syndromes, such as Lambert-Eaton myasthenic syndrome [103], opsoclonus-ataxia syndrome [104], and paraneoplastic encephalomyelitis [105] have been described in association with TCC of the bladder. Paraneoplastic cerebellar degeneration has also been described in patients affected by bladder urothelial carcinoma [106]. In two case reports, opsoclonus has been described in the presence of bladder cancer [107, 108].

Stauffer syndrome, a constellation of signs and symptoms of liver dysfunction that is usually due to presence of renal cell carcinoma, and, more rarely, in connection with other malignant neoplasms, has been described once in association with TCC of the bladder [109].

Testicular Cancer-Related Syndromes

Primary testicular tumors are the most common solid malignant tumor in men between the ages of 20 and 35 years in United States. Approximately 9,000 new cases are diagnosed in the United States each year. From 2002–2006, the median age at diagnosis was 34 years of age. In the United States, the incidence increased by 100% from 1988 to 2001. Diagnoses of seminomas increased 124% during the same period and diagnoses of nonseminomas increased by 64%. The most common presentation of testicular cancer is a painless swelling or nodule of one testicle. On the physical examination, this mass/nodule cannot be separated from the testis. Testicular cancers are highly curable, even in patients with metastatic disease at diagnosis. The prognosis depends upon the histologic type of cancer (seminoma vs nonseminoma), stage, and other features such as tumor marker and type of metastatic disease.

A paraneoplastic syndrome due to testicular cancer is a rare condition, and is often a neurological PNS. Paraneoplastic limbic encephalitis has been related to a testicular neoplasm. In general, patients with anti-Ma2 reactivity tend to be young and most have paraneoplastic limbic encephalitis associated with germ cell tumor of the testis. Neurological symptoms preceded the tumor diagnosis in the majority of patients. Identification of the tumor is particularly important in Ma-2associated paraneoplastic syndrome as the neurologic complications responds to treatment of the tumor in over one third of the patients, although the outcome of the treatment of the testicular cancer on the paraneoplastic syndrome is variable [60-62].

Dermatomyiositis (DM) has also been reported in literature as a paraneoplastic syndrome associated with testicular cancer. DM is a disease of unknown aetiology characterized by the association of progressive, proximal muscle weakness and pathognomonic or specific cutaneous findings. The first two cases of malignancy-associated DM were reported in 1916 by Stertz, who described a patient with gastric carcinoma, and Kankeleit, who reported on a female with DM associated with breast carcinoma. Since then, many case reports and multicenter, retrospective, and case-control studies have been published in the literature focusing on the incidence, type of tumors, possible predictive factors, and prognosis in paraneoplastic DM. Malignancy was associated with DM in 23% to 43% of patients, highly supporting the paraneoplastic nature of the disease. Symptoms of DM may appear before malignancy, after orchiectomy, or after orchiectomy and chemotherapy. Half of the patients diagnosed with DM and testicular cancer presented metastasis at diagnosis. Disappearance of the DM was totally different from case to case reported in literature [110-112].

Leydig cell tumors are rare testicular tumors of the male gonadal interstitium that may be hormonally active and lead to feminizing or virilising syndromes. Although uncommon, Leydig cell tumors comprise 1-3% of all testicular neoplasms. These tumors can be pure or can be mixed with other sex cord-stromal or germ cell tumors. Leydig cell tumors are usually benign, but malignant variants also occur [113]. Prepubertal boys affected by androgen-secreting Leydig tumors may present with precocious puberty; features may include prominent external genitalia, pubic hair growth, accelerated skeletal and muscle development, and mature masculine voice. In cases of oestrogen-secreting tumors clinical presentation is characterized by feminizing symptoms such as gynecomastia, breast tenderness, and gonadogenital underdevelopment. In general, adults with androgen-secreting tumors are asymptomatic, while in adults with oestrogen-secreting tumors, symptoms such as loss of libido, erectile dysfunction, and infertility have be reported [114, 115].

Gonadoblastoma is a rare benign tumor that has the potential for malignant transformation and affects a subset of patients with an intersex disorder or disorder of sex development. Gonadoblastoma is an uncommon tumor occurring almost exclusively in patients with disorder of sex development (DSD), who have either molecular evidence of a Y chromosome or a Y chromosome on karyotype analysis. The karyotype of these individuals is most often 46,XY; 45,X/46,XY; or 45,XO. Phenotypically, 80% of patients with gonadoblastoma are females and 20% are males [116, 117]. In patient history, a symptom of primary amenorrhea is often the first clue to the diagnosis of an intersex disorder. Additionally, any developmental delay of the genitalia or secondary sexual characteristics should also initiate a prompt search for an intersex abnormality with a karyotype analysis. Females usually present with a normal phenotype but with virilising features (eg, clitoromegaly, abnormal hirsutism); all phenotypic males present with undescended testis and hypospadiac urethra. In these cases, a karyotype analysis should be obtained to exclude an intersex disorder. Other important physical findings in males include phallic size, the existence of an inguinal hernia, and the presence of a uterus on the bimanual examination [118].

References

[1] Tarin, D. Update on clinical and mechanistic aspects of paraneoplastic syndromes. *Cancer and Metastasis Review,* 2013, 32(3-4):707-21.

[2] Sacco, E; Pinto, F; Sasso, F; Racioppi, M; Gulino, G; Volpe, A; Bassi, P. Paraneoplastic syndromes in patients with urological malignancies. *Urologia Internationalis*, 2009, 83(1):1-11.

[3] Alberti, C. Sindromi disendocrine paraneoplastiche: produzione inappropriata di PTHrP, ACTH/CRH, ADH da tumori in ambito urologico. *Urologia Pratica*, 2004, 3:55-63.

[4] Pelosof, LC & Gerber, DE. Paraneoplastic Syndromes: An Approach to Diagnosis and Treatment. *Mayo Clinic Proceedings*, 2010, 85(9): 838–854.

[5] Birkeland, KI; Gallefoss, F; Olsson, S; Haug, E. Primary hyperparathyroidism or hypercalcemia of malignancy? *Scandinavian Journal of Clinical and Laboratory Investigation*, 1992, 52:347-349.

[6] Stewart, AF. Humoral hypercalcemia of malignancy, in: Favus, MJ; Christakos, S; Goldring, SR; et al: *Primer on the Metabolic Bone Diseases and Disorders of Mineral Metabolism (ed. 3).* Philadelphia, PA, Lippincott-Raven, 1996.

[7] Vassilopoulou-Sellin, R; Newman, BM; Taylor, SH; Guinee, VF. Incidence of hypercalcemia in patients with malignancy referred to a comprehensive cancer center. *Cancer,* 1993, 71: 1309–1312.

[8] Lumachi, F; Brunello, A; Roma, A; Basso, U. Cancer-induced hypercalcemia. *Anticancer Research*, 2009, 29(5):1551-5.

[9] Stewart, AF; Horst, R; Deftos, LJ; Cadman, EC; Lang, R; Broadus, AE. Biochemical evaluation of patients with cancer-associated hypercalcemia: evidence of humoral and non-humoral groups. *The New England Journal of Medicine*, 1980, 303:1377-1383.

[10] Nathanson, L; Hall, TC. Paraneoplastic Syndromes. *Seminars in Oncology*, 1997; 24;265-386.

[11] Philbrick, WM; Wysolmerski, JJ; Galbraith, S; Holt, E; Orloff, JJ; Yang, KH; Vasavada, RC; Weir, EC; Broadus, AE; Stewart, AF. Defining the roles of parathyroid hormone-related protein in normal physiology. *Physiological Reviews*, 1996 76:127-173.

[12] Sone, S; Yano, S. Molecular pathogenesis and its therapeutic modalities of lung cancer metastasis to bone. *Cancer and Metastasis Reviews,* 2007, 26: 685–689.

[13] Sourbier, C & Massfelder, T. Parathyroid hormone-related protein in human renal cell carcinoma. *Cancer Letters*, 2006 240: 170–182.

[14] Buckle, RM; McMillan, M; Mallinson, C. Ectopic secretion of parathyroid hormone by a renal adenocarcinoma in a patient with hypercalcemia. *British Medical Journal*, 1970; 4: 724–726.

[15] Chaudhary, UB; Milling, DL; Bissada, NK. Transitional cell carcinoma of the bladder producing parathyroid hormone-related protein (PTHrP). *The Canadian Journal of Urology*, 2004; 11: 2136–2138.

[16] Abou-Samra, AB; Jüppner, H; Force, T; Freeman, MW; Kong, XF; Schipani, E; Urena, P, Richards, J; Bonventre, JV; Potts, JT Jr. Expression cloning of a common receptor for parathyroid hormone and parathyroid hormone-related peptide from rat osteoblast-like cells: a single receptor stimulates intracellular accumulation of both cAMP and inositol trisphosphates and increases intracellular free calcium. *Proceedings of the National Academy of Sciences, USA*, 1992, 89: 2732–2736.

[17] Ross, JR; Saunders, Y; Edmonds, PM; Patel, S; Broadley, KE; Johnston, SRD. Systematic review of role of bisphosphonates on skeletal morbidity in metastatic cancer. *British Medical Journal*, 2003, 327: 469-471.

[18] Stopeck, A; Lipton, A; Body, JJ; Steger, GG; Tonkin, K; De Boer, RH; Lichinitser, M; Fujiwara, Y; Yardley, DA; Viniegra, M; Fan, M; Jiang, Q; Dansey, R; Jun, S; Braun, A. Denosumab compared with zoledronic acid for the treatment of bone metastases in patients with advanced breast cancer: a randomized, double-blind study. *Journal of Clinical Oncology*, 2010;28(35):5132–5139.

[19] Fizazi, K; Carducci, M; Smith, M; Damião, R; Brown, J; Karsh, L; Milecki, P; Shore, N; Rader, M; Wang, H; Jiang, Q; Tadros, S; Dansey, R; Goessl, C. Denosumab versus zoledronic acid for treatment of bone metastases in men with castration-resistant prostate cancer: a randomised, double-blind study. *Lancet*, 2011, 377(9768):813–822.

[20] Hu, MI; Glezerman, I; Leboulleux, S; Insogna, K; Gucalp, R; Misiorowski, W; Yu, B; Ying, W; Jain, RK. Denosumab for patients with persistent or relapsed hypercalcemia of malignancy despite recent bisphosphonate treatment. *Journal of the National Cancer Institute*, 2013, 18;105(18):1417-2.

[21] Castellano, D; Sepulveda, JM; Garcı´a-Escobar, I; Rodriguez-Antolı´n, A; Sundlo¨v, A; Cortes-Funes, H. The role of RANK-ligand inhibition in cancer: the story of denosumab. *Oncologist,* 2011, 16:136–145.

[22] Reagan, P; Pani, A; Rosner, MH. Approach to Diagnosis and Treatment of Hypercalcemia in a Patient With Malignancy. *American Journal of Kidney Disease*, 2014, 63(1):141-7.

[23] Slater, D. Carcinoid tumor of the prostate associated with inappropriate ACTH secretion. *British Journal of Urology*, 1985, 57: 591–592.

[24] Kataoka, K; Akasaka, Y; Nakajima, K; Nagao, K; Hara, H; Miura, K; Ishii, N. Cushing syndrome associated with prostatic tumor adrenocorticotropic hormone (ACTH) expression after maximal androgen blockade therapy. *International Journal of Urology*, 2007, 14:436–439.

[25] Teves, DA; Clinical approach of Cushing syndrome resulting from ACTH-producing metastatic neuroendocrine tumor. *Endocrinologist*, 2005, 15(6):401-404.

[26] Akamatsu, S; Takenawa, J; Kanamaru, S; Soeda, A. Ectopic adrenocorticotropic hormone syndrome in a case of small cell carcinoma of the bladder manifesting as severe muscle weakness. *Urology*, 2006; 68:e5–e8.

[27] Nimalasena, S; Freeman, A; Harland, S. Paraneoplastic Cushing's syndrome in prostate cancer: a difficult management problem. *BJU International*, 2008;101:424-427.

[28] Nieman, LK. Medical therapy of Cushing's disease. *Pituitary*, 2002, 5:77-82.

[29] Ishikawa, S; Koyama, T; Kumagai, A; Takeuchi, I; Ogawa, D. A case of small cell carcinoma of the ureter with SIADH-like symptoms. *Nippon Hinyokika Gakkai Zasshi*, 2004; 95: 725–728.

[30] Yamazaki, T; Suzuki, H; Tobe, T; Sekita, N; Kito, H; Ichikawa, T. Prostate adenocarcinoma producing syndrome of inappropriate secretion of antidiuretic hormone. *International Journal of Urology*, 2001, 8: 513–516.

[31] Garzotto, M; Beer, TM. Syndrome of inappropriate antidiuretic hormone secretion: a rare complication of prostate cancer. *The Journal of Urology*, 2001, 166: 1386.

[32] Shaaban, H; Thomas, D; Guron, G. A rare case of metastatic ductal type prostate adenocarcinoma presenting with syndrome of inappropriate secretion of antidiuretic hormone: a case report and review. *Journal of Cancer Research and Therapy*, 2012, 8(2):308-10.

[33] Sorensen, JB; Andersen, MK; Hansen, HH. Syndrome of inappropriate secretion of antidiuretic hormone (SIADH) in malignant disease. *Journal of Internal Medicine*, 1995, 238, 97–110.

[34] Bartter, FC; Schwartz, WB. The syndrome of inappropriate secretion of antidiuretic hormone. *The American Journal of Medicine*, 1967, 42(5):790-806.

[35] Raftopoulos, H. Diagnosis and management of hyponatremia in cancer patients. *Support Care Cancer*, 2007, 15:1341-1347.

[36] Ellison, DH; Berl, T. The syndrome of inappropriate antidiuresis. *The New England Journal of Medicine*, 2007, 356:2064-2072.

[37] Kulke, MH; Benson, AB; Bergsland, E; Berlin, JD; Blaszkowsky, LS; Choti, MA; Clark, OH; Doherty, GM; Eason, J; Emerson, L; Engstrom, PF; Goldner, WS; Heslin, MJ; Kandeel, F; Kunz, PL; Kuvshinoff, BW; Moley, JF; Pillarisetty, VG; Saltz, L; Schteingart, DE; Shah, MH; Shibata, S; Strosberg, JR; Vauthey, JN; White, R; Yao, JC; Freedman-Cass, DA; Dwyer, MA; National Comprehensive Cancer Networks. Neuroendocrine tumors. *Journal of the National Comprehensive Cancer Network*, 2012, 1;10(6):724-64.

[38] Murali, R; Kneale, K; Lalak, N; Delprado, W. Carcinoid Tumors of the Urinary Tract and Prostate. *Archives of Pathology & Laboratory Medicine*, 2006, 130(11):1693-706.

[39] Sundin, A; Eriksson, B; Bergström, M; Långström, B; Oberg, K; Orlefors, H. PET in the diagnosis of neuroendocrine tumors. *Annals of the New York Academy of Sciences*, 2004, 1014:246-57.

[40] Nayar, MK; Lombard, MG; Furlong, NJ; McNulty, SJ; Hardy, KJ; Vora, J. Diagnosis and management of nonislet cell tumor hypoglycemia: case series and review of the literature. *Endocrinologist*, 2006, 16(4):227-230.

[41] Anderson, N; Lokich, JJ. Mesenchymal tumors associated with hypoglycemia: case report and review of the literature. *Cancer*, 1979, 44: 785–790.

[42] Moscardi, JL; Macedo, NA; Espasandin, JA; Piñeyro, MI. Malignant acanthosis nigricans associated with a renal tumor. *International Journal of Dermatology*, 1993, 32: 893–894.

[43] Gohji, K; Hasunuma, Y; Gotoh, A; Shimogaki, H; Kamidono, S. Acanthosis nigricans associated with transitional cell carcinoma of the urinary bladder. *International Journal of Dermatology,* 1994, 33:433–435.

[44] Anderson, SH; Hudson-Peacock, M; Muller, AF. Malignant acanthosis nigricans: potential role of chemotherapy. *British Journal of Dermatology*, 1999, 141:714-716.

[45] Doraiswamy, VA; Biboa, J; Obafemi, A; Goldschmid, M. Leukocytosis and hypercalcemia: a rare combination of paraneoplastic features in squamous cell penile cancer. *Southern Medical Journal*, 2010, 103(5):474-6.

[46] Wang, YC; Yang, S; Tzen, CY; Lin, CC; Lin, J. Renal cell carcinoma producing granulocyte colony-stimulating factor. *Journal of the Formosal Medical Association*, 2006, 105: 414–417.

[47] McRae, SN; Gilbert, R; Deamant, FD; Reese, JH. Poorly differentiated carcinoma of bladder producing granulocyte colony-stimulating factor and parathyroid hormone related protein. *The Journal of Urology*, 2001, 165: 527–528.

[48] Lin, HC; Chai, CY; Su, YC; Wu, WJ; Huang, CH. Leukemoid reaction resulting from granulocyte colony-stimulating factor producing urothelial carcinoma of the renal pelvis. *The Kaohsiung Journal of Medical Sciences*, 2007; 23: 89–92.

[49] Todenhöfer, T; Wirths, S; von Weyhern, CH; Heckl, S; Horger, M; Hennenlotter, J; Stenzl, A; Kanz, L; Schwentner, C. Severe paraneoplastic hypereosinophilia in metastatic renal cell carcinoma. *BMC Urology*, 2012, 21;12:7.

[50] Jameson, JL; Johnson, BE. Paraneoplastic syndromes: endocrinologic/hematologic. In: Fauci, AS; Braunwald, E; Kasper, DL; Hauser, SL; Longo, DL; Jameson, JL; Loscalzo, J; editors. *Harrison's Principles of Internal Medicine. 17th ed.* New York, NY, McGraw Hill Medical, 2008, 617-622.

[51] Lowe, D; Jorizzo, J; Hutt, MS. Tumor-associated eosinophilia: a review. *Journal of Clincal Pathology*, 1981, 34:1343–1348.

[52] Granger, JM; Kontoyiannis, DP. Etiology and outcome of extreme leukocytosis in 758 nonhematologic cancer patients: a retrospective, single-institution study. *Cancer*, 2009, 115:3919-3923.

[53] Naschitz, JE; Boss, JH; Misselevich, I; Yeshurun, D; Rosner, I. The fasciitis-panniculitis syndromes. Clinical and pathologic features. *Medicine (Baltimore)*, 1996, 75(1):6-16.

[54] Shah, A; Jack, A; Liu, H; Hopkins, RS. Neoplastic/paraneoplastic dermatitis, fasciitis, and panniculitis. *Rheumatic Disease Clinic of North America*, 2011, 37(4):573-92.

[55] Naschitz, JE; Yeshurun, D; Zuckerman, E; Rosner, I; Shajrawi, I; Missellevitch, I; Boss, JH. The fasciitis-panniculitis syndrome: clinical spectrum and response to cimetidine. *Seminars in Arthritis and Rheumathism*, 1992, 21(4):211-20.

[56] Baird, AD; Cornford, PA; Helliwell, T; Woolfenden, KA. Small cell prostate cancer with anti-Hu positive peripheral neuropathy. *The Journal of Urology*, 2002, 168: 192.

[57] Graus, F; Keime-Guibert, F; Rene, R; Benvahia, B; Ribalta, T; Ascaso, C; Escaramis, G; Delattre, JY. Anti-Hu-associated paraneoplastic encephalomyelitis: analysis of 200 patients. *Brain,* 2001, 124: 1138–1148.

[58] Gultekin, SH; Rosenfeld, MR; Voltz, R; Eichen, J; Posner, JB; Dalmau, J. Paraneoplastic limbic encephalitis: neurologic symptoms, immunological findings and tumour association in 50 patients. *Brain*, 2000, 123: 1481–1494.

[59] Stern, RC; Hulette, CM. Paraneoplastic limbic encephalitis associated with small cell carcinoma of the prostate. *Modern Pathology*, 1999; 12:814–818.

[60] Almeras, C; Soussi, N; Molko, N; Azoulay-Cayla, A; Richard, F; Chartier-Kastler, EJ. Paraneoplastic limbic encephalitis, a complication of the testicular cancer. *Urology*, 2001, 58(1):105.

[61] Voltz, R; Gultekin, SH; Rosenfeld, MR; Gerstner, E; Eichen, J; Posner, JB; Dalmau, J. A serologic marker of paraneoplastic limbic and brain-stem encephalitis in patients with testicular cancer. *The New England Journal of Medicine*, 1999, 10;340(23):1788-95.

[62] Tenner, L; Einhorn, L. Ma-2 paraneoplastic encephalitis in the presence of bilateral testicular cancer: diagnostic and therapeutic approach. *Journal of Clinical Oncology*, 2009, 10;27(23):e57-8.

[63] Clouston, PD; Saper, CB; Arbizu, T; Johnston, I; Lang, B; Newsom-Davis, J; Posner, JB. Paraneoplastic cerebellar degeneration. III.

Cerebellar degeneration, cancer, and the Lambert-Eaton myasthenic syndrome. *Neurology,* 1992, 42, 1944-1950.

[64] Prestigiacomo, CJ; Balmaceda, C; Dalmau, J. Anti-Ri-associated paraneoplastic opsoclonus-ataxia syndrome in a man with transitional cell carcinoma. *Cancer*, 2001, 15;91(8):1423-8.

[65] Delahunt, B; Abernethy, DA; Johnson, CA; Nacey, JN. Prostate carcinoma and the Lambert-Eaton myasthenic syndrome. *The Journal of Urology*, 2003, 169, 278-279.

[66] Henson, RA; Urich, H. Encephalomyelitis with carcinoma. In: Henson, RA; Urich, H. *Cancer and the nervous system.* Oxford: Blackwell Scientific, 1982. p. 314–45.

[67] Uchuya, M; Graus, F; Vega, F; Reñé, R; Delattre, JY. Intravenous immunoglobulin treatment in paraneoplastic neurologic syndromes with antineuronal antibodies. *Journal of Neurology, Neurosurgery and Psychiatry*, 1996, 60:388–392.

[68] Keime-Guibert, F; Graus, F; Broët, P; Reñé, R; Molinuevo, JL; Ascaso, C; Delattre, JY. Clinical outcome of patients with anti-Hu–associated encephalomyelitis after treatment of the tumor. *Neurology*, 1999.

[69] American Cancer Society. Kidney cancer (adult) – Renal cell carcinoma. Available from http://www.cancer.org/acs/groups/cid/ documents/ webcontent/003107-pdf.pdf.

[70] Chow, WH; Devesa, SS; Warren, JL; Fraumeni, JF Jr. Rising incidence of renal cell cancer in the United States. *Journal of the American Medical Association*, 1999, 281(17), 1628–1631.

[71] Gold, PJ; Fefer, A; Thompson, JA. Paraneoplastic manifestations of renal cell carcinoma. *Seminars in Urologic Oncology*, 1996, 14, 216–222.

[72] Campbell, SC & Lane, BR. Malignant renal tumors. In Wein, A; Kavoussi, L; Novick, A; Partin, A; Peters, C. (Eds.) *Campbell-Walsh urology (10th ed.)*, Philadelphia: Elsevier Saunders, 2012.

[73] Palapattu, GS; Kristo, B; Rajfer, J. Paraneoplastic syndromes in urologic malignancy: the many faces of renal cell carcinoma. *Reviews in Urology*, 2002;4: 163–170.

[74] Ding, GX; Feng, CC; Song, NH; Fang, ZJ; Xia, GW; Jiang, HW; Hua, LX; Ding, Q. Paraneoplastic symptoms: Cachexia, polycythemia, and hypercalcemia are, respectively, related to vascular endothelial growth factor (VEGF) expression in renal clear cell carcinoma. *Urologic Oncology*, 2013, 31(8):1820-5.

[75] Feng, CC; Ding, GX; Song, NH; Li, X; Wu, Z; Jiang, HW; Ding, Q. Paraneoplastic hormones: parathyroid hormone-related protein (PTHrP) and erythropoietin (EPO) are related to vascular endothelial growth factor (VEGF) expression in clear cell renal cell carcinoma. *Tumour Biology*, 2013, 34(6):3471-6.

[76] Odell, WD. Paraendocrine syndromes of cancer. *Advances in Internal Medicine*, 1989, 34:325–352.

[77] Kim, HL; Belldegrun, AS; Freitas, DG; Bui, MH; Han, KR; Dorey, FJ; Figlin, RA. Paraneoplastic signs and symptoms of renal cell carcinoma: implications for prognosis. *Journal of Urology*, 2003; 170: 1742–1746.

[78] Michael, A; Politi, E; Havranek, E; Corbishley, C; Karapanagiotou, L; Anderson, C; Relph, K; Syrigos, KN; Pandha, H. Prognostic significance of erythropoietin expression in human renal cell carcinoma. *BJU International,* 2007, 100:291–294.

[79] Giannakos, G; Papanicolaou, X; Trafalis, D; Michaelidis, I; Margaritis, G; Christofilakis, C. Stauffer's syndrome variant associated with renal cell carcinoma. *International Journal of Urology*, 2005, 12: 757–759.

[80] Boxer, RJ; Waisman, J; Lieber, MM; Mampaso, FM; Skinner, DG. Non-metastatic hepatic dysfunction associated with renal carcinoma. *The Journal of Urology*, 1978, 119:468–471.

[81] Blay, JY; Rossi, JF; Wijdenes, J; Menetrier-Caux, C; Schemann, S; Négrier, S; Philip, T; Favrot, M. Role of interleukin-6 in the paraneoplastic inflammatory syndrome associated with renal-cell carcinoma. *International Journal of Cancer*, 1997, 72:424–430.

[82] Gold, PJ; Fefer, A; Thompson, JA. Paraneoplastic manifestations of renal cell carcinoma. *Seminars in Urological Oncology*, 1996, 14(4):216-22.

[83] Kimura, M; Tomita, Y; Imai, T; Saito, T; Katagiri, A; Ohara-Mikami, Y; Matsudo, T; Takahashi, K. Significance of serum amyloid A on the prognosis in patients with renal cell carcinoma. *Cancer*, 2001, 15;92(8):2072-5.

[84] Vanatta, PR; Silva, FG; Taylor, WE; Costa, JC. Renal cell carcinoma and systemic amyloidosis: demonstration of AA protein and review of the literature. *Human Pathology*, 1983, 14(3):195-201.

[85] Evans, BK; Fagan, C; Arnold, T; Dropcho, EJ; Oh, SJ. Paraneoplastic motor neuron disease and renal cell carcinoma: improvement after nephrectomy. *Neurology*, 1990, 40:960–962.

[86] Swan, CHJ; Wharton, BA. Polyneuritis and renal cell carcinoma. *Lancet*, 1963, 2:383–384.

[87] Pavelic, K; Popovic, M. Insulin and glucagon secretion by renal adenocarcinoma. *Cancer*, 1981, 48:98.

[88] National Cancer Institute. Prostate Cancer Screening (PDQ®). Available online at http://www.cancer.gov/cancertopics/pdq/screening/ prostate/ HealthProfessional/allpages.

[89] 89. Smith, DC; Tucker, JA; Trump, D. L. Hypercalcemia and neuroendocrine carcinoma of the prostate: a report of three cases and a review of the literature. *Journal of Clinical Oncology,* 1992, 10,499-505.

[90] Cramer, SD; Chen, Z; Peehl, D. Prostate specific antigen cleaves PTHrP in the PTH-like domain. *The Journal of Urology*, 1996; 156: 526–530.

[91] Hong, MK; Kong, J; Namdarian, B; Longano, A; Grummet, J; Hovens, CM; Costello, AJ; Corcoran, NM. Paraneoplastic syndromes in prostate cancer. *Nature Reviews. Urology*, 2010, 7:681–92.

[92] Pinto, F; Brescia, A; Sacco, E; Volpe, A; Gardi, M; Gulino, G; Bassi, P. Disseminated intravascular coagulation secondary to metastatic prostate cancer: case report and review of the literature. *Archivio Italiano di Urologia, Andrologia*, 2009, 81, 212-214.

[93] Duran, I & Tannock, IF. Disseminated intravascular coagulation as the presenting sign of metastatic prostate cancer. *Journal of General Internal Medicine*, 2006, 21, C6-C8.

[94] Gakiya, M; Naka, H; Saito, S. Paraneoplastic neurological and hematological syndromes associated with prostate cancer. *International Journal of Urology*, 2012, 19(5):471-4.

[95] Kuramoto, T; Senzaki, H; Koike, H; Yamagiwa, K; Tamura, S; Fujimoto, T; Inagaki, T. Cholestatic jaundice as a paraneoplastic manifestation of prostate cancer. *Case Reports in Urology,* 2013.

[96] Harper, DG; Arsura EL; Bobba, RK; Reddy, CM; Sawh, AK. Acquired color blindness in an elderly male patient from recurrent metastatic prostate cancer. *Journal of the American Geriatric Society*, 2005, 53:1265-1267.

[97] Siegel, R; Naishadham, D; Jemal, A. Cancer statistics, 2013. *CA: A Cancer Journal for Clinicians*, 2013, 63(1):11-30.

[98] Brennan, P; Bogillot, O; Cordier, S; Greiser, E; Schill, W; Vineis, P. Cigarette smoking and bladder cancer in men: a pooled analysis of 11 case-control studies. *International Journal of Cancer*, 2000, 86(2):289-94.

[99] Talanin, NY; Bushore, D; Rasberry, R; Rudolph, T; Tuli, M; Friedman-Musicante, R. Dermatomyositis with the features of inclusion body

myositis associated with carcinoma of the bladder. *The British Journal of Dermatology*, 1999, 141(5):926-30.
[100] Kaji, K; Fujimoto, M; Hasegawa, M; Kondo, M; Saito, Y; Komura, K. Identification of a novel autoantibody reactive with 155 and 140 kDa nuclear proteins in patients with dermatomyositis: an association with malignancy. *Rheumatology*, 2007;46(1):25-8.
[101] Lin, JT; Wang, WH; Yen, CC; Yu, IT; Chen, PM. Prurigo nodularis as initial presentation of metastatic transitional cell carcinoma of the bladder. *The Journal of Urology*, 2002,168(2):631.
[102] Patel, AB; Wilson, L; Blick, C; Meffan, P. Paraneoplastic hypercalcaemia associated with TCC of bladder. *The Scientific World Journal*, 2004, 10;4:1069-70.
[103] Collins, DR; Connolly, S; Burns, M; Offiah, L; Grainger, R; Walsh, JB. Lambert-eaton myasthenic syndrome in association with transitional cell carcinoma: a previously unrecognized association. *Urology*, 1999, 54(1):162.
[104] Prestigiacomo, CJ; Balmaceda, C; Dalmau, J. Anti-Ri-associated paraneoplastic opsoclonus-ataxia syndrome in a man with transitional cell carcinoma. *Cancer*, 2001, 15;91(8):1423-8.
[105] Lukacs, S; Szabo, N; Woodhams, S. Rare association of anti-hu antibody positive paraneoplastic neurological syndrome and transitional cell bladder carcinoma. *Case Reports in Urology*, 2012.
[106] Greenlee, JE; Dalmau, J; Lyons, T; Clawson, S; Smith, RH; Pirch, HR. Association of anti-Yo (type 1) antibody with paraneoplastic cerebellar degeneration in the setting of transitional cell carcinoma of the bladder: detection of Yo antigen in tumor tissue and fall in antibody titers following tumor removal. *Annals of Neurology*, 1999, 45:805–809.
[107] Lowe, BA; Mershon, C; Mangalik, A. Paraneoplastic neurological syndrome in transitional cell carcinoma of the bladder. *Journal of Urology*, 1992, 147:462–4.
[108] Young, RH; Scully, RE. Clear cell adenocarcinoma of the bladder and urethra. A report of three cases and a review of the literature. *The American Journal of Surgical Pathology*, 1985, 9:816–26.
[109] Moreno-Palacios, J; Wingartz-Plata, H; Pardo-Belasteguigoitia, P; Moreno-Aranda, J. Stauffer syndrome in transitional cell carcinoma of the bladder. *Archivos Espanoles de Urologia*, 2011, 64(9):911-3.
[110] Norrenberg, S; Gangji, V; Del Marmol, V; Soyfoo, MS. Diffuse Muscular Pain, Skin Tightening, and Nodular Regenerative Hyperplasia

Revealing Paraneoplastic Amyopathic Dermatomyositis due to Testicular Cancer. *Case Reports in Rheumatology*, 2012, 2012:534236.

[111] Dourmishev, LA; Popov, JM; Rusinova, D. Paraneoplastic dermatomyositis associated with testicular cancer: a case report and literature review. *Acta Dermatovenerologica Alpina, Panonica et Adriatica*, 2010, 19(1):39-43.

[112] Hayami, S; Kubota, Y; Sasagawa, I; Suzuki, H; Nakada, T; Motoyama, T. Dermatomyositis associated with intratubular germ cell tumor and metastatic germ cell cancer. *The Journal of Urology*, 1998, 159(6):2096-7.

[113] Leonhartsberger, N; Ramoner, R; Aigner, F; Stoehr, B; Pichler, R; Zangerl, F; Fritzer, A; Steiner, H. Increased incidence of Leydig cell tumours of the testis in the era of improved imaging techniques. *BJU International,* 2011, 108(10):1603-7.

[114] Kaufman, E; Akiya, F; Foucar, E; Grambort, F; Cartwright, KC. Viralization due to Leydig cell tumor diagnosis by magnetic resonance imaging. Case management report. *Clinical Pediatrics,* 1990, 29(7): 414-7.

[115] Mineur, P; De Cooman, S; Hustin, J; Verhoeven, G; De Hertogh, R. Feminizing testicular Leydig cell tumor: hormonal profile before and after unilateral orchidectomy. *The Journal of Clinical Endocrinology and Metabolism,* 1987, 64(4):686-91.

[116] Page, DC. Hypothesis: a Y-chromosomal gene causes gonadoblastoma in dysgenetic gonads. *Development*, 1987, 101 Suppl:151-5.

[117] Lau, YF; Li, Y; Kido, T. Gonadoblastoma locus and the TSPY gene on the human Y chromosome. *Birth Defects Res C Embryo Today*, 2009, 87(1):114-22.

[118] Gourlay, WA; Johnson, HW; Pantzar, JT; McGillivray, B; Crawford, R; Nielsen, WR. Gonadal tumors in disorders of sexual differentiation. *Urology*, 1994,43(4):537-40.

In: Paraneoplastic Syndromes
Editor: Lora H. Winter
ISBN: 978-1-63117-878-8

Chapter IV

Paraneoplastic Polyneuropathies: Searching in the Mist

Antonios Kerasnoudis*, M.D.
Neuroimmunological Department, St. Luke Hospital, Panorama, Thessaloniki, Greece
Neurological Private Practice, Serres, Greece

Abstract

Paraneoplastic neurologic syndromes are a heterogeneous group of neurologic disorders associated with systemic cancer and caused by mechanisms other than metastases, metabolic and nutritional deficits, infections, coagulopathy, or side effects of cancer treatment. These syndromes may affect any part of the nervous system from cerebral cortex to neuromuscular junction and muscle, either damaging one area or multiple areas.

The clinical importance of paraneoplastic polyneuropathies is high, as in most patients the neurologic symptoms are the presenting feature of an otherwise undiagnosed tumor. In addition, paraneoplastic polyneuropathies often cause severe and permanent neurologic morbidity. On the other hand, prompt recognition of this disorder may maximize the

* Email: antonis.kerasnoudis@gmail.com. Tel: 00306974994379.

likelihood of successful tumor treatment and a favorable neurologic outcome.

For patients without a known neoplasm who present with a peripheral neuropathy, the likelihood of a paraneoplastic etiology is difficult to quantitate and depends on the particular clinical syndrome. For example, severe rapidly progressive sensory neuronopathy is much more likely to be paraneoplastic than a mild, distal, slowly progressive axonal polyneuropathy. Among the most common paraneoplastic polyneuropathies are included: a) subacute sensory neuronopathy, b) demyelinating polyneuropathies, c) autonomic insufficiency, d) motor neuronopathy, e) vasculitic neuropathy.

This review provides an update on the clinical, paraclinical and electrophysiological presentation of the most common paraneoplastic polyneuropathies and fresh insight to the pathomechanism of peripheral nerve injury.

Introduction

The first report of a paraneoplastic syndrome dates back to the 19th century. The description of the relationship between neurological disorders and systemic tumors has been attributed to a French physician, M. Auchè, who described peripheral nervous system involvement in cancer patients in 1890 [1].

Peripheral neuropathies are among the most common neurologic complications of cancer. Depending on diagnostic criteria, up to 50% of patients with carcinoma develop peripheral neuropathy [2]. The differential diagnosis of peripheral nervous system dysfunction in cancer patients is broad and includes: direct nerve compression or infiltration by tumor; neurotoxicity of cancer treatment; nutritional deficiencies; metabolic derangements; and paraneoplastic disorders. Immunologic factors are believed to be important in the pathogenesis of PNS because antibodies and T-cell responses against nervous system antigens have been defined for many of these disorders [3, 4]. Presumably, the immunologic response is elicited by the ectopic expression of neuronal antigens by the tumor. Expression of these "onconeural" antigens is limited to the tumor and the nervous system, and sometimes also the testis. At the time of presentation of the neurological symptoms, most patients have not yet been diagnosed with cancer [5-9].

Paraneoplastic disorders may affect any part of the peripheral nervous systems. The incidence of PNS varies with the neurological syndrome and with the tumor. Approximately 10% of patients with plasma cell disorders accompanied by malignant monoclonal gammopathies are affected by a paraneoplastic peripheral neuropathy. More than half of the patients with the rare osteosclerotic form of myeloma develop a severe predominantly motor paraneoplastic peripheral neuropathy. In other hematological malignancies, the incidence of PNS is very low, with the exception of Hodgkin's disease. However, the incidence of PNS even in Hodgkin's disease is well below 1%. In solid tumors, the more common neurological syndromes are myasthenia gravis, which occurs in 15% of patients with a thymoma, and LEMS, which affects 3% of patients with SCLC. For other solid tumors, the incidence of PNS is <1% [1]. For patients without a known neoplasm who present with a peripheral neuropathy, the likelihood of a paraneoplastic etiology is difficult to quantitate and depends on the particular neuropathy syndrome. For example, severe rapidly progressive sensory neuronopathy is much more likely to be paraneoplastic than a mild, distal, slowly progressive axonal polyneuropathy [10-12].

1. Sensory Neuronopathy

In 1948 Denny-Brown reported 2 patients with sensory neuropathy in whom autopsy revealed severe neuronal loss in the dorsal root ganglia and a previously undiagnosed bronchial carcinoma [13]. Acquired sensory neuronopathies or ganglionopathies encompass different disorders characterized by a primary degeneration of sensory neurons in dorsal root ganglia. Subsequent reports established, that in most patients, paraneoplastic sensory neuronopathy is part of a multifocal encephalomyeloneuritis.

In the majority of patients with paraneoplastic sensory neuronopathy, the neurologic symptoms are the presenting feature of the associated neoplasm, preceding discovery of the tumor by intervals ranging from several months up to 2 years or more [14-15]. Early symptoms are patchy or asymmetric numbness and paresthesias, often involving face, trunk, or proximal limbs. The symptoms eventually spread to involve all limbs. Burning dysesthesias and severe aching or lancinating pain are common and may be the most distressing feature of the disease. Neurological examination reveals severe sensory ataxia, predominant impairment of vibration sense and proprioception, frequent pseudoathetosis, and hypoactive or absent muscle stretch reflexes [16]. Most patients with paraneoplastic sensory neuronopathy have additional signs and symptoms, that reflect a multifocal encephalomyeloneuritis. These include varied combinations of altered sensorium, confusion, memory loss, personality change, ocular dysmotility, dysarthria, dysphagia, cerebellar ataxia, corticospinal tract findings, asymmetric lower motor neuron weakness, intestinal pseudo-obstruction, or autonomic system degeneration [17-20].

The neuropathologic hallmark of paraneoplastic sensory neuronopathy is severe loss of primary sensory neurons in the dorsal root ganglia and gasserian ganglia. The neuronal loss is not only diffuse but also patchy and asymmetric, reflecting patients' clinical presentation [21]. In addition, a highly variable degree of peivascular infiltration by T and B lymphocytes, plasma cells, and macrophages is often documented [22, 23].

The diagnostic evaluation of patients with paraneoplastic sensory neuronopathy reveals in cerebrospinal fluid (CSF): elevated protein levels, mild mononuclear pleocytosis, elevated IgG index, and/or oligoclonal bands, while only 10% of patients have normal CSF findings [24]. Nerve conduction studies may depict an axonal affection of sensory nerve fibers (reduced amplitude or complete absence of sensory nerve action potentials, with normal or only slightly reduced sensory nerve conduction velocities), while motor nerve fibers may still be slightly affected. Needle EMG often reveals denervation, especially in patients with a component of motor neuropathy or encephalomyelitis and anterior horn cell involvement. Sural nerve biopsy shows usually nonspecific axonal degeneration and reduced population of myelinated fibers [25].

The most common circulating antibodies found in patients with paraneoplastic sensory neuronopathy are polyclonal IgG anti-Hu antibodies. More than 90% of reported patients with anti-Hu antibodies and sensory neuronopathy have small cell lung carcinoma, while neuroblastoma, non–small cell lung carcinoma, carcinoma of the breast or prostate, or thymoma may be also linked to this syndrome [24]. In rare cases, patients with paraneoplastic sensory neuronopathy and small cell lung carcinoma may have no detectable antineuronal antibodies, or antibodies with patterns of immunoreactivity distinct to Hu-antibodies (like anti-CV2, anti-amphiphysin, ANNA-3, anti-Ma) [26-31] (Table 1).

Considering the diagnostic workup, Chest CT, MR scanning or FDG-PET are more sensitive compared to conventional X-rays in detecting the underlying lung neoplasm in patients with a suspected paraneoplstic sensory neuronopathy [32, 33]. It should be mentioned though, that the initial evaluation for the underlying malignancy may not reveal any pathological findings, therefore the same workup should be repeated every several months. In view of the prognosis, the great majority of patients with paraneoplastic sensory neuronopathy or encephalomyeloneuritis deteriorate over weeks to months and then stabilize at a level of severe disability. Less commonly, patients have stepwise deterioration or exhibit a relentlessly progressive course leading to coma and death. Exceptional patients may have few, if any, overt central nervous system manifestations and a relatively indolent sensory neuronopathy that does not progress to neurologic disability even over several years [21].

Table 1.

Clinical syndrome	Tumors	Antibodies
Sensory neuronopathy	SCLC, lymphoma, adenocarcinoma	Hu, anti-CV2, anti-Amphiphysin, ANNA-3, anti-Ma
Demyelinating polyneuropathies	Lymphomas, adenocarcinomas, SCLC	anti-CV2, MAG
Autonomic neuropathies	SCLC, lymphoma, adenocarcinomas, thymoma	Hu, ganglionic AChR
Motor neuronopathy	SCLC, lymphoma	Hu, CV2, Yo b4 spectrin
Vasculitic neuropathy	Prostate, kidney, gastrointestinal and lung cancers, lymphomas	No known antibodies

2. Demyelinating Neuropathies

Paraneoplastic sensorimotor neuropathies may fulfill the diagnostic criteria of GBS, CIDP, Miller–Fisher syndrome, or multifocal motor neuropathy [34-37]. Both the clinical features, and the electrophysiological, CSF findings can be indistinguishable from those of idiopathic acute (AIDP) or chronic inflammatory demyelinating polyneuropathy (CIDP) or MMN [34, 35]. All these clinical syndromes may precede the discovery of the neoplasm by up to several years. Nerve conduction studies show marked slowing of motor and sensory conduction, prolonged or absent F-waves and temporal dispersion or focal conduction block. Signs of partial denervation may also be present in EMG. Sural nerve biopsy may show acute or chronic perivascular inflammatory infiltrates not only in the endoneurium, but also in the epineurium, without accompanying evidence of vasculitis.

According to the literature, paraneoplastic GBS is more frequently associated with Hodgkin disease and SCLC [38, 39]. On the other hand, paraneoplastic CIDP may occur in the setting of gastrointestinal cancer, Hodgkin and non-Hodgkin lymphomas (NHL) with monoclonal bands (Table 1) [40-42]. Patients with a CIDP variant characterized by predominant sensory symptoms, absence of anti-myelin-associated glycoprotein (MAG) antibodies and disproportionately prolonged distal motor latencies are sometimes associated with chronic lymphocytic leukemia and NHL owing to secondary axonal degeneration [42].

Neurologic improvement may follow tumor resection, IVIg, or corticosteroid therapy. Several recently reported patients with CIDP and melanoma had vitiligo or serum antibodies against gangliosides and other antigens shared by tumor cell and peripheral nerves [43, 44].

3. Autonomic Neuropathies

Paraneoplastic autonomic neuropathies are usually characterized by gastrointestinal dysmotility, due to loss of neurons of the enteric plexuses. This syndrome, is also defined as chronic intestinal pseudo-obstruction and is usually associated in the literature with SCLC [46]. The most common symptoms and signs are nausea, early satiety, persistent constipation, weight loss, and abdominal distention. Imaging studies demonstrate dilated intestinal loops without evidence of obstruction.

On the other hand, a less common cinical syndrome is a autonomic neuronopathy characterized by subacute pandysautonomia with impairment of the sympathetic (orthostatic hypotension, anhydrosis) and parasympathetic function (impaired pupillary responses, dry mouth, gastrointestinal dysmotility, urinary retention, erectile dysfunction, and fixed heart rate). The syndrome, also known as autoimmune autonomic ganglionopathy, usually is not paraneoplastic [47].

The diagnosis of paraneoplastic autonomic neuropathy is based on the detection of Hu antibodies, that are in most cased indicative of underlying SCLC [48]. Up to 20% of patients with paraneoplastic autonomic neuronopathy harbor ganglionic acetylcholine receptor (AChR) antibodies [47, 49].

4. Motor Neuronopathy

Various literature reports exist on the coexistence of motor neuronopathy and neoplasia [50, 51]. In addition, there are several well-described patients with a lower or combined upper and lower motor neuron syndrome, who had significant neurologic improvement after resection of lung or renal carcinomas [52, 53].

The typical clinical presentation of paraneoplastic motor neuronopathy is a subacute clinical syndrome compatible with a lower motor neuron disease and sparing of the bulbar muscles. Especially in cases with underlying lymphoma the weakness usually appears after the diagnosis of the tumor, tends to be asymmetric, and greater in the legs. Muscle weakness is rarely severe and sometimes stabilizes or improves without any specific treatment [54, 55]. On the other hand, patients with breast cancer may present only with an upper motor neuron disease [56].

The most frequent antibodies found in paraneoplastic motor neuronopathy are the Hu or CV2 (both of which are highly associated with SCLC) [57]. Other described antibodies are Yo (PCA1) (by patients who also develop cerebellar ataxia) or b4 spectrin [58, 59]

5. Vasculitic Neuropathy

Paraneoplastic vasculitis is mainly characterized by nerve and/or muscle involvement, without clinical or paraclinical evidence of systemic involvement. The most common tumors causing paraneoplastic vasculitis are solid tumors, particularly prostate, kidney, gastrointestinal and lung cancers, and lymphomas [60-62]. The clinical syndrome is mainly characterized by a progressive, often asymmetric and painful sensorimotor neuropathy. The classical clinical syndrome of mononeuritis multiplex is less common in clinical practice. The proximal muscle weakness observed in some patients probably reflects the coincident muscle vasculitis.

The paraclinical diagnostic reveals typically elevated erythrocyte sedimentation rate and elevated CSF protein level. Nerve conduction studies usually depict a multifocal mononeuropathy, or a diffuse axonal polyneuropathy with asymmetric involvement [63]. Sural nerve biopsy shows intra- and perivascular inflammation with CD8 cells, usually without signs of necrosis.

Conclusion

Paraneoplastic neuropathies may mimic almost every type of peripheral nerve disease. They usually present with clinical and electrophysiological features that do not raise the suspicion of a paraneoplastic origin. Most neurologic paraneoplastic disorders are believed to be autoimmune diseases, as tumor cells express "onconeural" antigen(s) identical or antigenically related to molecules normally expressed by neurons, and that in rare instances an autoimmune response initially arising against the tumor subsequently attacks neurons expressing the same or related antigen(s).

However, recent studies indicate that a careful clinical evaluation helps and electrophysiological studies can assist to differentiate paraneoplastic from idiopathic polyneuropathies. The definition of the typical distribution pattern of electrophysiological, ultrasound and clinical findings will be a challenging future aspect of research.

References

[1] Auche M. Des nevrites peripheriques chez les cancereux. *Rev Med.* 1890;10:785-807.

[2] Posner JB. *Neurologic complications of cancer:* Philadelphia: FA Davis, 1995.

[3] Dropcho EJ. Remote neurologic manifestations of cancer. *Neurol Clin* 2002;20 (1):85-122.

[4] Darnell RB, Posner JB. Paraneoplastic syndromes involving the nervous system. *N Engl J Med* 2003;349:1543–1554.

[5] Graus F, Keime-Guibert F, Rene R et al. Anti-Hu-associated paraneoplastic encephalomyelitis: analysis of 200 patients. *Brain* 2001;124: 1138–1148.

[6] Sillevis Smitt P, Grefkens J, De Leeuw B et al. Survival and outcome in 73 anti-Hu positive patients with paraneoplastic encephalomyelitis/ sensory neuronopathy. *J Neurol* 2002;249:745–753.

[7] Shams'ili S, Grefkens J, de Leeuw B et al. Paraneoplastic cerebellar degeneration associated with antineuronal antibodies: analysis of 50 patients. *Brain* 2003;126:1409–1418.

[8] Rojas I, Graus F, Keime-Guibert F et al. Long-term clinical outcome of paraneoplastic cerebellar degeneration and anti-Yo antibodies. *Neurology* 2000;55:713–715.
[9] Denny-Brown D. Primary sensory neuropathy with muscular changes associated with carcinoma. *J Neurol Neurosurg Psychiatry* 1948;11: 73–87.
[10] Camerlingo M, Nemni R, Ferraro B, et al. Malignancy and sensory neuropathy of unexplained cause: a prospective study of 51 patients. *Arch Neurol* 1998;55:981-984.
[11] Antoine JC, Mosnier JF, Absi L, et al. Carcinoma associated paraneoplastic peripheral neuropathies in patients with and without anti-onconeural antibodies. *J Neurol Neurosurg Psychiatr* 1999;67:7
[12] Molinuevo JL, Graus F, Serrano C, et al. Utility of anti-Hu antibodies in the diagnosis of paraneoplastic sensory neuropathy. *Ann Neurol* 1998;44:976-980.
[13] Denny-Brown D. Primary sensory neuropathy with muscular changes associated with carcinoma. *J Neurol Neurosurg Psychiatry.* 1948 May;11(2):73-87
[14] Horwich MS, Cho L, Porro RS, Posner JB. Subacute sensory neuropathy: a remote effect of carcinoma. *Ann Neurol* 1977;2:7-19.
[15] Sillevis Smitt P, Grefkens J, de Leeuw B, et al. Survival and outcome in 73 anti-Hu positive patients with paraneoplastic encephalomyelitis/ sensory neuronopathy. *J Neurol* 2002,249.745-53.
[16] Oki Y, Koike H, Iijima M, et al. Ataxic vs painful form of paraneoplastic neuropathy. *Neurology* 2007;69:564-72.
[17] Dalmau J, Graus F, Rosenblum MK, Posner JB. Anti-Hu-associated paraneoplastic encephalomyelitis/sensory neuronopathy. A clinical study of 71 patients. *Medicine (Baltimore)* 1992;71(2):59-72
[18] Lucchinetti CF, Kimmel DW, Lennon VA. Paraneoplastic and oncologic profiles of patients seropositive for type I antineuronal nuclear autoantibodies. *Neurology* 1998;50:652-7.
[19] Keime-Guibert F, Graus F, Broet P, et al. Clinical outcome of patients with anti-Hu-associated encephalomyelitis after treatment of the tumor. *Neurology* 1999;53:1719-23
[20] Poepel A, Jarius S, Heukamp LC, et al. Neurological course of long-term surviving patients with SCLC and anti-Hu syndrome. *J Neurol Sci* 2007;263:145-8.
[21] Ohnishi Y, Ohara S, Sakamoto T, et al. Cancer-associated retinopathy with retinal phlebitis. *Brit J Ophthalmol* 1993;77:795-798.

[22] Wanschitz J, Hainfellner JA, Kristoferitsch W, et al. Ganglionitis in paraneoplastic subacute sensory neuronopathy: a morphologic study. *Neurology* 1997;49:1156-1159.
[23] Bernal F, Graus F, Pifarre A, Saiz A, et al. Immunohistochemical analysis of anti-Hu-associated paraneoplastic encephalomyelitis. *Acta Neuropathol* 2002;103:509-515.
[24] Dalmau J, Graus F, Rosenblum MK, Posner JB. Anti-Hu-associated paraneoplastic encephalomyelitis/sensory neuronopathy: a clinical study of 71 patients. *Medicine* 1992;71:59-72.
[25] Camdessanche JP, Antoine JC, Honnorat J, et al. Paraneoplastic peripheral neuropathy associated with anti-Hu antibodies: a clinical and electrophysiological study of 20 patients. *Brain* 2002;125:166-175
[26] Honnorat J, Antoine JC, Derrington E, Aguera M, Belin MF. Antibodies to a subpopulation of glial cells and a 66 kDa developmental protein in patients with paraneoplastic neurological syndromes. *J Neurol Neurosurg Psychiatr* 1996;61:270-278.
[27] Yu Z, Kryzer TJ, Griesmann GE, et al. CRMP-5 neuronal antoantibody: marker of lung cancer and thymoma-related autoimmunity. *Ann Neurol* 2001;49:146-154.
[28] Dropcho EJ. Antiamphiphysin antibodies with small cell lung carcinoma and paraneoplastic encephalomyelitis. *Ann Neurol* 1996;39:659-667.
[29] Antoine JC, Absi L, Honnorat J, et al. Antiamphiphysin antibodies are associated with various paraneoplastic neurological syndromes and tumors. *Arch Neurol* 1999;56:172-177.
[30] Saiz A, Dalmau J, Butler MH, et al. Anti-amphiphysin I antibodies in patients with paraneoplastic neurologic disorders associated with small cell lung carcinoma. *J Neurol Neurosurg Psychiatr* 1999;66:214-217.
[31] Dalmau J, Gultekin SH, Voltz R, et al. Ma1, a novel neuron- and testis-specific protein, is recognized by the serum of patients with paraneoplastic neurological disorders. *Brain* 1999;122:27-39.
[32] Antoine JC, Cinotti L, Tilikete C, et al. Fluorodeoxyglucose positron emission tomography in the diagnosis of cancer in patients with paraneoplastic neurological syndrome and anti-Hu antibodies. *Ann Neurol* 2000;48:105-108.
[33] Rees JH, Hain SF, Johnson MR, et al. The role of 18F-fluoro-deoxyglucose-PET scanning in the diagnosis of paraneoplastic neurological disorders. *Brain* 2001;124:2223-2231.

[34] Vital C, Vital A, Julien J, et al. Peripheral neuropathies and lymphoma without monoclonal gammopathy: a new classification. *J Neurol* 1990;237:177-185.

[35] Vallat JM, De Mascarel HA, Bordessoule D, et al. Non-Hodgkin's malignant lymphomas and peripheral neuropathies-13 cases. *Brain* 1995;118:1233-1245.

[36] Usmani N, Bhatia R, Ikpatt OF, Sharma KR. Diffuse large B-cell lymphoma presenting as Miller–Fisher syndrome. *Muscle Nerve* 2012; 45:138–143.

[37] Rigamonti A, Lauria G, Stanzani L, et al. A case of multifocal motor neuropathy with conduction block associated with gastric and lung adenocarcinoma. *J Peripher Nerv Syst* 2012; 17:226–228.

[38] Lisak RP, Mitchell M, Zweiman B, et al. Guillain-Barre´ syndrome and Hodgkin's disease: three cases with immunological studies. *Ann Neurol* 1977;1:72–78.

[39] Naveed S, Okoli K, Hollingsworth J, Kasmani R. Guillain-Barre´ syndrome as a paraneoplastic manifestation of small-cell carcinoma of lung. *South Med J* 2010; 103:156–158.

[40] Antoine JC, Mosnier JF, Lapras J, et al. Chronic inflammatory demyelinating polyneuropathy associated with carcinoma. *J Neurol Neurosurg Psychiatry* 1996; 60:188–190.

[41] Viala K, Behin A, Maisonobe T, et al. Neuropathy in lymphoma: a relationship between the pattern of neuropathy, type of lymphoma and prognosis? *J Neurol Neurosurg Psychiatry* 2008; 79:778–782

[42] Larue S, Bombelli F, Viala K, et al. Nonanti-MAG DADS neuropathy as a variant of CIDP: clinical, electrophysiological, laboratory features and response to treatment in 10 cases. *Eur J Neurol* 2011; 18:899–905.

[43] Bird SJ, Brown MJ, Shy ME, Scherer SS. Chronic inflammatory demyelinating polyneuropathy associated with malignant melanoma. *Neurology* 1996;46:822-824.

[44] Weiss MD, Luciano CA, Semino-Mora C, Dalakas MC, Quarles RH. Molecular mimicry in chronic inflammatory demyelinating polyneuropathy and melanoma. *Neurology* 1998;51:1738-1741

[45] Nobile-Orazio E, Francomano E, Daverio R, et al. Antimyelin-associated glycoprotein IgM antibody titers in neuropathy associated with macroglobulinemia. *Ann Neurol* 1989; 26:543–550.

[46] Chinn JS, Schuffler MD. Paraneoplastic visceral neuropathy as a cause of severe gastrointestinal motor dysfunction. *Gastroenterology* 1988; 95:1279–1286.

[47] Graus F, Dalmau J. Paraneoplastic neuropathies. *Curr Opin Neurol* 2013, 26:489–495.

[48] Graus F, Delattre JY, Antoine JC, et al. Recommended diagnostic criteria for paraneoplastic neurological syndromes. *J Neurol Neurosurg Psychiatry* 2004; 75:1135–1140.

[49] Vernino S, Adamski J, Kryzer TJ, et al. Neuronal nicotinic ACh receptor antibody in subacute autonomic neuropathy and cancer-related syndromes. *Neurology* 1998; 50:1806–1813.

[50] Rosenfeld MR, Posner JB. Paraneoplastic motor neuron disease. *Adv Neurol* 1991;56:445-459.

[51] Verma A, Berger JR, Snodgrass S, Petito C. Motor neuron disease: a paraneoplastic process associated with anti-Hu antibody and small-cell lung carcinoma. *Ann Neurol* 1996;40:112-116.

[52] Evans BK, Fagan C, Arnold T, Dropcho EJ, Oh SJ. Paraneoplastic motor neuron disease and renal cell carcinoma: improvement after nephrectomy. *Neurology* 1990;40:960-962.

[53] Forman D, Rae-Grant AD, Matchett SC, Cowen JS. A reversible cause of hypercapnic respiratory failure: lower motor neuronopathy associated with renal cell carcinoma. *Chest* 1999;115:899-901.

[54] Schold SC, Cho ES, Somasundaram M, Posner JB. Subacute motor neuronopathy: a remote effect of lymphoma. *Ann Neurol* 1979; 5:271–287.

[55] Briani C, Vitaliani R, Grisold W, et al. Spectrum of paraneoplastic disease associated with lymphoma. *Neurology* 2011; 76:705–710

[56] Forsyth PA, Dalmau J, Graus F, et al. Motor neuron syndromes in cancer patients. *Ann Neurol* 1997; 41:722–730

[57] Ducray F, Graus F, Vigliani MC, et al. Delayed onset of a second paraneoplastic neurological syndrome in eight patients. *J Neurol Neurosurg Psychiatry* 2010; 81:937–939.

[58] Distad BJ, Weiss MD. Paraneoplastic motor neuron disease associated with Purkinje cell autoantibody type 1. *J Clin Neuromuscul Dis* 2010; 12: 36–41.

[59] Berghs S, Ferracci F, Maksimova E, et al. Autoimmunity to beta IV spectrin in paraneoplastic lower motor neuron syndrome. *Proc Natl Acad Sci U S A.* 2001; 98:6945–6950

[60] Oh SJ. Paraneoplastic vasculitis of the peripheral nervous system. *Neurol Clin* 1997; 15:849–863.

[61] Choi HS, Kim DH, Yang SN, et al. A case of paraneoplastic vasculitic neuropathy associated with gastric cancer. *Clin Neurol Neurosurg* 2013; 115:218–221.

[62] Vasku M, Papathemelis T, Maass N, et al. Endometrial carcinoma presenting as vasculitic sensorimotor polyneuropathy. *Case Rep Obstet Gynecol* 2011; 2011:968756. doi: 10.1155/2011/968756.

[63] Zivkovic SA, Ascherman D, Lacomis D. Vasculitic neuropathy–electrodiagnostic findings and association with malignancies. *Acta Neurol Scand* 2007; 115:432–436.

In: Paraneoplastic Syndromes
Editor: Lora H. Winter

ISBN: 978-1-63117-878-8

Chapter V

Correction of Cancer-Related Anemia with Oxyresveratrol

G. I. Solyanik*[*], *O. N. Pyaskovskaya and N. K. Rodionova
R. E. Kavetsky Institute of Experimental Pathology, Oncology and Radiobiology of National Academy of Sciences of Ukraine, Kyiv, Ukraine

Abstract

It is well-known that malignant tumor exerts nonmetastatic systemic effects on organism caused the development of paraneoplastic syndrome (PNS). The symptomatic manifestations of PNS may pose the most troublesome and life threatening problems for cancer patients. Treatments of paraneoplastic conditions are frequently based on beneficial anti-cancer therapy. Unfortunately such therapy can not be carried out against resistant form of tumors and also in case of serious symptoms of PNS (paraneoplastic disorders of hemapoiesis, liver and kidney). Development of tumor-specific and/or tumor non-specific therapeutics against organism disorder PNS symptoms is of great importance to improve qualify of life, and in some cases, prolong life of cancer patients.

Despite the onrush of molecular biology and chemistry providing fast escalation of synthesized *de novo* drugs, plants still remain traditional

[*] Corresponding author: Dr G. Solyanik, Department of experimental cancer therapeutics; E-mail: gsolyanik@gmail.com.

sources of medicinal compounds. Widely distributed plant polyphenols are today among the most studied classes of phytochemicals.

In recent years stilbenes, naturally occurring polyphenolic compounds, have come to the attention because of their potential use as prophylactic and therapeutic agents in many diseases. The most well-known stilbenes are resveratrol and oxyresveratrol (OXY). Resveratrol, a representative of this group, has been widely investigated for its protecting and therapeutic effects against a number of pathological processes including cancer. Although OXY is characterized by better water solubility, higher bioavailability and less cytotoxicity (as compared to resveratrol) yet it is pharmacologically less investigated and the most study of OXY are applied to non-cancer diseases.

In this chapter the data concerning the pharmacological activity of OXY against both cancer-related anemia and tumor growth and metastasis are presented and discussed.

In order to evaluate an ability of OXY to correct cancer-related anemia without increasing risk of tumor progression the research was carried out using highly angiogenic and metastatic variant of Lewis lung carcinoma which growth in tumor-bearing mice is accompanied by an extensive manifestation of anemia and thrombopenia. Metronomic administration of OXY resulted in considerable elevation of erythrocyte counts, hemoglobin content and number of platelets.

At the same time the efficacy of OXY to inhibit tumor growth and metastasis has been revealed.

Introduction

In recent years plentiful results of research have demonstrated that progress in understanding the mechanisms of uncontrolled tumor growth and progression is impossible without deep analysis of interplay between cancer cells and normal cells of an organism. Such interactions play a crucial role in many processes underlying invasion and metastasis of malignant tumors.

Further, tumor exerts a systemic action toward organism which leads to significant changes in normal tissues as well as damages of functional body systems. Systemic effect of tumor on an organism causes the formation of paraneoplastic syndrome (PNS), i.e., systemic nonmetastatic manifestations accompanying the development of tumor process.

PNS development is characterized by large diversity (Figure 1). Therewith practically each PNS has a broad spectrum of clinical manifestations that in many cases are unique to a given cancer patient.

This, in turn, complicates PNS diagnostics and as a consequence, hampers an adequate evaluation of the rate of its manifestations.

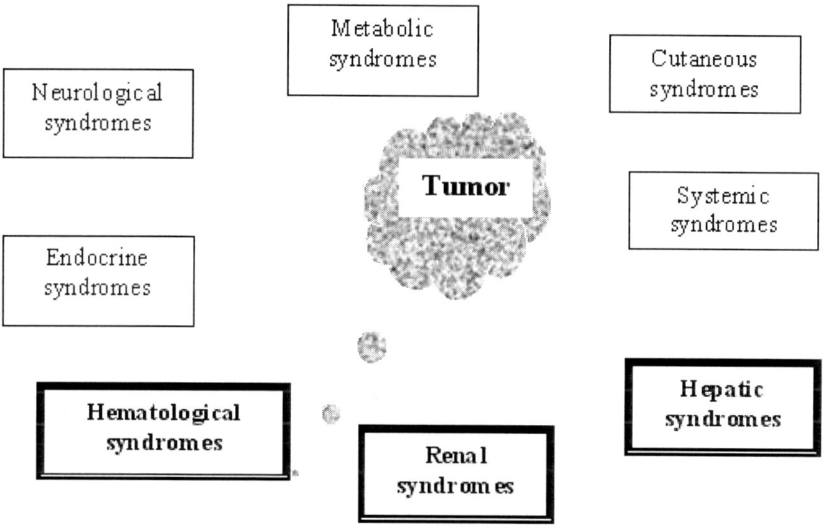

Figure 1. Diversity of paraneoplastic syndrome manifestation.

At the same time, according to the different estimates, the number of cancer patients being affected by some form of PNS ranged from 15% up to 70% [1, 2].

The phenomenon of PNS is mediated by humoral factors of tumor origin (hormones, cytokines) or cytokines produced by effector cells of antitumor immune response [3, 4].

It should be noted that PNS manifestations represent a severe and often life-threatening problem for cancer patients. The performance of effective cancer therapy is the most widely used PNS treatment option providing significant reduction of tumor material, consequently decreasing an influence of tumor of an organism. Unfortunately, this therapy can not be performed in the case of chemoresistant tumor forms.

Furthermore, some PNS manifestations including malfunction of hemopoiesis, liver and kidney failure, significantly limits the use of conventional cytotoxic cancer therapy and sometimes present a direct contraindication for its initiation.

As an example of this PNS form one could mention anemia caused by tumor development [5, 6].

Nearly 30% of primary cancer patients suffer from anemia of different severity stages, and at the moment of diagnosis half of them have hemoglobin level below 9.0 g/dl, what does not allow starting radio- and/or chemotherapy.

In other half of cancer patients the manifestation of anemia stipulates the reduction of cancer drug dosage and as a result decreases an expected effectiveness of the therapy.

In another case when treatment of underlying malignancy is impossible or its efficacy is questionable, the correction of cancer-related anemia include red blood cell transfusion, therapy with iron containing drugs and/or erythropoiesis-stimulating agents (ESA) [7]. The introduction of ESA as a treatment option represented a significant advance in the treatment of anemia [8].

However, ESA therapy of patients with cancer is characterized by moderate response rates (50%-60%) and slow time to response. Moreover, administration of ESAs was significantly associated with increased risks of venous thromboembolism and mortality in cancer patients receiving these drugs [9].

That is s why the search of agents providing the correction of paraneoplastic anemia and characterized with low toxicity toward normal tissues and body systems, is an urgent problem of modern experimental and clinical oncology.

Paraneoplastic Symptoms in Mice Bearing High Angiogenic Variant of Lewis Lung Carcinoma

Among diverse biologically active mediators of tumor origin an important place is occupied by angiogenesis-associated cytokines, in particular, vascular endothelial growth factor (VEGF). It is well-known that in contrast to majority of the normal cells (for instance, epithelial cells) cancer cells were shown to secrete VEGF in a constant way due to up-regulation of this growth factor in the tumor cell compartment [10]. Such alterations of VEGF expression in cancer cells cause an uncontrolled angiogenesis that promotes tumor growth. Elevated VEGF expression in tumor cells is associated with tumor progression and poor prognosis [11].

VEGF is also a potent biologically active mediator able to exert numerous physiologic and pathologic effects on vascular and other physiological systems of organism. At present time, it is supposed that VEGF is involved in the formation of renal, hepatic and hematological PNS. It was shown that increased serum levels of VEGF in VEGF-expressing RAS melanoma-bearing mice are associated with a lethal hepatic syndrome characterized by massive sinusoidal dilation, endothelial cell proliferation and apoptosis.

Systemic levels of VEGF in these animals correlate with the severity of liver pathology and overall clinical compromise. Moreover, this VEGF-induced syndrome resembles peliosis hepatis, a rare human condition that is encountered in the setting of advanced malignancies [12]. VEGF is one of the factors that are considered to contribute to the pathogenesis of paraneoplastic glomerulonephritis. The role of VEGF in the pathogenesis of paraneoplastic glomerulonephritis and focal segmental glomerulosclerosis is supported by the findings that overexpression of VEGF in podocytes induces collapsing focal segmental glomerulosclerosis in experimental animal models, and that serum VEGF levels are elevated in children with renal syndrome [13].

VEGF regulates the development of vasculature and hemopoiesis, significantly effecting the differentiation of erythroid progenitors. It was revealed that conditional deletion of VEGF within erythroid lineage was associated with an increased erythroid differentiation [14]. In adults, VEGF is involved in the support of vascular integrity, hemopoiesis regulation in bone marrow, wound healing and control of reproductive functions [15]. High levels of serum VEGF may increase micro-vascular hyperpermeability as well as a number of circulating endothelial progenitor cells in the peripheral blood [16].

Tumor-derived VEGF modulates the hematopoietic system by suppression of bone marrow hematopoiesis, leading to activation of extramedullary hematopoiesis in liver and spleen in mice bearing T241 fibrosarcoma transfected with DNA constructs which stably express human VEGF [17].

High correlation was revealed between cancer-related anemia and the increased serum-VEGF levels in patients [18, 19].

An important role of VEGF in formation of cancer-related anemia is confirmed also by the results of study on the symptoms of PNS development in mice with transplanted Lewis lung carcinoma variants which differ significantly by VEGF production levels. Just an availability of high- (LLC/R9) and low-angiogenic (LLC) Lewis lung carcinoma variants has prompted us to analyze the role of VEGF in pathogenesis of tumor-induced anemia.

The investigation was carried out using C57Bl/6 female mice weighting 19-22 g and aged 2.0-2.5 months, which were fed diets with normal protein contents. Mice were bred at animal facility of R.E. Kavetsky Institute of Experimental Pathology, Oncology and Radiobiology (IEPOR). Animal study protocols and operation procedures were approved by the Animal Ethics Committee of IEPOR.

LLC/R9 and LLC cells were kindly provided by Ukrainian National Bank of Cell Lines and Transplanted Tumors. LLC/R9 was derived from wild-type LLC strain as a result of experimental progression of LLC towards the development of drug resistance to cis-diamminedichloroplatinum (cis-DDP) and following in vitro growth adaptation of cis-DDP resistant cells.

Experimental progression of LLC included 9 sequential stages of tumor transplantation to experimental animals with cis-DDP therapy at each stage [20, 21].

LLC/R9 and LLC cells were maintained in RPMI medium (Sigma, US) supplemented with 10% fetal calf serum (Sigma, US), 2 mM L-glutamine, and 40 μg/ml gentamycin at 37°C in humidified atmosphere with 5% CO_2.

For in vivo study both variants of tumor cells were expanded in vitro in standard conditions and inoculated in the thigh muscle of the right hind leg of mice ($1.2x10^6$ cells in 0.1 ml of Hank's solution).

VEGF level in culture medium and in blood plasma was determined using mouse VEGF ELISA kit (R and D Systems, US) following the manufacturer's protocol adapted for blood plasma. Plasma samples were collected into tubes with EDTA, centrifuged for 20 min at 2000 g at 10°C and stored at -20°C until assayed.

Hematological and bone marrow indices of experimental animals were investigated during tumor growth on 0th, 14th, 20th, and 26th day after tumor cell inoculation (5-7 animals per each time point). The counts of erythrocytes, platelets, and leukocytes, cell sizes, hemoglobin content, hematocrit value in blood of animals with LLC/R9 and LLC, and also in intact animals were determined using hematological analyzer "Particle counter model PCE 210" (ERMA, Japan) adapted for the estimation of mouse blood cells.

Bone marrow was isolated from femoral bone of mice with LLC/R9 and LLC, and also intact (tumor-free) mice. Suspension for determination of total cellularity and imprint smears were prepared. Myelograms were calculated from imprint smears stained by Pappenheim, in an amount of 200 cells. Proliferative activity of erythroid and granulocytic cells was evaluated by the number of mitoses per 1000 cells in myelogram.

Statistical analysis of obtained results included descriptive statistics, Student's t-test, and Mann-Whitney u-test and was performed using Statistica v.8.5.

The obtained data displayed that LLC/R9 was characterized by significantly higher angiogenic potential compared with LLC (Table 1). The rate of VEGF production as one of the main attribute of cancer cell angiogenic potential, was 1.5 times higher ($p<0.05$) in LLC/R9 cells than in LLC cells. Such activity of VEGF production by LLC/R9 cells caused sharp increase of the circulating VEGF level at early stages of tumor growth (up to 14th day).

Table 1. Production of VEGF by LLC/R9 and LLC cells

Tumor variant	Rate of VEGF production *in vitro* (pg/h/10^6 cells)	Concentration of circulating VEGF on 14th day of tumor growth (pg/ml)
LLC/R9	38.4 ± 3.3*	76.0 ± 13.0*
LLC	25.1 ± 2.1	39.0 ± 5.0

Note: $^*p < 0.05$ vs. corresponding value of LLC.

On 14th day, the circulating VEGF level in mice with LLC/R9 was nearly twice higher ($p < 0.05$) than that in mice with LLC.

The study of hematological indexes of peripheral blood in mice with LLC/R9 confirmed that high angiogenic potential of tumor is associated with the development of anemia in tumor-bearing animals registered on 20th day after tumor cell inoculation with further progression at later terms. In blood of mice with LLC/R9 on 20th day after tumor cell inoculation there were detected significant decrease of erythrocyte counts (by 46.5%, $p<0.05$), hemoglobin content (by 42.3%, $p<0.05$) and hematocrit level (by 34.4%, $p<0.05$) comparing to tumor-free mice (intact animals) (Figure 2).

Herewith, the average hemoglobin content per one erythrocyte did not change significantly, while the average erythrocyte volume was significantly larger. During examination of blood smears there were significant aniso- and/or poikilocytosis (with the presence of large number of spherocytes), and also erythrocyte polychromatosis; sometimes immature erythroid cells: polychromatophilic and oxyphilic normocytes were also detected.

In other words, the events typical for the development of anemia of hemolytic type were observed. Later on, in mice with LLC/R9 the negative alterations of cellular composition of peripheral blood progressed and on 26th day after tumor cell inoculation the erythrocyte count and hemoglobin level did not exceed 35% from corresponding values in tumor-free mice.

These changes in peripheral blood indices were not observed during the growth of wild-type variant of Lewis lung carcinoma (LLC) [22].

The literature data gives grounds to hypothesize that anemia which develops in mice during LLC/R9 growth may originate from on the ability of VEGF to suppress bone marrow hemopoiesis [17, 23].

The results of the study confirmed this assumption. It has been shown that in vivo growth of LLC/R9 tumor was accompanied with significant decrease of total number of myelocytes (Figure 3).

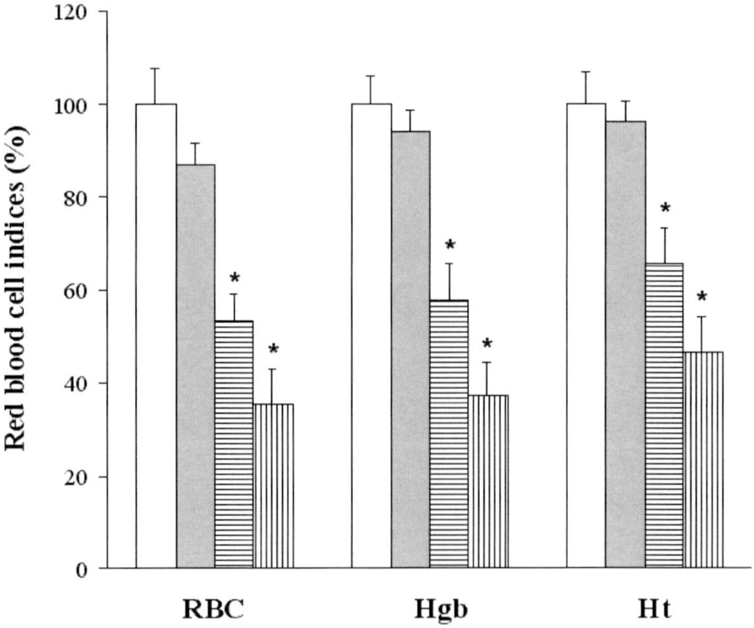

RBC – erythrocyte number, Hgb – hemoglobin content, Ht – hematocrit. Column represents the corresponding data on 14th day of tumor growth (grey column), on 20th day (column with horizontal lines), on 26th day (column with vertical lines). White column – intact mice. *p < 0.05 vs. corresponding value of intact mice.

Figure 2. Changes of red blood cell indices during LLC/R9 growth in percent of that of intact mice.

At early stages of LLC/R9 growth, 1.5-fold decrease ($p<0.05$) of bone marrow cellularity in mice with LLC/R9 compared to corresponding values in intact control, most likely, is determined by direct inhibition of mitotic activity of cells of both hemopoietic lines (Table 2).

Low myelocyte content at the later stages of tumor growth (on 20th and 26th days) despite significant activation of mitotic activity is, most likely, resulted from a substantial departure of the cells from the bone marrow into the peripheral blood as a compensatory response to anemia development.

The study of LLC/R9-bearing mice myelogram has shown that significant suppression of bone marrow hemopoiesis preceded the decrease of erythropoiesis indices in peripheral blood.

Such suppression of bone marrow hemopoiesis was accompanied by significant changes of erythroid cell indices which anticipated the failure of other cell pools of bone marrow (Table 2).

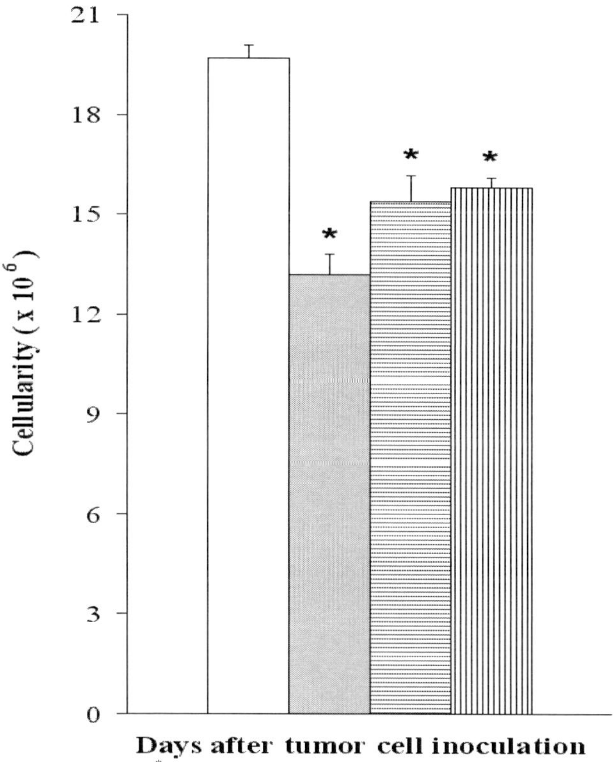

Designations as in Figure 2 $^{*}p < 0.05$ vs. corresponding value of intact mice.

Figure 3. Changes of bone marrow cellularity during LLC/R9 growth.

On 14th day, in bone marrow of animals the count of immature erythroid elements was significantly lower as compared with that of intact mice.

Erythroblasts were detected extremely rarely, the major part was composed from polychromatophilic and oxyphilic normoblasts, the number of erythroid cells in mitosis was very low.

These alterations in erythroid line of hemopoiesis led to the development of anemia which was revealed during the study of blood indices on 20th day after LLC/R9 cell inoculation and progressed at later terms. The drastic decrease of erythrocyte counts was accompanied with corresponding changes of their morphometric characteristics and decrease of hemoglobin content.

Table 2. Changes of bone marrow cellular composition of LLC/R9-bearing mice during tumor growth

Myelogram indices (%)	Days after tumor cell inoculation			
	0	14	20	26
Undifferentiated blasts	0.83±0.17	0.50±0.29	1.17±0.44	0.17±0.17*
Neutrophilic cells: - myeloblasts	0.83±0.44	0.83±0.60	1.50±0.50	0.17±0.17*
- promyelocytes	2.00±0.76	2.50±1.04	5.17±1.09	3.75±0.66
- myelocytes	4.50±1.61	7.33±1.01	13.8±2.7	12.4±1.7
- metamyelocytes	7.33±1.92	11.0±0.9	12.7±1.8	15.6±0.5
- stab cells	19.7±3.2	20.33±2.33	16.2±3.8	11.8±3.0
- segmentated	23.0±1.6	21.5±4.2	6.33±0.33*	5.00±1.04*
Eosinophilic cells: - pro- and myelocytes	0.50±0.29	0.67±0.44	0.83±0.33	-
- metamyelocytes	0.33±0.23	1.00±0.29	1.33±0.33	0.33±0.17
- stab and segmentated cells	0.50±0.29	0.83±0.44	0.33±0.33	0.75±0.25
Granulocytes: - young	18.5±6.7	23.3±2.7	35.2±2.9	32.4±2.0
- adult	43.8±2.2	42.7±5.7	22.8±4.0	21.8±3.2
All granulocytes	62.3±8.9	66.0±8.3	58.0±6.5	54.0±4.1
Erythroblasts	0.67±0.17	0.17±0.17*	0.17±0.17*	0.0
Pronormocytes	1.50±1.26	0.50±0.29*	0.50±0.29*	0.67±0.17*
Normocytes: - basophilic	3.50±1.04	1.50±0.29*	5.33±1.88	3.17±0.44
- polychromatophilic	9.50±2.75	5.83±2.62	10.0±1.7	12.3±3.4
- oxyphilic	10.8±3.4	10.0±4.1	5.67±0.60*	4.50±0.87*
All erythroid cells	26.0±7.5	17.7±6.9	21.0±3.5	19.9±4.2
Myelo-erythroid ratio	2.47±1.10	3.72±1.53	2.82±0.25	2.87±0.38
Lymphocytes	8.00±1.00	11.5±0.9	19.0±6.0*	24.0±7.7*
Megakaryoblasts, -cytes	0.33±0.17	0.67±0.17	0.50±0.29	0.17±0.17
Total mitotic index (MI), ‰	5.67±1.20	1.00±0.01*	8.00±1.15	5.33±1.45
MI of red cells, ‰	1.67±1.20	0.67±0.33*	4.67±1.76	2.67±1.67
MI of white cells, ‰	4.00±0.58	0.33±0.33*	3.33±1.33	2.67±0.67

Note: *$p < 0.05$ vs. corresponding value of intact mice.

Analysis of the state of granulocytic line of hemopoiesis on 14th day of tumor growth showed an extremely low mitotic activity of granulocytes despite the fact that cellular composition of granulocytes with various type of differentiation did not differ between LLC/R9 bearing mice and intact animals.

Apparently it caused the observed leukopenia in these terms in the peripheral blood (Table 3).

Table 3. Changes of leukogram indices of LLC/R9 bearing mice during tumor growth

Cell number ×1000/μl	Days after tumor cell inoculation			
	0	14	20	26
WBC	9.8 ± 1.5	5.7 ± 0.2*	12.7 ±1.1	14.9 ± 2.5
LY	7.15 ± 0.95	4.1 ± 0.8*	8.3 ±0.8	10.5 ± 2.0
Mo	1.1 ± 0.2	0.72± 0.2	1.6 ±0.2	1.7 ± 0.4
Gr	1.6 ± 0.2	0.95 ± 0.3	2.9 ±0.3*	2.7 ± 0.3*

Note: *difference vs. intact mice is statistically significant, $p<0.05$. WBC – white blood cells, LY - lymphocytes, Mo - monocytes, Gr – granulocytes.

Earlier registration of altered leukocyte counts in peripheral blood compared to erythrocytes directly depends on lifetime of the cells of these lines: it is known that lifetime of leukocytes is significantly shorter that that of erythrocytes.

Comparison of myelograms of animals with LLC/R9 on 20th day compared to earlier observation point has revealed activation of proliferation activity of bone marrow cells with a simultaneous increase in the proportion of younger generations of cells of both hemopoiesis lines. This observation is confirmed by an expressed tendency for significant increase of the mitoses number in erythroid line compared with that in intact control.

Comparing this fact with morphological changes of erythrocytes (presence of polychromatophils, appearance of spherocytes) one may suggest that not only suppression of erythropoiesis plays a role in anemia development during LLC/R9 growth, but also a direct destruction of erythrocytes in peripheral blood via autoimmune processes.

On 26th day in bone marrow there was revealed a high ratio of lymphocyte count (24% vs. 8% in intact mice) along with low number of mature granulocytic and erythroid cells which was stipulated by a necessity to restore the deficiency of circulating pools in peripheral blood and evidenced on decreased reserve blood system capacity. Noteworthy is the considerable left shift in granulocytic line of hemopoiesis and significant decrease of the mature granulocytes in cellular composition of bone marrow (up to 25% as compared to intact control). In contrast, at this observation time point the leukocyte count in peripheral blood increased significantly.

Possibly, this reaction of hemopoiesis is related to tumor tissue necrosis and development of inflammatory processes that require release of cells from their natural storage places, including bone marrow.

Considerable inhibition of erythropoiesis was displayed not only in the decrease of “young” erythroid cell portion in myelogram but also in marked reduction of the number of erythroid cells with different differentiation grade among total myelocariocyte count in femoral bone of LLC/R9-bearing mice (Figure 4).

It is known that insufficiency of hemopoiesis in bone marrow may cause compensatory activation of this process out of bone marrow (in liver and/or spleen) resulting in hepato- and splenomegaly (extramedullary hemopoiesis).

It was confirmed by earlier obtained data on histological study of PNS manifestations in mice with high angiogenic LLC/R9 variant [22].

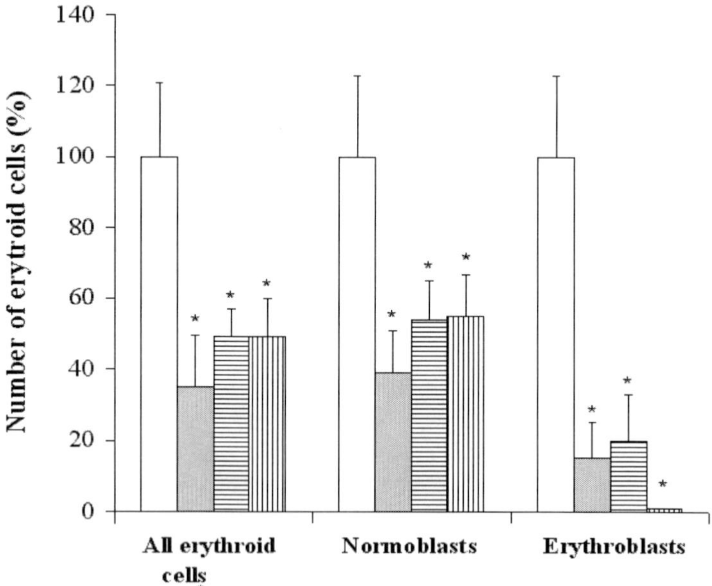

Designations as in Figure 2. *p < 0.05 vs. corresponding value of intact mice.

Figure 4. Changes of the number of erythroblasts, normoblasts and all erythroid cells in bone marrow during LLC/R9 growth in percent to that of intact animal (white column).

In this study hepatomegaly was revealed in statistically significant increase of weight and total cellularity of liver at the period of intense tumor growth (8-14 days), when maximal level of circulating VEGF was registered.

Morphological structure of the liver in animals with LLC/R9 on 14th day of tumor growth was characterized by vast number of small cell clusters of large blast-cells with basophilic cytoplasm, which represented the sites of extramedullary hematopoiesis. Moreover hepatic vasculature became highly dilated and was characterized by formation of new microvessels.

Simultaneously with hepatomegaly in animals with LLC/R9 there was found an expressed splenomegaly which was displayed in 2-fold increase of spleen weight and 3-fold increase of its cellularity. These changes in the weight and cellularity of the spleen in mice with LLC/R9 were accompanied by histological changes of the organ. Particularly, on 14th day apparent borders between the white pulp and red pulp were vanished and were replaced by a mixture of white pulp and red pulp without any distinctive borders throughout the entire spleen of LLC/R9-bearing mice, in contrast to LLC-bearing animals [22]. In addition the presence of a large number of blast-cells in the agglomerations of the lymphoid tissue in spleen of mice with LLC/R9 was observed.

An increase of proliferative activity of splenocytes in mice with high-angiogenic LLC/R9 variant was supported by the results of cytofluorometry analysis of the character of splenocyte distribution by cell cycle phases. As it is shown in Figure 5, proliferative activity of splenocytes in mice with LLC/R9 on 14th day of tumor growth was higher by 66% ($p<0.05$) than that in mice with LLC.

Enhanced proliferative activity of splenocytes in mice with LLC/R9 was accompanied by high level of antibody-genesis. Notably, the study of total level of circulating immunoglobulins IgG (which was carried out by immuno-enzyme method following the manufacturer's protocol) has shown that at 14th day after tumor cell inoculation in blood serum of mice with LLC/R9 this index was 10-fold ($p<0.05$) and 4-fold ($p<0.05$) higher than indices of intact animals and mice with LLC, respectively (Figure 6).

It is known that tumor process is characterized by activation of anticancer antibody-genesis. It is assumed that antibody-dependent cytotoxicity may cause an inhibiting effect on the tumor growth and metastasis.

Indeed, according to obtained data LLC/R9 variant was characterized by lower metastatic potential compared with LLC variant. As one may see in Table 4, on 26th day the number of lung metastases in mice with LLC/R9 was twice lower ($p < 0.05$) than in mice with LLC. The lower metastatic potential of LLC/R9 cells may partially result from antibody dependent cytotoxicity.

The presence of such a reverse relation between antibody-genesis and tumor metastatic potential was circumstantially confirmed by the study which results evidenced on increased metastasis in the case of splenectomy in animals with LLC/R9 (data not shown).

On the other side, in both cases tumor angiogenic potential correlated with its proliferative activity. Tumor growth rate in the case of high angiogenic variant was significantly higher than in the case of low angiogenic variant: on 26th day of tumor growth the volume of tumor in mice with LLC/R9 was more than 1.6-fold higher ($p < 0.05$) than that in mice with LLC (Table 4).

In this way, conducted study has demonstrated that the growth of high angiogenic variant of Lewis lung carcinoma (in contrast to low angiogenic variant) was accompanied with the development of hematologic PNS which was presented by anemia signs, in particular, decreased erythrocyte count, low hemoglobin and hematocrit level, development of extramedullary hemopoiesis including hepato- and splenomegaly, increased proliferative activity of splenocytes and enhancement of antibody genesis.

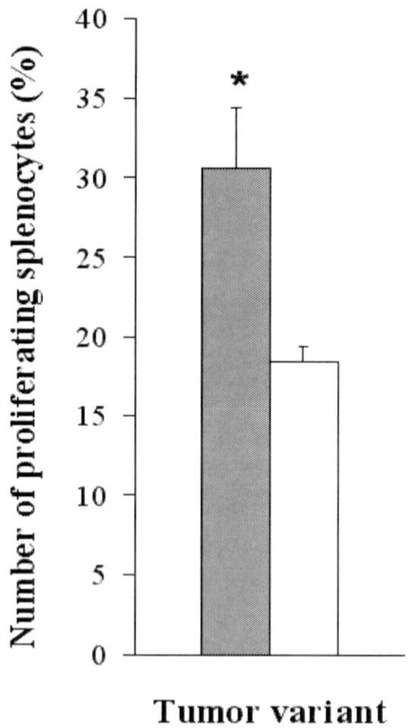

*$p < 0.05$ vs. corresponding value of LLC bearing mice.

Figure 5. Number of proliferating splenocytes of LLC/R9 bearing mice (grey column) and LLC bearing mice (white column) on 14th day of tumor growth.

Table 4. Parameters of LLC/R9 and LLC growth and metastasis on 26th day after tumor cell inoculation

Tumor variant	Tumor volume (cm^3)	Parameters of lung metastases	
		Number	Volume (mm^3)
LLC/R9	2.42±0.30*	13.4±1.8*	15.8±4.1
LLC	1.47±0.27	24.4±4.6	10.6±2.8

Note: *$p < 0.05$ vs. corresponding value of LLC-bearing mice.

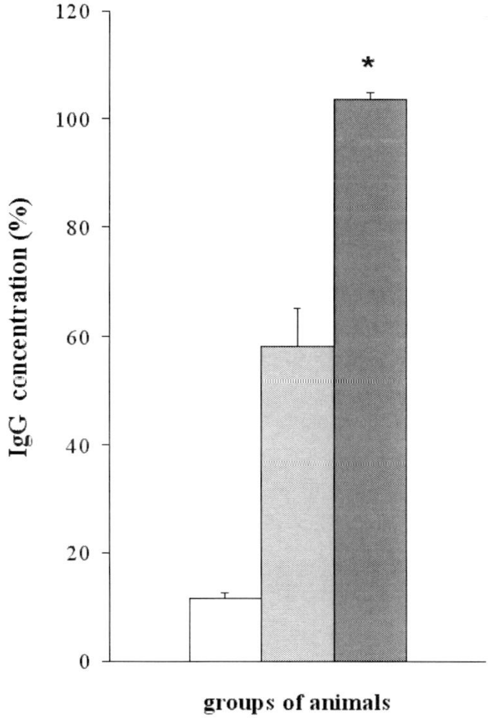

*$p < 0.05$ vs. corresponding value of intact mice.

Figure 6. Blood serum IgG level in LLC/R9 (dark grey column) and LLC (grey column) bearing mice on 14th day of tumor growth in percent of that of intact mice (white column).

It is necessary to note that these manifestations were induced at early stages of tumor growth, when in blood plasma high level of circulating VEGF was registered.

The presence of the mentioned symptoms in the case of high angiogenic LLC/R9 variant and their absence in the case of low angiogenic variant may illustrate an important role of VEGF in a complex multilevel interaction of tumor and organism and in formation of hematologic PNS in particular.

Hydroxystilbenes – Potential Modificator of Paraneoplastic Symptoms

Despite drastic development of molecular biology and chemistry providing quick escalation of de novo synthesized preparations, plants still represent a traditional source of medicinal compounds; up to 40% of modern drugs may directly or indirectly be related to natural compounds [24]. Lately the special attention is focused on grape polyphenols for some of which pleiotropic health beneficial effects and low toxicity have been shown [25].

Recent study revealed an ability of naturally occurring polyphenols selectively stimulate and protect erythropoiesis [26] particularly due to their ability to inhibit the oxidation of red cell membrane proteins and lipids induced by malignant neoplasm and/or anticancer agents [27].

The results of these investigations support the prospect for the use of polyphenols for correction of cancer associated and/or chemotherapy induced anemia.

Recently among many other polyphenol compounds a special interest has been drawn to stilbenes (hydroxystilbenes) [28]. Consumption of nutrients rich in hydroxystilbenes has been promoted because of their health benefits. Stilbene is hydrocarbon consisting of trans/cis ethene double bond substituted with phenyl group on both carbon atoms of the double bond.

A great number of stilbene derivates (stilbenoids) are naturally occurring agents. They are mainly synthesized in plants in response to various environmental disturbing factors such as UV irradiation and fungal infection.

It was revealed that stilbenes (stilbenoids) display a wide range of biological and pharmacological activities: antioxidant, antiinflammatory, cardiotropic, anticancer etc. [29-33]. The most widely investigated stilbene is resveratrol (3,5,4'-trans-tryhydroxystilbene) which preventive effects against chemical and biological agents received increasing attention of scientists [34].

These effects include cardioprotective activity, suppression of lipid peroxidation, inhibition of platelet aggregation, antioxidant, anti-inflammatory, antibacterial and antiviral activities [35].

Extensive research using in vitro and in vivo model systems also revealed that resveratrol (RES) exhibits anticancer activities [36]. RES has been shown to suppress proliferation of a wide variety of tumor cells and to induce apoptosis in cancer cells exhibiting variety of the mechanisms of anticancer activity [37]. RES may also ameliorate suppression of erythropoiesis via modulation of NF-κB signaling in CD34(+) cells [38].

Recent study have found that another hydroxystilbene oxyresveratrol (2,4,3',5'-transtrihydroxystilbene) in some cases manifests higher biological and pharmacological activities as compared with well-investigated RES [39, 40]. Oxyresveratrol (OXY) is widely present in wood and/or fruits of mulberry trees, jackfruits, cajeput trees and several other herbs.

An extra hydroxyl group in chemical structure of OXY makes it as active hydrogen-donor, which accounts for its notable antioxidant activity [41]. This hydroxystilbene is considered to be the most effective tyrosinase inhibitor of natural origin. Reports have documented high anti-inflammatory [42], hepato-protective [43], neuroprotective [44-46] and antiviral [47, 48] activities of OXY. The results of experimental study suggest that certain pharmacological properties of OXY might be correlated with inhibition of the iNOS expression through down-regulation of NF-kappaB binding activity and significant inhibition of COX-2 activity [42]. OXY was shown to decrease the LPS-induced plasma cytokines and tumor necrosis factor (TNF)-alpha which may mediate the formation of some paraneoplastic symptoms [44].

In terms of pharmacology, OXY possesses an advantage in comparison with RES by its higher bioavailability [49] and water solubility (about 0.3 mg/ml for OXY versus 0.03 mg/ml for RES). It should be noted that unlike resveratrol, the activity of which has been widely studied with respect to tumor associated processes, investigation of OXY was negligible, and was limited by study of pathologies not related to the cancer process.

Meanwhile, even the relatively few research results concerning possible mechanisms of OXY biological activity indicate its ability to influence both the development of the tumor process, and the manifestations of PNS.

Correction of Cancer Related Anemia by Oxyresveratrol

Study of OXY effect on hemopoiesis of tumor-bearing mice was carried out using two variants of Lewis lung carcinoma: LLC/R9 and LLC.

As it was shown earlier, these experimental tumor models are of the same genesis. At the same time, they differ significantly by the growth rate of primary tumors, angiogenic and metastatic potential and the spectrum of manifestation of paraneoplastic syndrome.

In contrast to wild-type strain of Lewis lung carcinoma (LLC), the growth of LLC/R9 in mice is accompanied by formation of an expressed anemia, splenomegaly, hepatomegaly and thymus involution.

OXY was obtained by extraction of crushed wood of Maclura pomifera and white mulberry (Morus alba), in which OXY content is 2% of the dry weight. The crushed wood was macerated in the extragent at 50° C for 24 hours followed by separation of the extragent. Acetonitrile was used as extragent as it produces the best results. The vacuum-dried extract was applied on silicagel for column chromatography, and separation was performed in a gradient system which consisted of a polar and nonpolar solvent. The best results were achieved using the acetonitrile-benzene (1:1) system.

This system provided the highest separation efficacy and allowed to receive anhydrous crystal OXY via removal of water traces using azeotropic distillation with benzene during concentration.

Purity control of prepared OXY (which was 98%) was carried out by the method of high-performance liquid chromatography on a column Nucleosil C18 2*250 mm with sorbent granularity of 5 µm at gradient elution regimen in water-acetonitrile system. Pike of OXY was identified by characteristic spectrum in UV range. The structure of isolated OXY was confirmed using NMR-C13 and mass-spectrometry.

The investigation was carried out using C57Bl/6 female mice weighting 19-22 g and aged 2.0-2.5 months, which were fed diets with normal protein contents. Mice were bred at animal facility of R. E. Kavetsky Institute of Experimental Pathology, Oncology and Radiobiology (IEPOR).

Animal study protocols and operation procedures were approved by the Animal Ethics Committee of IEPOR.

LLC/R9 and LLC cells were cultured in vitro in RPMI medium (Sigma, US) supplemented with 10% fetal calf serum (FCS), 2 mM L-glutamine, and 40 µg/ml gentamycin at 37°C in humidified atmosphere with 5% CO_2.

After intramuscular inoculation of tumor cells ($1.2x10^6$ cells per animal in 0.1 ml of Hanks' solution) all animals were randomized by weight and assigned to 4 groups (20 animals per group): two groups of animals (experimental and control) for each tumor model. Mice of experimental groups were treated with OXY while mice of control groups received water. OXY was administered per os by orogastric gavage technique daily, five times a week, during three weeks, starting from 2th day after tumor cell inoculation (total dose was 0.2 g/kg of mouse weight). It should be noted that single dose as well as the total dose of OXY used in the study were significantly lower than the maximum tolerated dose (MTD). In practice, MTD determined in the frame of study on acute OXY toxicity after its single oral administration to C57Bl/6 mice was higher than 0.7 g/kg of animal body weight.

One-half fraction of mice of every group was sacrificed in a day after the end of OXY treatment (on the 20th day after tumor cell inoculation) while the mice of the second half were sacrificed in a eight days after therapy completion (on the 26th day after tumor cell inoculation). The volume of primary tumor as well as the total volume of lung metastases and the number of metastatic nodules was estimated. The sampling of bone marrow from mouse femur was carried out and cellular content of marrow tissue was analyzed. Hematological indices were determined using the hematological analyzer «Particle counter model PCE 210» (ERMA, Japan), adapted for the study of mouse blood cells.

Administration of OXY into mice with transplanted LLC/R9 resulted in significant positive changes in erythropoiesis (Table 5). On the 20th day of tumor growth after completion of OXY therapy, the erythrocyte count, hemoglobin content and hematocrit level were significantly higher by 49.6%, 57.5% and 41.6% respectively as compared to control animals.

Unfortunately, in 8 days after the end of OXY therapy (26 days after cancer cell inoculation) anti-anemia effect of OXY decreased significantly. However, during this observation period the indexes of erythroid cells of peripheral blood of OXY-treated mice remained at higher levels than that of untreated animals (it should be noted that the mentioned differences were statistically insignificant due to their variability and had a type of tendency).

OXY did not exert significant effects on the parameters of thrombocytes and white blood cell group of peripheral blood. Meanwhile, on the 20th day of tumor growth after completion of OXY therapy a statistically significant normalization of neutrophilic leukocytosis (which was typical for OXY untreated LLC/R9 bearing mice) was observed. However, this positive effect was not preserved without further drug administration, and on the 26th day of tumor growth the number of granulocytes in OXY-treated mice did not differ from this index in the control group of mice and was nearly twice higher than that of animals without tumors (Table 6).

Despite significant positive influence of OXY on erythropoiesis in LLC/R9-bearing mice, administration of OXY to animals with transplanted LLC had practically no effect on peripheral blood indices.

Table 5. Hematological indices of LLC/R9-bearing mice after therapy with OXY

Blood indices	Intact mice	LLC/R9-bearing mice			
		In a day after therapy completion		In 8 days after therapy completion	
		Control	OXY treated	Control	OXY treated
RBC, x10^6/µl	10.5±0.8	05.6±0.6	08.4±1.0*	03.7±0.8	04.9±0.9
Hgb, g/dl	13.7±0.8	07.9±1.1	12.4±1.4*	05.1±1.0	7.6±1.8
HCT, %	35.8±2.5	23.5±2.7	33.3±2.9*	16.7±2.7	22.6±4.4
MCV, fl	34.4±1.8	41.9±0.3	40.2±1.5	46.0±3	45.9±1.6
MCH, pg	13.3±1.3	13.9±0.2	14.8±0.1	13.9±0.9	14.9±0.9
MCHC, g/dl	37.9±2.9	33.2±0.8	36.9±1.1	30.2±0.9	32.6±1.4
RDW, %	22.9±1.2	26.8±1.1	22.6±2.8	22.4±1.7	26.1±1.7
PLT, x1000/µl	214.3±28.2	162.0±22.5	188.3±15.1	174.0±40.4	144.3±38.3

Note: *difference vs. OXY free mice is statistically significant, $p<0.05$. RBC – erythrocyte number, Hgb – hemoglobin content, Ht – hematocrit, MCV –volume of erythrocyte, MCH – hemoglobin content in erythrocytes, MCHC – hemoglobin concentration in erythrocyte, RDW – red blood cell distribution width, PLT – platelet number.

Table 6. Leukogram of LLC/R9-bearing mice after therapy with OXY

Blood indices	Intact mice	LLC/R9-bearing mice			
		In a day after therapy completion		In 8 days after therapy completion	
		Control	OXY treated	Control	OXY treated
WBC, x1000/	9.8±1.5	12.7±1.2	09.3±2.0	14.7±2.4	11.8±0.8
LY, x1000/µl	7.2±0.95	8.3±0.8	6.4±1.3	10.5±2.0	7.6±1.1
Mo, x1000/µl	1.1±0.2	1.57±0.1	1.05±0.2	1.7±0.4	1.2±0.2
Gr, x1000/µl	1.6±0.2	2.85±0.3	1.8±0.4*	2.7±0.3	3.1±0.6

Note: *difference vs. OXY free mice is statistically significant, $p<0.05$. WBC – white blood cells, LY - lymphocytes, Mo - monocytes, Gr – granulocytes.

This fact points on protective mechanism of paraneoplastic anemia correction exerted by OXY, rather than its direct stimulating action toward erythropoiesis.

Significant difference in the degree of blood system changes between the animals treated or untreated with OXY was found during analysis of myelograms. It was revealed that the use of OXY in LLC/R9-bearing mice improved the processes of differentiation and maturation of erythroid cells. After completion of OXY therapy the count ratio of erythroid cells of different differentiation grade was significantly higher than the corresponding indices of untreated mice and practically did not differ from that of intact animals (Table 7). At this observation time point mitotic index of erythroid cells in animals with LLC/R9 treated with OXY was 3 fold higher compared with tumor-free control but did not exceed this index in tumor-bearing animals without therapy. Meanwhile, significant increase of erythrocyte count in bone marrow and peripheral blood of mice administered with OXY indicated high efficacy of compensatory processes induced by the therapy performed.

Table 7. Myelogram of LLC/R9-bearing mice after therapy with OXY

Myelogram indices (%)	Intact mice	LLC/R9-bearing mice			
		In a day after therapy completion		In 8 days after therapy completion	
		Control	OXY treated	Control	OXY treated
Undifferentiated blasts	0.83±0.17	1.17±0.44	1.17±0.17	0.17±0.17	1.17±0.44*
Neutrophilic cells: - myeloblasts	0.83±0.44	1.50±0.50	1.50±0.58	0.17±0.17	1.83±1.09*
- ppomyelocytes	2.00±0.76	5.17±1.09	4.00±1.15	3.75±0.66	2.33±1.09
- myelocytes	4.50±1.61	13.8±2.7	14.3±2.3	12.4±1.7	13.2±1.6
- metamyelocytes	7.33±1.92	12.7±1.8	12.7±2.2	15.6±0.5	15.3±1.3
- stab cells	19.7±3.2	16.2±3.8	11.8±3.0	11.8±3.0	8.00±0.58
- segmentated	23.00±1.6	6.33±0.33	7.92±2.62	5.00±1.04	4.00±0.50
Eosinophilic cells: - pro-, myelocytes	0.50±0.29	0.83±0.33	1.00±0.58	0.0	1.00±0.34
- metamyelocytes	0.33±0.33	1.33±0.33	1.00±0.01	0.33±0.17	0.33±0.33
- segmentated and stab cells	0.50±0.29	0.33±0.33	1.00±0.29	0.75±0.25	0.67±0.17
Granulocytes: - young	18.5±6.7	35.2±2.9	34.1±5.0	32.4±2.0	37.0±3.6
- adult	43.8±2.2	22.8±4.0	20.8±4.8	21.8±3.2	12.7±1.1
All granulocytes	62.3±8.9	58.0±6.5	51.7±1.2	54.0±4.1	49.7±4.5

Table 7. (Continued)

Myelogram indices (%)	Intact mice	LLC/R9-bearing mice			
		In a day after therapy completion		In 8 days after therapy completion	
		Control	OXY treated	Control	OXY treated
Erythroblasts	0.67±0.17	0.17±0.17	0.67±0.17*	0.0	3.67±0.88*
Pronormocytes	1.50±1.26	0.50±0.29	0.42±0.08	0.67±0.17	1.17±0.44
Normocytes: - basophilic	3.50±1.04	5.33±1.88	6.08±1.72	3.17±0.44	14.3±4.1*
- polychromatophilic	9.50±2.75	10.0±1.7	10.8±2.0	12.3±3.4	13.5±1.3
- oxyphilic	10.8±3.4	5.67±0.60	11.2±2.0*	4.50±0.87	9.50±0.50*
All erythroid cells	26.0±7.5	21.0±3.5	29.2±2.4	19.9±4.2	39.5±7.0*
Myelo-erythroid ratio	2.47±1.10	2.82±0.25	1.78±0.11*	2.87±0.38	1.40±0.41*
Lymphocytes	8.0±1.0	19.0±6.0	12.6±2.2	24.0±7.7	7.00±0.76*
Megakaryoblasts, megakaryocytes	0.33±0.17	0.50±0.29	0.33±0.33	0.17±0.17	0.33±0.33
Total mitotic index (MI), ‰	5.67±1.20	8.00±1.15	10.7±0.9	5.33±1.45	21.3±4.7*
MI of red cells, ‰	1.67±1.20	4.67±1.76	5.00±0.58	2.67±1.67	13.3±4.7*
MI of white cells, ‰	4.00±0.58	3.33±1.33	5.67±1.20	2.67±0.67	8.00±3.46*

Note: *difference vs. OXY free mice is statistically significant, $p<0.05$.

In 8 days after the end of OXY treatment, analysis of bone marrow allowed to register even more expressed activation of compensatory-restorative processes not only in erythroid but in granulocytic line as well (Table 7). In myelograms there were detected high number of undifferentiated blasts, myeloblasts, erythroblasts (which were nearly absent in myelograms of untreated animals). Erythroid cell ratio in bone marrow was by 1.5 times higher than that in intact mice, and proliferative activity was by 8 fold higher.

Figures 7, 8 demonstrate the data on the number of erythroblasts and normocytes in the total myelocariocyte count in femoral bone of animals. One may see an effectiveness of OXY therapy: the number of blast and maturating erythroid cells is significantly higher than in control group.

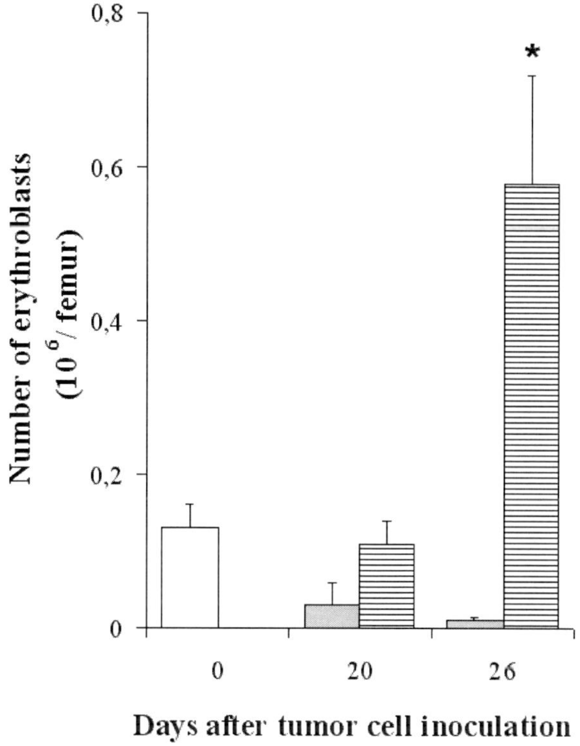

Columns with horizontal lines – corresponding indices of LLC/R9 bearing mice treated with OXY; grey columns – corresponding indices of OXY-free mice with LLC/R9; white column – corresponding index of OXY-free intact mice. $^{*}p < 0.05$ vs. corresponding value of OXY- free mice.

Figure 7. Total number of erythroblasts in a day (20th day of tumor growth) and in 8 days (26th day of tumor growth) after OXY therapy completion.

It is necessary to note that in 8 days after the end of OXY treatment, the count of erythroid cells was restored practically up to its level in tumor-free group. However, despite intense work of hematopoietic system it is still not sufficient enough to support number of circulating pools, and in peripheral blood we have again registered anemia development accompanied with significant decrease of practically all erythropoiesis indices.

The obtained results revealed that the use of OXY at the background of paraneoplastic anemia contributes to the activation of erythropoiesis and significantly elevates compensatory capacity of blood.

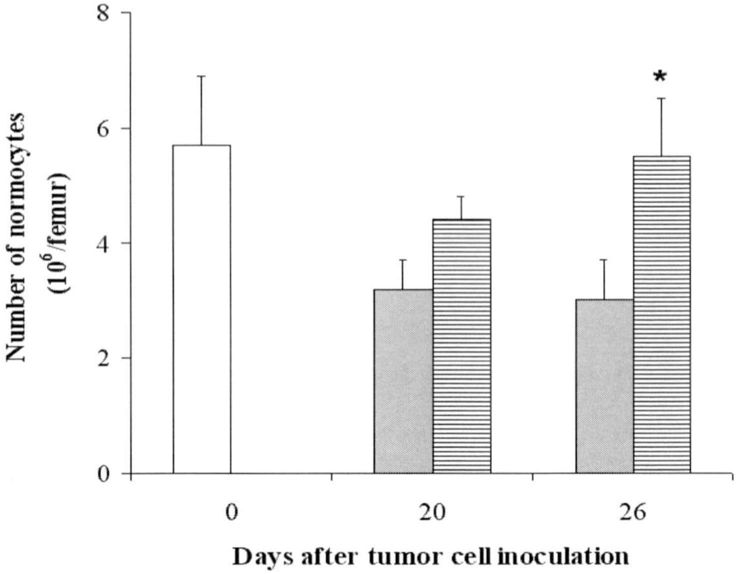

Designations as in Figure 7. *$p < 0.05$ vs. corresponding value of OXY-free mice.

Figure 8. Total number of normocytes in a day (20th day of tumor growth) and in 8 days (26th day of tumor growth) after OXY therapy completion.

Effect of Oxyresveratrol on Tumor Growth and Metastasis

The risk of stimulation of tumor progression is an important factor sometimes limiting the clinical use of agents capable to decrease PNS manifestations (especially paraneoplastic anemia). Therefore the investigation of OXY influence on the growth and metastasis of both Lewis lung carcinoma variants (LLC/R9 and LLC) has been performed. It was shown that metronomic administration of OXY to mice with transplanted tumors resulted in suppression of tumor growth of both variants of Lewis lung carcinoma.

As it is seen in (Table 8), the inhibition of primary tumor growth in a day after completion of OXY therapy was similar in the cases of LLC/R9 and LLC and yielded nearly 36%. Apparently, an observed anticancer activity of OXY can be partially related to its cytotoxic/cytostatic action toward LLC/R9 and LLC cells, and the results of the study of OXY effect on in vitro cell viability (MTT-test) support this assumption.

Table 8. Antitumor activity of OXY against LLC/R9 and LLC

Tumor strain	Time after cancer cell inoculation/day after the end of OXY treatment	Tumor volume (cm^3)		Tumor growth inhibition
		Control mice	Oxy treated mice	
LLC/R9	20 day/2 day	1.62±0.15	1.04±0.15*	35.8 %
	26 day/8 day	2.42±0.30	1.22±0.32*	49.6 %
LLC	20 day/2 day	0.89±0.11	0.57±0.09*	36.0 %
	26 day/8 day	1.47±0.27	1.11±0.22	

Note: *difference vs. OXY free mice is statistically significant, $p<0.05$.

It has been shown that OXY exerts cytotoxic/cytostatic action toward cells of both Lewis lung carcinoma variants. Herewith the sensitivity of LLC/R9 cells to the action of OXY was significantly lower by 17% compared with LLC cells (after 24 hours incubation of tumor cells with the agent IC_{50} was 0.068 ± 0.002 mg/ml and 0.058 ± 0.001 mg/ml for LLC/R9 and LLC respectively). Despite lower sensitivity of LLC/R9 cells to the action of OXY in vitro, its anticancer activity in vivo toward this tumor model was increased and in 8 days after therapy completion tumor growth inhibition was about 50%. This elevation of OXY anticancer efficacy was resulted from stabilization of the growth of primary LLC/R9 tumor which occurred after treatment completion (Figure 9). Such feature of anticancer action of OXY toward LLC/R9 may be partially related to the capability of this agent to inhibit tumor angiogenesis. According to preliminary data obtained in vitro, OXY decreased VEGF production of these cells.

In contrast to LLC/R9, anticancer benefit of OXY against LLC was not preserved due to increased tumor growth rate after the end of OXY administration (Figure 10). Interestingly, inhibition of VEGF production in LLC cells upon the action of OXY in vitro was not observed.

Moreover, if OXY was used in low noncytotoxic concentrations, there was observed a tendency for stimulation of VEGF production in LLC cells.

The performed study has shown that OXY exerted also a notable anti-metastatic action. In a week after treatment completion, the number and volume of lung metastases in animals treated with OXY were significantly lower by 55.0%-71.0% compared with animals from control groups (Table 9).

It is known that metastasis is a complex multistage process the result of which depends on multiple interactions between metastatically active tumor cells with nonmetastatic tumor counterparts and body as a whole [50].

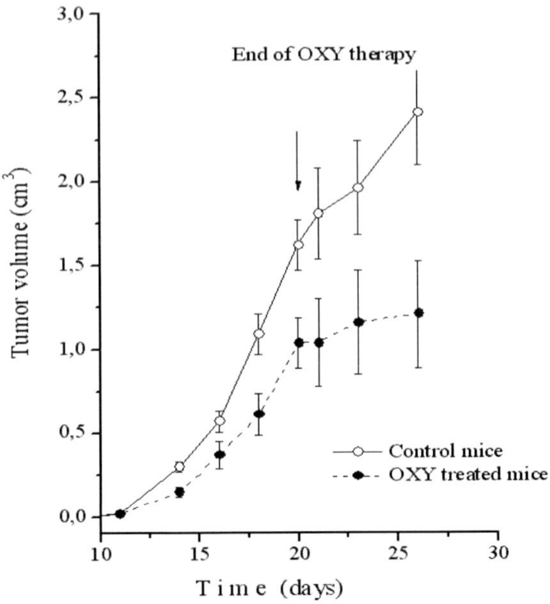

Figure 9. Influence of OXY on growth kinetics of LLC/R9.

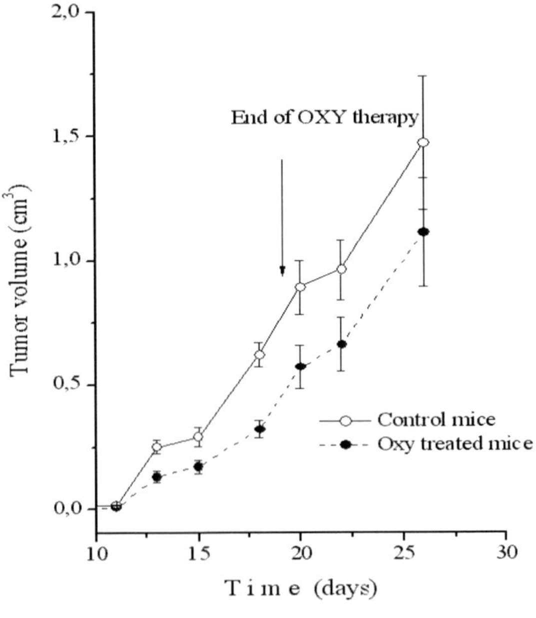

Figure 10. Influence of OXY on growth kinetics of LLC.

Table 9. Antimetastatic activity of OXY against LLC/R9 and LLC

Tumor strain	Time interval after the end of OXY treatment	Number and volume (mm^3) of metastases	Tumor volume (cm^3)		Inhibition of lung metastases
			Control mice	Oxy treated mice	
LLC/R9	1 day	Number	7.4±1.8	4.56±0.92	-
		Volume	2.9±1.0	2.32±0.77	-
	8 days	Number	13.4±1.8	5.9±2.0*	56.0 %
		Volume	15.8±4.0	5.4±3.4*	66.1%
LLC	1 day	Number	5.3±1.1	4.4±1.4	-
		Volume	1.6±0.5	1.9±0.6	-
	8 days	Number	24.4±4.6	7.0±1.4*	71.3 %
		Volume	10.6±2.8	3.1±1.1*	70.8%

Note: *difference vs. OXY free mice is statistically significant, $p<0.05$.

Among many functional, structural and molecular characteristics of tumor cells providing their survival in a complex and aggressive cascade of interactions, their migration capacity play the most important role.

Migration activity is typical only to metastatic tumor cells.

This property underlies the domination of metastatic clones in primary tumor, tumor invasion, intravasation, and extravasation [51].

To understand the mechanisms of antimetastatic action an effect of OXY on migration activity of LLC/R9 cells has been studied. Thereto the tumors were derived from non-treated LLC/R9 bearing mice on 17th day of tumor growth [52]. Tumor tissue was triply washed with PBS to remove blood and debris and cut into tumor tissue sections (TTS) with the weight of 2.0 ± 0.2g. TTS were placed on 0.22 μm nitrocellulose filters and cultured in DMEM supplemented with 10% fetal calf serum, 2% L-glutamine and 20 μg/ml of gentamicin in 5% CO_2 atmosphere at 37°C. After 1 hour of adaptation of LLC/R9 bioptates, OXY was added into incubation medium at different concentrations, and incubation was continued for three days. Eighteen TTS for each OXY concentration were used. After incubation filters were fixed in ethanol-formalin mixture, stained by Karacchi hematoxylin and embedded in cedar seed oil. The cell migration area (in mm^2) around TTS were estimated and used as a characteristic of LLC/R9 migration capacity. It was shown that OXY in noncytotoxic concentrations significantly suppressed migration of LLC/R9 cells.

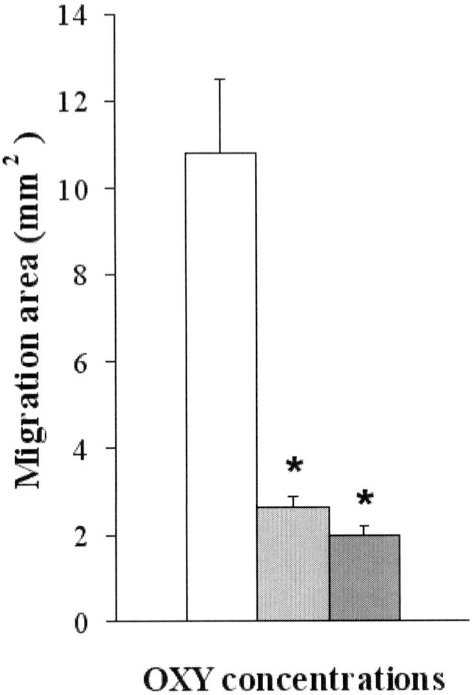

*p < 0.05 vs. corresponding value of OXY-free cells.

Figure 11. Effect of OXY (at different concentrations) on migrating capacity of LLC/R9 cells. OXY concentrations: 0.0 mg/ml – white column; 0.01 mg/ml – grey column; 0.04 mg/ml – dark grey column.

As it is seen in Figure 11 the area of tumor cell migration upon treatment with OXY was decreased by more than 70%. Therewith, a part of cytotoxic components at these concentrations did not exceed 30%.

It should be noted that the ability of agents with antioxidant properties to inhibit metastatic process has been documented by many authors [53-56]. In such a case antimetastatic action of antioxidants is mediated by reactive oxygen species (ROS). It is known that tumor cells are producers of ROS which in turn significantly promote tumor cell migration and realization of their metastatic potential [57]. It is confirmed by the study showing that higher metastatic activity of LLC cells directly correlated with higher level of ROS production by these cells (as compared with that of LLC/R9 cells) (Figure 12). ROS intracellular level was determined using 2,7-dichlorofluorescein diacetate (Sigma, US) and was recalculated on 10^6 cancer cells.

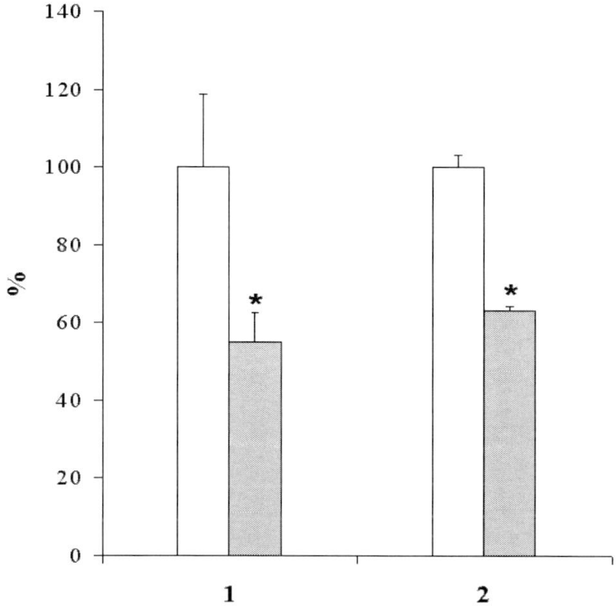

*p < 0.05 vs. corresponding value of LLC bearing mice.

Figure 12. Number of metastasis on 26th day of tumor growth (1) and ROS intracellular level (2) of LLC/R9 (grey column) in a percents of that of LLC (white column).

An expressed antioxidant activity of OXY has been revealed at wide concentration range (from 0.005mg/ml to 0.6 mg/ml) in a dose-dependent manner. Importantly, OXY at a concentration of 0.01 mg/ml, which is lower than IC_{50} by more than 80% ($p<0.01$) for both cell lines, reduced intracellular ROS level by more than 60% (Figure 13). At higher concentrations, OXY completely neutralized ROS in tumor cells.

Thereby, the administration of OXY to mice with LLC/R9 and LLC at a dose which is sufficient for correction of paraneoplastic anemia in mice with high-angiogenic variant of Lewis lung carcinoma, leads to significant inhibition of growth and metastasis of malignant tumors.

Conclusion

It is well-known that the most important part of PNS treatment is to get a proper and rapid diagnosis of both the underlying cancer and the type of paraneoplastic disorder involved.

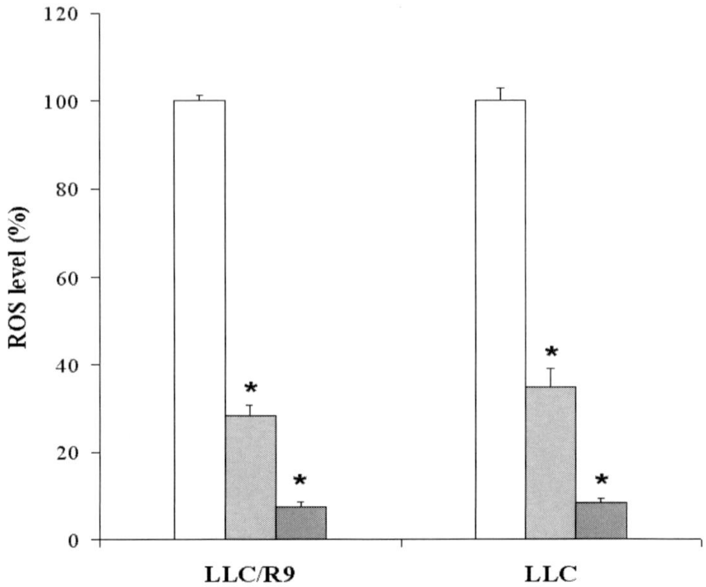

*p < 0.05 vs. corresponding value of OXY-free cells.

Figure 13. Effect of OXY (at different concentrations) on intracellular level of ROS (calculated per 10^6 cancer cells in % of control). OXY concentrations: 0.0 mg/ml (control) – white column; 0.01 mg/ml – grey column; 0.1 mg/ml – dark grey column.

This knowledge can help to provide more targeted and effective treatment that can ultimately improve both life expectancy and quality of life.

There are two main approaches taken in the treatment of paraneoplastic syndromes. One of them is to suppress the mediator which is identified to cause the paraneoplastic syndrome. An important advantage of such an approach is a possibility of its effective use in the case of resistant forms of malignant tumors. Second and the most common approach is directed toward the treatment of the cancer (not the PNS) using surgery, radiation, chemotherapy, biotherapy or by some combination of the previously listed.

In this case, it is assumed that reduction of tumor tissue leads to decreased level of PNS mediators produced by tumor cells and, accordingly, decreases an intensity of symptoms. High toxicity of the majority of therapeutic approaches toward normal tissues and organs is a limiting factor in this case. It is known that hemopoiesis damage is among the most common side effects of cancer cytotoxic therapy. Performance of this therapy can enhance hematological symptoms of PNS.

It is necessary to note that the use of any approach for PNS therapy could be ineffective due to irreversible damage of the target organ developing at early stages of tumor growth before the beginning of any treatment.

The results of the study presented in this chapter have shown that OXY administration to mice with high angiogenic LLCR9 variant of Lewis lung carcinoma promoted significant activation of erythroid line of hemopoiesis, significant suppression of which has been caused by the development of this tumor at early stages of its growth. Correction of paraneoplastic anemia by OXY was accompanied also with its anticancer and antimetastatic action, what predicates a possible direct relation between these effects.

However, such a relation is opposed by the fact, that despite the stability of anticancer effect for 8 days after OXY therapy completion (when primary tumor volume remained unaltered) the indices of erythropoiesis of mice were reduced.

In other words, correction of anemia by OXY had a reversible character and after treatment completion, a positive pharmacological effect receded.

In this situation it is possible to suppose on protective but not corrective action of hydrooxystylbene toward mechanisms determining the formation of tumor-associated anemia in mice with LLCR9. What is the basis of this protective effect of OXY remains to be explored.

Despite the above mentioned data, high antianemic effectiveness of OXY toward LLCR9 combined with its anticancer and antimetastatic activity is of utmost importance. Here, administration of OXY to tumor-bearing mice without PNS symptoms did not lead to stimulation of erythropoiesis.

Moreover, irrespectively of tumor type, treatment with OXY did not cause inhibiting or stimulating effect on other blood indices of experimental animals. This fact positively differs OXY from conventional drugs directed on the reduction of underlying cancer, anticancer activity of which is achieved, as a rule, at high doses (close to MTD) and often correlates with their ability to suppress hemopoiesis. Meanwhile, as it has been revealed, OXY displays its sufficiently high pharmacologic activity at a total dose which is 3.5-fold lower than MTD. The daily dose of OXY was more than 50-fold lower than MTD that in combination with its low cumulative toxicity, explains the absence of significant toxic manifestations of OXY treatment (at least toward hemopoiesis system).

In conclusion, the results of the performed study have shown that OXY can be considered as an effective, safe and challenging agent for treatment of cancer-related anemia.

References

[1] Berardi, R., Grilli, G., Romagnoli, E., Saladino, T., Freddari, F., Tamburrano, T., Galizia, E., Carbonari, G., Mariani, C., Braconi, C., Pierantoni, C., Battelli, N., Scartozzi, M., Cascinu, S. Paraneoplastic syndromes: a review. *Clin. Ter.*, 2005 156, 281-288.

[2] Tarin, D. Update on clinical and mechanistic aspects of paraneoplastic syndromes. *Cancer Metastasis Rev.*, 2013 32, 707-721. doi: 10.1007/s 10555-013-9446-4.

[3] Ngonga, G. F., Ferrari, D., Lorusso, L., Gasparetto, C., Neznama, E., D'Abramo, M., Ricevuti, G. Paraneoplastic syndromes: pathogenetic theories, clinical aspects and therapeutic approach. *Ann. Ital. Med. Int.,* 2005 20, 28-38.

[4] Pelosof, L. C., Gerber, D. E. Paraneoplastic syndromes: an approach to diagnosis and treatment. *Mayo Clin. Proc.*, 2010 85, 838-854. doi: 10. 4065/mcp.2010.0099.

[5] Lechner, K., Obermeier, H. L. Cancer-related microangiopathic hemolytic anemia: clinical and laboratory features in 168 reported cases. *Medicine (Baltimore)*. 2012 91, 195-205. doi: 10.1097/MD.0b013e3182 603598.

[6] Qiu, M. Z., Xu, R. H., Ruan, D. Y., Li, Z. H., Luo, H. Y., Teng, K. Y., Wang, Z. Q., Li, Y. H., Jiang, W. Q. Incidence of anemia, leukocytosis, and thrombocytosis in patients with solid tumors in China. *Tumour Biol.,* 2010 31, 633-641. doi: 10.1007/s13277-010-0079-8.

[7] Gordon, M. S. Managing anemia in the cancer patient: old problems, future solutions. *Oncologist*, 2002 7, 331-341.

[8] Gilreath, J. A., Stenehjem, D. D., Rodgers, G. M. Diagnosis and treatment of cancer-related anemia. *Am. J. Hematol.,* 2014 89, 203-212. doi: 10.1002/ajh.23628.

[9] Bennett, C. L., Silver, S. M., Djulbegovic, B., Samaras, A. T., Blau, C. A., Gleason, K. J., Barnato, S. E., Elverman, K. M., Courtney, D. M., McKoy, J. M., Edwards, B. J., Tigue, C. C., Raisch, D. W., Yarnold, P. R., Dorr, D. A., Kuzel, T. M., Tallman, M. S., Trifilio, S. M., West, D. P., Lai, S. Y., Henke, M. Venous thromboembolism and mortality associated with recombinant erythropoietin and darbepoetin administration for the treatment of cancer-associated anemia. *JAMA*, 2008 299, 914-924. doi: 10.1001/jama.299.8.914.

[10] Folkman, J. Angiogenesis. *Annu. Rev. Med.,* 2006 57, 1-18.

[11] Jain, L., Vargo, C. A., Danesi, R., Sissung, T. M., Price, D. K., Venzon, D., Venitz, J., Figg, W. D. The role of vascular endothelial growth factor SNPs as predictive and prognostic markers for major solid tumors. *Mol. Cancer Ther.*, 2009 8, 2496-2508. doi: 10.1158/1535-7163. MCT-09-030 2.

[12] Wong, A. K., Alfert, M., Castrillon, D. H., Shen, Q., Holash, J., Yancopoulos, G. D., Chin, L. Excessive tumor-elaborated VEGF and its neutralization define a lethal paraneoplastic syndrome. *Proc. Natl. Acad. Sci. US,* 2001 98, 7481–7486.

[13] Lien, Y. H., Lai, L. W. Pathogenesis diagnosis and management of paraneoplastic glomerulonephritis. *Nat. Rev. Nephrol.*, 2011 7, 85–95. doi: 10.1038/nrneph.2010.171.

[14] Drogat, B., Kalucka, J., Gutiérrez, L., Hammad, H., Goossens, S., Ghahremani, M. F., Bartunkova, S., Haigh, K., Deswarte, K., Nyabi, O., Naessens, M., Ferrara, N., Klingmüller, U., Lambrecht, B. N., Nagy, A., Philipsen, S., Haigh, J. J. VEGF regulates embryonic erythroid development through Gata1 modulation. *Blood,* 2010 116, 2141-2151. doi: 10. 1182/blood-2010-01-264143.

[15] Ferrara, N., Gerber, H. P., LeCouter, J. The biology of VEGF and its receptors. *Nat. Med.*, 2003 9, 669-676.

[16] Rosti, V., Massa, M., Campanelli, R., De Amici, M., Piccolo, G., Perfetti, V. Vascular endothelial growth factor promoted endothelial progenitor cell mobilization into the peripheral blood of a patient with POEMS syndrome. *Haematologica,* 2007 92, 1291-1292.

[17] Xue, Y., Chen, F., Zhang, D., Lim, S., Cao, Y. Tumor-derived VEGF modulates hematopoiesis. *J. Angiogenes. Res.,* 2009 1, 9. doi: 10.1186/ 2040-2384-1-9.

[18] Dunst, J., Becker, A., Lautenschläger, C., Markau, S., Becker, H., Fischer, K., Haensgen, G. Anemia and elevated systemic levels of vascular endothelial growth factor (VEGF). *Strahlenther. Onkol.,* 2002 178, 436-441.

[19] Tschirch, E., Weber, B., Koehne, P., Guthmann, F., Gise, A., von Wauer, R. R., Rudiger, M. Vascular Endothelial growth factor as marker for tissue hypoxia and transfusion need in anemic infants: a prospective clinical study. *Pediatrics,* 2009 123, 784-790. doi: 10.1542/peds.2007-2304.

[20] Solyanik, G. I., Pyaskovskaya, O. N., Garmanchouk, L. V. Cisplatin-resistant Lewis lung carcinoma cells possess increased level of VEGF secretion. *Exp. Oncol.,* 2003 25, 260-265.

[21] Pyaskovskaya, O. N., Dasyukevich, O. I., Kolesnik, D. L., Garmanchouk, L. V., Todor, I. N., Solyanik, G. I. Changes in VEGF level and tumor growth characteristics during Lewis lung carcinoma progression towards cis-DDP resistance. *Exp. Oncol.*, 2007 29, 197-202.

[22] Fedorchuk, O. G., Pyaskovskaya, O. M., Skivka, L. M., Gorbik, G. V., Trompak, O. O., Solyanik, G. I. Paraneoplastic syndrome in mice bearing high-angiogenic variant of Lewis lung carcinoma: relations with tumor derived VEGF. *Cytokine,* 2012 57, 81-88. doi: 10.1016/j.cyto.2011.10.022.

[23] Xue, Y., Religa, P., Cao, R., Hansen, A. J., Lucchini, F., Jones, B., Wu, Y., Zhu, Z., Pytowski, B., Liang, Y., Zhong, W., Vezzoni, P., Rozell, B., Cao, Y. Anti-VEGF agents confer survival advantages to tumor-bearing mice by improving cancer-associated systemic syndrome. *Proc. Natl. Acad. Sci. US,* 2008 105, 18513–18518. doi: 10.1073/pnas.0807967105.

[24] Kimura, Y. New anticancer agents: in vitro and in vivo evaluation of the antitumor and antimetastatic actions of various compounds isolated from medicinal plants. *In Vivo*, 2005 19, 37-60.

[25] Curin, Y., Andriantsitohaina, R. Polyphenols as potential therapeutical agents against cardiovascular diseases. *Pharmacol. Rep.*, 2005 57, 97-107.

[26] Sen, G., Mandal, S., Saha Roy, S., Mukhopadhyay, S., Biswas, T. Therapeutic use of quercetin in the control of infection and anemia associated with visceral leishmaniasis. *Free Radic. Biol. Med.,* 2005 38, 1257-1264.

[27] Mikstacka, R., Rimando, A. M., Ignatowicz, E. Antioxidant effect of trans-resveratrol, pterostilbene, quercetin and their combinations in human erythrocytes in vitro. *Plant Foods Hum. Nutr.*, 2010 65, 57-63. doi: 10.1007/s11130-010-0154-8.

[28] Roupe, K. A., Remsberg, C. M., Yanez, J. A., Davies, N. M. Pharmacometrics of stilbenes: seguing towards the clinic. *Curr. Clin. Pharmacol.,* 2006 1, 81-101.

[29] Jung, J. C., Lim, E., Lee, Y., Kang, J. M., Kim, H., Jang, S., Oh, S., Jung, M. Synthesis of novel trans-stilbene derivatives. *Eur. J. Med. Chem.,* 2009 4, 3166-3174. doi: 10.1016/j.ejmech.2009.03.011.

[30] Shang, Y. J., Qian, Y. P., Liu, X. D., Dai, F., Shang, X. L., Jia, W. Q., Liu, Q., Fang, J. G., Zhou, B. Radical-scavenging activity and mechanism of resveratrol. *J. Org. Chem.*, 2009 74, 5025-5031.

[31] Celimene, C. C., Smith, D. R., Young, R. A., Stanosz, G. R. In vitro inhibition of Sphaeropsis sapinea by natural stilbenes. *Phytochemistry*, 2001 56, 161–165.

[32] Aburjai, T. A. Anti-platelet stilbenes from aerial parts of Rheum palaestinum. *Phytochemistry,* 2000 55, 407–410.

[33] Kimura, Y., Sumiyoshi, M., Baba, K. Antitumor activities of synthetic and natural stilbenes through antiangiogenic action. *Cancer Sci.*, 2008 99, 2083–2096. doi: 10.1111/j.1349-7006.2008.00948.x.

[34] Raederstorff, D., Kunz, I., Schwager, J. Resveratrol, from experimental data to nutritional evidence: the emergence of a new food ingredient. *Ann. N Y Acad. Sci.*, 2013 1290, 136-141. doi: 10.1111/nyas.12147.

[35] Bhat, K. P. L., Kosmeder, J. W. 2nd., Pezzuto, J. M. Biological effects of resveratrol. *Antioxid. Redox Signal*, 2001 3, 1041-1064.

[36] Singh, C. K., George, J., Ahmad, N. Resveratrol-based combinatorial strategies for cancer management. *Ann. N Y Acad. Sci.*, 2013 1290, 113-121. doi: 10.1111/nyas.12160.

[37] Aggarwal, B. B., Bhardwaj, A., Aggarwal, R. S., Seeram, N. P., Shishodia, S., Takada, Y. Role of resveratrol in prevention and therapy of cancer: preclinical and clinical studies. *Anticancer Res.,* 2004 24, 2783-2840.

[38] Jeong, J. Y., Silver, M., Parnes., Nikiforow, S., Berliner, N., Vanasse, G. J. Resveratrol ameliorates TNFα-mediated suppression of erythropoiesis in human CD34(+) cells via modulation of NF-κB signaling. *Br. J. Haematol.,* 2011 155, 93-101. doi: 10.1111/j.1365-2141.2011.08800.x.

[39] Aftab, N., Likhitwitayawuid, K., Vieira, A. Comparative antioxidant activities and synergism of resveratrol and oxyresveratrol. *Nat. Prod. Res.*, 2010 24, 1726-1733. doi: 10.1080/14786410902990797.

[40] Galindo, I., Hernáez, B., Berná, J., Fenoll, J., Cenis, J. L., Escribano, J. M., Alonso, C. Comparative inhibitory activity of the stilbenes resveratrol and oxyresveratrol on African swine fever virus replication. *Antiviral Res.*, 2011 91, 57-63. doi: 10.1016/j.antiviral.2011.04.013.

[41] Lorenz, P., Roychowdhury, S., Engelmann, M., Wolf, G., Horn, T. F. Oxyresveratrol and resveratrol are potent antioxidants and free radical scavengers: effect on nitrosative and oxidative stress derived from microglial cells. *Nitric Oxide*, 2003 9, 64–76.

[42] Chung, K. O., Kim, B. Y., Lee, M. H., Kim, Y. R., Chung, H. Y., Park, J. H., Moon, J. O. In-vitro and in-vivo anti-inflammatory effect of oxyresveratrol from Morus alba L. *J. Pharm. Pharmacol.*, 2003 55, 1695-1700.

[43] Oh, H., Ko, E. K., Jun, J. Y., Oh, M. H., Park, S. U., Kang, K. H., Lee, H. S., Kim, Y. C. Hepatoprotective and free radical scavenging activities

of prenylflavonoids, coumarin, and stilbene from Morus alba. *Planta Med.*, 2002 68, 932-934.

[44] Mouihate, A., Horn, T. F., Pittman, Q. J. Oxyresveratrol dampens neuro-immune responses in vivo: a selective effect on TNF-alpha. *Am. J. Physiol. Regul. Integr. Comp. Physiol.*, 2006 291, R1215-1221.

[45] Andrabi, S. A., Spina, M. G., Lorenz, P., Ebmeyer, U., Wolf, G., Horn, T. F. Oxyresveratrol (trans-2,3',4,5'-tetrahydroxystilbene) is neuroprotective and inhibits the apoptotic cell death in transient cerebral ischemia. *Brain Res.*, 2004 1017, 98–107.

[46] Weber, J. T., Lamont, M., Chibrikova, L., Fekkes, D., Vlug, A. S., Lorenz, P., Kreutzmann, P., Slemmer, J. E. Potential neuroprotective effects of oxyresveratrol against traumatic injury. *Eur. J. Pharmacol.*, 2012 680, 55-62.

[47] Sasivimolphan, P., Lipipun, V., Ritthidej, G., Chitphet, K., Yoshida, Y., Daikoku, T., Sritularak, B., Likhitwitayawuid, K., Pramyothin, P., Hattori, M., Shiraki, K. Microemulsion-based oxyresveratrol for topical treatment of herpes simplex virus (HSV) infection: physicochemical properties and efficacy in cutaneous HSV-1 infection in mice. *AAPS Pharm. Sci. Tech.*, 2012 13, 1266-1275. doi: 10.1208/s12249-012-9828-x.

[48] Chuanasa, T., Phromjai, J., Lipipun, V., Likhitwitayawuid, K., Suzuki, M., Pramyothin, P., Hattori, M., Shiraki, K. Anti-herpes simplex virus (HSV-1) activity of oxyresveratrol derived from Thai medicinal plant: mechanism of action and therapeutic efficacy on cutaneous HSV-1 infection in mice. *Antiviral Res.*, 2008 80, 62–70. doi: 10.1016/j.antiviral.2008.05.002.

[49] Huang, H. L., Zhang, J., Chen, G., Lu, Z., Wang, X., Sha, N., Shao, B., Li, P., Guo, D. A. High performance liquid chromatographic method for the determination and pharmacokinetic studies of oxyresveratrol and resveratrol in rat plasma after oral administration of Smilax china extract. *Biomed. Chromatogr.*, 2008 22, 421-427.

[50] Langley, R. R., Fidler, I. J. Tumor cell-organ microenvironment interactions in the pathogenesis of cancer metastasis. *Endocr. Rev.*, 2007 28, 297–321.

[51] Kolobov, A. V., Polezhaev, A. A., Solyanik, G. I. The role of cell motility in metastatic cell dominance phenomenon: analysis by mathematical model. *J. Theor. Medicine*, 2000 3, 63-77.

[52] Yakshibaeva, Yu. R., Pyaskovskaya, O. N., Solyanik, G. I., Chekhun, V. F. Decrease in migration capacity of Lewis lung carcinoma cells during tumor growth and metastasis. *Exp. Oncol.*, 2002 24, 155-156.

[53] Shimojo, Y., Akimoto, M., Hisanaga, T., Tanaka, T., Tajima, Y., Honma, Y., Takenaga, K. Attenuation of reactive oxygen species by antioxidants suppresses hypoxia-induced epithelial-mesenchymal transition and metastasis of pancreatic cancer cells. *Clin. Exp. Metastasis*, 2013 30, 143-154. doi: 10.1007/s10585-012-9519-8.

[54] Watson, J. Oxidants, antioxidants and the current incurability of metastatic cancers. *Open Biol.*, 2013 3, 120144. doi: 10.1098/rsob.120144.

[55] Ogasawara, M., Matsunaga, T., Suzuki, H. Differential effects of antioxidants on the in vitro invasion, growth and lung metastasis of murine colon cancer cells. *Biol. Pharm. Bull.*, 2007 30, 200-204.

[56] Solyanik, G., Misin, V., Pyaskovskaya, O. N., Banakchevich, N., Ogay, Yu. Correction of the cancer therapy-induced anemia by the grape polyphenol concentrate Enoant. In: Pierce, G. N., Mizin, V. I., Omelchenko, A., editors. *Advanced bioactive compounds countering the effects of radiological, chemical and biological agents: Strategies to counter biological damage.* Series: NATO Science for Peace and Security Series A: Chemistry and Biology. Dordrecht, The Netherlands: Springer; 2013; 43-54.

[57] Nishikawa, M. Reactive oxygen species in tumor metastasis. *Cancer Lett.*, 2008 266, 53-59. doi: 10.1016/j.canlet.2008.02.031.

In: Paraneoplastic Syndromes
Editor: Lora H. Winter

ISBN: 978-1-63117-878-8

Chapter VI

Paraneoplastic Syndromes Associated with Lung Cancer

***Neven Z. Rakusic* [1,*] *and Nevena Rakusic* [2]**
[1]Clinical Hospital Centre Zagreb, University Hospital for Lung Diseases „Jordanovac", Zagreb, Croatia
[2]General Practice and Family Medicine Unit, Zagreb, Croatia

Abstract

A spectrum of paraneoplastic syndromes occur in 10-20% of patients with lung cancer, ranging from mild to severe manifestations including cutaneous, skeletal, neuromuscular, endocrine, hematological, renal, vascular, collagenous, metabolic and systemic features.

A paraneoplastic symptoms and signs occur distant from the primary tumor or metastasis, and are caused by the underlying pathogenic mechanisms which include immunologic cross-reaction of tumor associated antigens with normal tissue directed by antibody, or cellular cytotoxic response. Besides, production of systemic factors by the tumor, such as hormones, hormone-like peptides, cytokines and prostaglandins cause variety of paraneoplastic spectrum. However, all pathogenic mechanisms and some new paraneoplastic features associated with lung cancer are not yet fully understood and recognized.

* Email: neven.rakusic@zg.t-com.hr.

Paraneoplastic extent of symptoms and signs may precede the diagnosis and be the first sign of underlying lung cancer, as well as the first sign of its recurrence; or may occur in the later phase of disease irrespectively of tumor mass.

The understanding and early recognition of paraneoplastic symptoms may speed-up the proper diagnosis and in some cases correspond with the therapy effect in the follow-up.

Endocrine Syndromes

Paraneoplastic syndromes due to ectopic production of hormones are associated with lung cancer, especially with type of small cell lung cancer (SCLC), the most common being Cushing's syndrome [1, 2, 3]. The spectrum of endocrine syndromes (Table 1.) includes Cushing's syndrome due to ectopic production of adrenocorticotrophic hormone (ACTH) [4, 5, 6], the syndrome of inappropriate antidiuretic secretion (SIADH) due to ectopic synthesis of arginine-vasopressin [7, 8], non-metastatic hypercalcemia [9, 10], gynecomastia, hyperproduction of calcitonin, human chorionic gonadotropin (HCG) and luteinizing hormone (LH), melanocyte-stimulating hormone (MSH) with skin darkening, and carcinoid syndrome [11, 12, 13]. The presence of paraneoplastic syndromes of endocrine ectopic origin is not always a negative prognostic factor.

Table 1. Endocrine paraneoplastic syndromes

Cushing' syndrome
Syndrome of inappropriate antidiuretic hormone (SIADH)
Hypercalcemia
Gynecomastia
Hypoglycemia
Carcinoid syndrome
Hypercalcitoninemia
Hyperproduction of luteinizing hormone (LH)
Hyperproduction of follicle stimulating hormone (FSH)
Hyperthyroidism

Cushing's syndrome. The most commonly produced ectopic hormone in lung cancer is adrenocorticotropic hormone (ACTH), being mostly associated and restricted to SCLC and carcinoids. Due to short natural history of extensive form of SCLC and better response to novel therapy of SCLC, patients with SCLC do not manifest classical signs and symptoms of Cushing's syndrome, but rather moderate forms of Cushing's syndrome. Cushing's syndrome in lung cancer may appear before, concomitant and after the diagnosis is established, as well as relapse of paraneoplastic Cushing's syndrome may herald the recurrence of tumor [4, 12]. Tumor cells secrete adrenocorticotropic hormone or corticotrophin-releasing factor, resulting in production and release of adrenal glands hormone cortisol [5, 11, 14]. Diagnosis is suggested by muscle weakness, hyperglycemia, mild hypertension and hypokalemia. Patients have difficulties in walking, standing, and getting out of the chair or bed. Varying degrees of confusion, drowsiness and depression can occur. Confirmation of diagnosis can be achieved by laboratory findings of elevated serum level of ACTH and elevated serum and urinary levels of 17-hydroxycorticosteroid; baseline cortisol level greater than 29 μg/dL, midnight adrenocorticotropic hormone greater than 100 ng/L, and urinary free cortisol level greater than 47 μg/24h [15]. There is no suppression effect on ACTH by corticosteroid administration.

When symptoms appear before the primary tumor, imaging studies including computed tomography (CT), magnetic resonance (MR), F18 FDG positron emission tomography (PET scan) and octreotide scan are valuable in discovering and locating the tumor.

Steroid production inhibition by variety of drugs including ketoconazole, metyrapone, mitotane and aminoglutethimideis is pharmacologic option for treatment of paraneoplastic Cushing's syndrome. Octreotide blocks the adrenocorticotropic hormone release and lead to symptom improvement [16].

Patients with Cushing's syndrome in lung cancer are at greater risk of opportunistic bacterial and fungal infection.

Syndrome of inappropriate antidiuretic hormone (SIADH). The most frequently occurrence of this syndrome is in the patients with small cell lung cancer (SCLC), but occasionally SIADH also occur in the different pulmonary diseases, including sarcoidosis, tuberculosis and pulmonary embolism [5, 7, 11]. Antidiuretic hormone (arginine-vasopressin) is normally secreted in the supraoptic nuclei of the hypothalamus, then carried and stored to the posterior pituitary gland lobe [17]. Antidiuretic hormone (ADH) controls water excretion by the kidney, and it is normally secreted and released into blood circulation when serum osmolarity exceeds 280 mOsm/kg; on contrary, serum osmolarity below this level inhibits secretion of ADH, thus enhancing diuresis and excretion of water.

Diagnosis is based on the common symptoms including anorexia, nausea and vomiting, or more severe manifestations of altered consciousness, such as confusion, lethargy, psychotic behavior, seizures and coma, which is associated with severe hyponatremia resulting in water intoxication, and ultimately if untreated to death.

Besides of paraneoplastic ectopic secretion of antidiuretic hormone in patients with lung cancer and SIADH, which can be attributed to the half of cases, the remainder of SIADH is a result of altered or defective chemoreceptor control of the posterior lobe of pituitary with abnormal release of ADH, or occasionally because of metastatic involvement of posterior pituitary [11].

Diagnostic (laboratory) confirmation is by finding of low serum sodium and serum osmolarity below 280 mOsm/kg, simultaneously with the high urine sodium concentration and urine osmolarity greater than 500 mOsm/kg. Serum urea, creatinine and total proteins can be low with normal renal, adrenal and thyroid function. Severe hyponatremia with serum sodium below 110 mmol/L is associated with seizures and ultimately with cerebral coma.

Treatment should focus on the underlying lung cancer, and monitoring the degree and speed of hyponatremia development. If there are no symptoms, and level of serum sodium is not below 130 mEq/L, treatment can be free water restriction to 500 ml/day, along with diuretic medication with furosemide. In the conditions of symptomatic patient and very low serum sodium, it is necessary to elevate sodium level above 130 mEq/L. That can be achieved by infusion of hypertonic saline solution, along with furosemide and potassium replacement. Chemotherapy of the underlying lung cancer can be administered only after correction of serum irregularities of electrolytes and osmolarity.

Hypercalcemia. The presence of hypercalcemia in a malignant disease indicate a poor prognosis and shortens patient's life expectancy. It occurs in up to 10% of all patients with underlying malignancy [9]. In lung cancer it is most common in squamous cell type, with approximately 15% of patients developing hypercalcemia in the terminal stage. In small cell lung cancer is extremely rare (less than 1 %) [10, 18, 19].

Mechanism of hypercalcemia in cancer patients is commonly due to humoral causes with secretion of parathyroid hormone (PTH)-related protein (PTHrP), in which level of serum calcium is elevated in the absence of bone metastasis, known as non-metastatic hypercalcemia, and occurs most often in squamous cell carcinoma. Only about 20% of cases of hypercalcemia arise directly from osteolytic activity of bone metastasis and it's destruction, which is underlying mechanism of hypercalcemia in plasmocytoma, breast cancer and lymphomas [20, 21, 22, 23].

Ionized serum calcium causes symptoms on a number of organs, mostly prominent on central nervous system, gastrointestinal and renal system. Neurologic symptoms include progressive weakness and lethargy, occasionally leading to seizures and coma. Gastrointestinal complications of hypercalcemia consist of anorexia, nausea, vomiting, pancreatitis and constipation. Renal complications include tubular damage leading to metabolic alkalosis, polyuria, hyperuricemia and elevated serum urea and creatinine.

Severity of symptoms depends on degree of hypercalcemia; usually serum calcium concentration exceeds values of 4,0 mmol/L, with normal or low phosphate concentration. The rapidity of onset of hypercalcemia and patient's baseline renal and neurological function contribute also to the symptom severity.

The clinical state is deteriorating by combination of impaired consciousness, reduced oral intake and vomiting, all resulting to dehydration, with secondary serum calcium elevation and progressive renal function impairment.

The laboratory evaluation of hypercalcemia includes complete blood count, blood urea nitrogen, creatinine, serum electrolytes including calcium and phosphorus levels, and evaluation of overall dehydration. In patients with non-metastatic hypercalcemia, typical laboratory findings show elevated level of calcium, low to normal level of phosphorus, low to normal PTH levels and high PTHrP level.

Treatment modalities depend on urgency of situation. Eliminating of contributing factors such as high dietary calcium food, thiazide diuretics and drugs that affect calcium levels is logical step. Patients with no or mild symptoms can be treated by oral fluid intake. If symptoms persist and serum calcium level is rising, approach should be fluid repletion with normal saline and potassium replacement, which increases the glomerular filtration rate and inhibits renal calcium reabsorption. Loop diuretics such as furosemide, added after adequate fluid replacement, can induce rapid but transient drop of serum calcium level [9, 18].

Intravenous bisphosphonates with favorable efficacy and toxicity profile are widely used in the treatment of hypercalcemia; serum calcium levels will decline within 2 days and remain suppressed after infusion treatment up to 3 weeks. Hemodialysis is an effective procedure in the patients with underlying cardiac or renal disease who cannot tolerate large fluid infusions or bisphosphonates.

Gynecomastia. Unilateral or bilateral enlargement of male breast (gynecomastia) as a paraneoplastic feature occurs in lung cancer, predominantly in association of adenocarcinoma and large cell carcinoma. When unilateral, it is usually on the same sides as the primary tumor. It is painful and associated with increased serum levels of human chorionic gonadotropin (HCG) or its subunits (β-HCG) [11].

Gynecomastia as an asymptomatic non-paraneoplastic feature can occur in up to 35% of normal males. It can be found in puberty and old age, after intake of numerous drugs and in alcoholic cirrhosis. Number of malignant neoplasms such as pancreatic carcinoma, testicular tumors, hepatomas and adrenocortical carcinoma are causes of gynecomastia [11, 25].

Neurologic Syndromes

Paraneoplastic neurologic syndromes are observed in about 5% of all the patients with different malignancies, mostly in lung, ovarian, breast and gastric cancer, of which half is found in lung carcinoma, almost exclusively with small cell lung carcinoma (SCLC) [26, 27].

Neurological paraneoplastic manifestations in patients with lung cancer result from autoimmune reactions of tumor cells cross-reactivity with components of nervous tissue [28]. Patient produces tumor-directed antibodies known as *onconeural antibodies* in response to cancer presence and development, which attack antigenic targets on cancer cells and similar components of nervous system. Not all the mechanisms of onconeural antibodies are fully understood, but there are basically 3 main categories: 1) those occurring in cancer and cancer-associated syndromes, 2) those that are partly and 3) those fully and well molecularly characterized with a firm association to cancer. Some onconeural antibodies interfere with synaptic acetylcholine binding, so resulting in dysfunction of neuromuscular junction; the majority of onconeural antibodies are directed against intracellular antigens with likely T-cell mediated cellular immunity [28, 29, 30].

Paraneoplastic neurological syndromes (Table 2.) can involve any part of nervous system: cerebrum, cerebellum, spinal cord and peripheral nerves [31]. Involvement is usually limited to the one part of nervous system, but occasionally the same patient can have involvement in more than one area. Depending on affection of nervous system area, symptoms vary and may include cognitive and personality changes, cranial nerve deficit, instability, weakness, ataxia and numbness. Affection of neuromuscular junction manifests as Lambert-Eaton myasthenia syndrome; limbic encephalitis and paraneoplastic cerebellar degeneration occur in central nervous system affection. Subacute sensory neuropathy and autonomic neuropathy are due to peripheral nervous system affection [31, 32].

Table 2. Neurologic paraneoplastic syndromes

Lambert-Eaton myasthenic syndrome
Subacute sensory-motor neuropathy
Limbic encephalitis
Subacute necrotizing myelopathy
Cerebellar degeneration
Opsoclonus-myoclonus
Autonomic neuropathy

Lambert-Eaton myasthenic syndrome. This syndrome is rare but exclusively associated with SCLC, predominantly in females and caused by autoimmune reaction that happen with IgG autoantibodies directed against voltage-gated calcium channels which has been demonstrated both at the neuromuscular junction and in the cancer [33]. It is characterized by muscle weakness which begins in the proximal muscles of lower extremities and is more pronounced in the thighs and pelvic girdle, then moving to the upper extremities and making it difficult to get up from the bed and out of the chair, and climb the stairs. The other associated features include autonomic symptoms of eye and mouth dryness, dysphagia, dysarthria, ptosis, diplopia, blurred vision, impotence and paresthesias. On contrary to the true myasthenia gravis, oculobulbar muscles are usually spared, tendon reflexes are depressed or absent, and muscle strength is rising after exercise. There is poor response to administration of endrophonum chloride and anticholinergic drugs.

Differential diagnosis includes toxic, infectious, metabolic and vascular etiologies, because neurologic symptoms can arise from electrolyte and fluid disturbances, infection, metastases to central or peripheral nervous system, leptomeningeal diseases, cerebral and spinal vascular diseases, spinal cord and nerve compression, treatment toxicity and adverse effects by cytotoxic agents and radiation. Established diagnosis of paraneoplastic syndrome should be by exclusion of former criteria [32].

Diagnostic procedures include serology, imaging such as computed tomography (CT), magnetic resonance (MR) and F-fluoroglucose positron emission tomography (PET), electromyography, electroencephalography and in-vitro immunologic tests for onconeural antibodies.

Treatment is directed to underlying tumor, but may or may not modify the paraneoplastic syndrome. Assuming that paraneoplastic syndrome is immuno-mediated, immunomodulation therapy can be beneficial: corticosteroids, azathioprine, cyclophosphamide, methotrexate and anti-CD 20 monoclonal antibody rituximab. Intravenous immunoglobulins have been shown to improve muscle strength. Plasmapheresis directly removes antineuronal antibody from the circulation with prompt effect which lasts 3 to 4 weeks. Administration of potassium channel blocker 3,4 diaminopyridone can be beneficial. All of these treatment modalities produce effect on symptom stabilization rather than symptom improvement, because of irreversible pathologic changes on nervous components [34, 35, 36, 37, 38].

Peripheral Nerve Involvement

Peripheral nerves involvement in various paraneoplastic syndromes manifests as *sensory* or *motor* affection. Pure sensory neuropathy known as *subacute sensory neuropathy* is only occasionally observed, while mixed *sensory-motor neuropathy* is quite common and most characteristic neuropathy in SCLC. It may occur before, during and after the diagnosis of lung cancer, with acute onset mimicking Guillain-Barre syndrome, or may be of chronic form with progressive weakness and loss of tendon reflexes and sensation, mostly in the lower limbs. The associated symptoms consist of paresthesias, pain and numbness, while involvement of autonomic system may be presented by constipation, orthostatic hypotension, hypothermia, sleep apnea, cardiac arrhythmias and impotence [31, 32, 39, 40].

Central Nerve Involvement

The various syndromes of central nervous system are characterized by similar processes that occur on different levels and consist of neuronal loss and inflammatory reaction with perivascular lymphocytic infiltration of spinal cord, cerebellum and brainstem [26].

Limbic encephalitis. The limbic system consists of hypothalamus, rhinencephalon, amygdaloid-hippocampal complex and cingulate gyrus. Limbic encephalitis consists of profound memory impairment and subsequent dementia, with psychiatric disturbances including anxiety, depression and personality changes. Seizures, delusions and hallucination can occur. Anti–Hu antibody can be detected in the serum [11, 41, 42].

Subacute necrotizing myelopathy is characterized by severe tissue destruction and necrosis of spinal cord in the form of patchy multifocal lesions or massive involvement. Symptoms consist of ascending sensory and motor paralysis to the thoracic level [11].

Cerebellar degeneration. Atrophy and loss of Purkinje cells with degeneration of cerebellar cortex and brainstem nuclei lead to signs and symptoms such as nystagmus, vertigo, progressive dysarthria, and symmetrical bilateral ataxia of extremities and trunk [11, 43].

Opsoclonus-myoclonus. Opsoclonus is characterized by irregular, continual eyes movement in spontaneous and conjugate motions at about 10 times/sec. When accompanied with other symptoms of central nervous system involvement (e.g., ataxia), constitutes opsoclonus-myoclonus syndrome [44, 45].

Autonomic neuropathy is rarely seen, mostly in SCLC. Patients may have dysfunction of autonomic system, such as neurogenic bladder and orthostatic hypotension. Abdominal pain, nausea and vomiting may be the signs of intestinal pseudo-obstruction (Ogilvie's syndrome) [46].

Skeletal Syndromes

Hypertrophic pulmonary osteoarthropathy (HPOA) has been observed and mentioned by Hippocrates since antiquity, but nearly completely understood nowadays. It is characterized by periostitis and periostal new bone formation along the phalanges („finger clubbing“) and long bones, joint swelling and pain (arthritis). There is also connective tissue proliferation beneath nail matrix with excessive osteoblast and fibroblast proliferation. Periosteum becomes elevated above new bone deposits, along with reabsorption of endosteal bone beneath it. The prominent changes are at the distal phalanges of hands and feet on the junction of nail's bed. Swelling on that sites leads to clubbing of fingers and disappearance of angle between nail bed and nail [47, 48, 49].

Clubbing may be an isolated feature, but also accompanied by thickening of the skin on the legs and increased sweating of feet and palms. Patients experience deep seated aching pain and burning in the affected area of long bones, knees, ankles and wrists due to periostitis and arthritis. Lung cancer accounts for more than 80% of HPOA in adults, the majority of cases are observed in adenocarcinoma, less frequently in squamous cell carcinoma and none in small cell lung carcinoma [48].

Various vascular, humoral, endocrine, neural and immunologic factors of HPOA have been proposed; platelet-derived growth factor, vascular endothelial growth factor and prostaglandine E2 have been identified to contribute in HPOA onset and development [50, 51].

Differential diagnosis includes hereditary form, hereditary cyanotic heart diseases, suppurative lung diseases, malignancies of esophagus, thyroid and thymus, inflammatory bowel diseases, cirrhosis of the liver, acromegaly and various arthritides. Plain radiography shows periostal thickening of long bones, and nuclear bone scans demonstrate symmetric and high uptake of radioactive tracers along these bones in the areas of periostal hypertrophy [47].

Treatment consists of tumor resection, or if not possible other different modes of cancer therapy, after which symptoms and sings of HPOA may resolve. Symptomatic treatment options include non-steroidal anti-inflammatory agents, bisphosphonates, opiate analgesics and localized radiation [47, 52].

Collagen-Vascular Syndromes

Dermatomyositis-polymyositis. This disorder is inflammatory myopathy characterized by progressive weakness of proximal musculature of neck, shoulders and pelvis, with inability to firmly raise the head and keep it in proper position, or stand up from sitting position. Multiple cutaneous changes precede the muscle weakness and are typically of heliotrope eruption on the upper eyelids, erythema of the face, neck, chest, back, arms and hands with periorbital and periungual telangiectasia. Gottron's papules over the phalangeal joints mimic psoriatic changes. Raynaud phenomena and arthritis can occasionally be found. Aside from lung cancer, dermatomyositis as a paraneoplastic feature can be found in ovarian, breast and prostate cancer [48, 53, 54].

Histologically, dermatomyositis is characterized by mixed B and T-cell perivascular inflammatory infiltrate, infarcts, perifascicular muscle fiber atrophy and necrosis, endothelial cell swelling and vessel wall membrane complex deposition [54, 55].

The diagnosis of dermatomyositis and polymyositis is suggested by elevation of serum creatinine, creatinine phosphokinase and lactate dehydrogenase, electromyographic findings, and muscle biopsy showing perifascicular muscle fiber atrophy and B and T-cell perivascular inflammatory infiltrate [54].

Successful tumor management will also ameliorate symptoms, but up to one-third of patients remain symptoms of substantial residual motor impairment. The mainstay of dermatomyositic therapy are glucocorticoids, but additional immune-modulating therapies such as azathioprine, methotrexate, cyclosporine A and cyclophosphamide are often required [48, 54].

Hematologic Syndromes

Hematologic abnormalities including anemia, thrombocytosis, leukocytosis and eosinophilia are frequently observed late in the natural history of lung cancer, rarely require specific therapy and may show improvement with successful treatment of the underlying malignancy. The pathogenesis is multifactorial including iron deficiency, chronic disease, bone marrow infiltration, toxic effect of chemotherapy and radiation, and pure red cell aplasia [15, 56].

Leukocytosis is frequently seen in patients with lung cancer either during the course of the disease or at the time of diagnosis. About 15% patients with non-small cell lung cancer (NSCLC) have leukocytosis which does not reflect an active infection. The white blood cell count usually ranges from 12 to 30x109/L, but values exceeding 50x109/L are occasionally observed. Leukocytosis may be due to overproduction of granulocyte-colony stimulating factor [57] and interleukin-6 production by the lung cancer [58, 59], or result from metastatic bone marrow involvement. Paraneoplastic leukocytosis does not need specific therapy.

Eosinophilia. Paraneoplastic eosinophilia is commonly observed in lymphomas and leukemias, but also with lung cancer, gynecological and gastrointestinal malignancies. It appears to be due to tumor production of eosinophil growth factor interleukin (IL)-3, IL-5, and granulocyte-macrophage colony stimulating factor (GM-CSF). Patients have elevated serum levels of former factors, as well as elevated eosinophil chemoattractant IL-2 [61, 62].

Paraneoplastic eosinophilia is typically asymptomatic; when symptoms as dyspnea and wheezing do occur, corticosteroids are beneficial for symptom resolving.

Thrombocytosis. Paraneoplastic thrombocytosis occur in cancers of lung, gastrointestinal, gynecological and renal systems, prostate, head and neck, mesothelioma and lymphoma. It is thought to be due to tumor production of cytokines such as IL-6. Usually, thrombocytosis is marked in advanced disease and associated with worse prognosis and clinical outcomes [63, 64, 65, 66].

Coagulopathic Syndromes

A variety of coagulation disorders such as migratory superficial thrombophlebitis (Trousseau's syndrome), deep venous thrombosis, disseminated intravascular coagulopathy (DIC), thrombotic microangiopathy and non-bacterial thrombotic endocarditis have been observed in lung cancer [67, 68].

Thrombophlebitis. Patients have frequent episodes of migratory thrombophlebitis on unusual sites such as arms, jugular venous system, trunk veins and inferior vena cava. Initially observed in association with cancers of gastrointestinal organs, mostly pancreas, syndrome is now found more in lung adenocarcinoma [11]. Approximately 3% patients with lung cancer develop venous thromboembolism, including poor prognosis and higher risk for death. In the pathogenesis of venous thrombosis decisive role is activation of clotting mechanism by tumor cells through the procoagulants: tissue factor and cancer procoagulant [69].

Treatment should be the same as in thrombophlebitis of non-malignant patients, with preference of low molecular heparin comparing to unfractionated heparin and oral anticoagulant therapy with coumarides [70].

Disseminated intravascular coagulation (DIC) is characterized by skin bleeding such as petechiae, ecchymoses and hematomas all over the body and bleeding into internal organs, accompanied with thrombosis. It is caused by the activation of intravascular coagulation and fibrinolysis. Serum levels of fibrinogen and platelet are elevated. The clinical state may be complicated by neurologic findings related to intracranial bleeding and thrombosis, pulmonary and intestinal hemorrhage, respiratory distress syndrome, and skin infarctions of purpura fulminans. Treatment option is heparin administration [11].

Non-bacterial thrombotic endocarditis occurs in lung adenocarcinoma but can also be found in adenocarcinoma of prostate. Syndrome is characterized by vegetations and sterile verrucuos deposition of fibrin and platelets on mitral and aortic valves, usually mitral, which may break off and cause embolization of multiple organs (brain, kidney, spleen, intestine) [11, 71].

Cutaneous Syndromes

Lung cancer is associated with variety of paraneoplastic cutaneous syndromes, that occur before, concurrent or after the established diagnosis, or herald the recurrence of previously treated malignancy (Table 3.). Cutaneous syndromes that commonly occur without underlying malignancy and are non-specific, have better response to therapy than true paraneoplastic equivalents [11, 48, 72, 73].

Table 3. Cutaneous paraneopalastic syndromes

Acanthosis nigricans
Laser-Trelat sign
Erythema gyratum repens
Acquired hypertrichosis lanuginosa
Acrokeratosis (Bazex's disease)
Acute febrile neutrophilic dermatosis (Sweet syndrome)
Rinophyma paraneoplasticum
Pruritus and urticaria
Pemphigus
Pityriasis rubra pilaris

Acanthosis nigricans has been observed in adenocarcinoma and squamous cell carcinoma of the lung, and in adenocarcinomas of abdominal organs, especially gastric adenocarcinoma. It is characterized by thickening of hyper-pigmented skin predominantly on neck and flexural regions of axilla and loins (Figure 1.); on palms termed *tripe palms* [74]. Mucosal involvement is found in half of these patients [75].

The proposed pathogenetic mechanisms are cytokine secretion by the tumor, tumor transforming growth factor-α and epidermal growth factor. The paraneoplastic acanthosis nigricans is poorly responsive to symptomatic treatment such as topical corticosteroids, but may result in certain improvement or even resolution of changes by the successful therapy of the underlying malignancy [75].

Leser-Trelat sign is sudden appearance of hyperpigmented seborrhoic keratosis on shoulders and trunk, and may be associated with pruritus. The syndrome is observed in lung adenocarcinoma preceding or simultaneous with tumor, and may regress with successful treatment of the tumor [11].

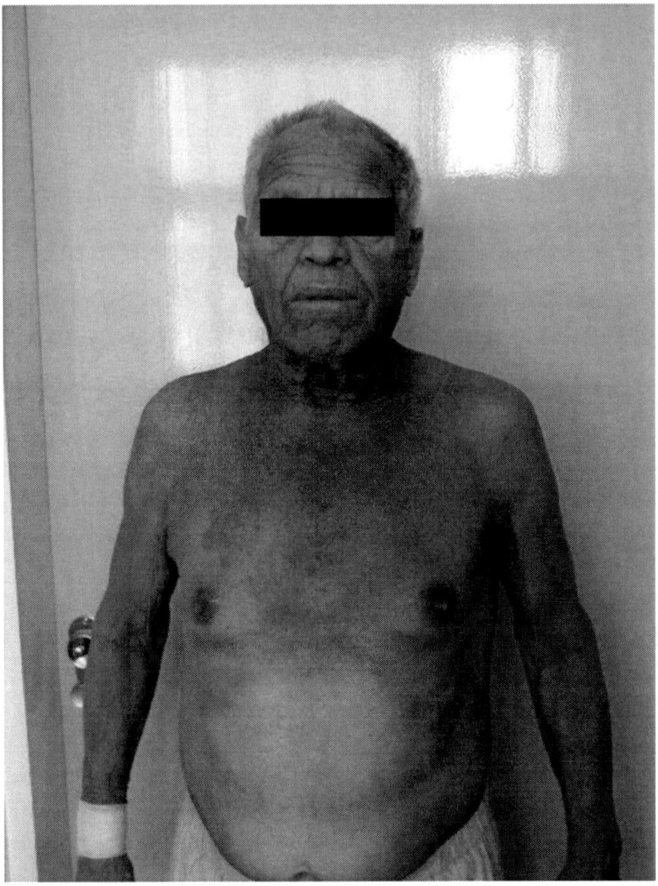

Figure 1. Acanthosis nigricans in a 66-year causcasian man.

Erythema gyratum repens is nearly always associated with various malignancies, mostly of the lung. The skin lesions consist of rapidly changing erythematous bands with scaling and pruritus. Histology shows dense perivascular lymphocytic infiltrate [11].

Acquired hypertrichosis lanuginosa is characterized by rapidly development of long tender and silky hair on forehead and ears, or occasionally on the trunk and entire body [11].

Acrokeratosis (Bazex's diasease) occurs predominantly on palms and soles in patients with squamous cell carcinoma of lung, mostly in men (Figures 2.,3.). Characteristic erythematous hyperkeratosis of palms and soles may resolve by removal or successful tumor treatment [76, 77].

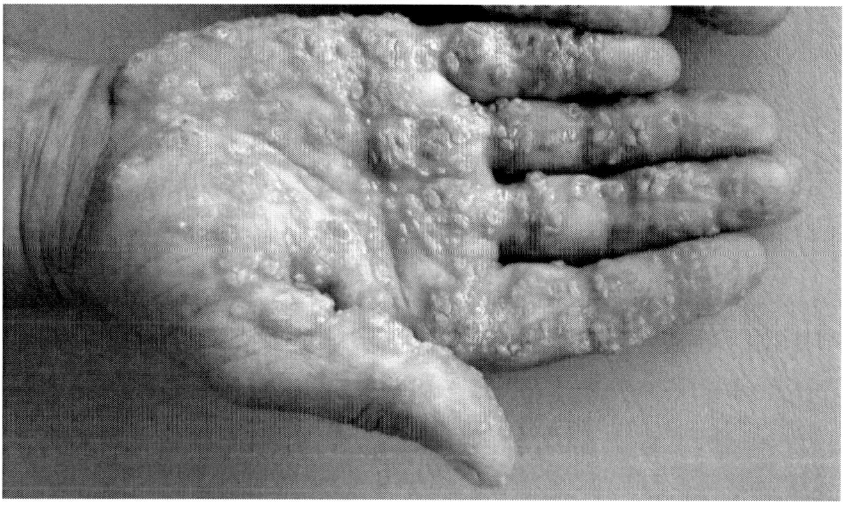

Figure 2. Acrokeratosis. (Bazex's disease)1

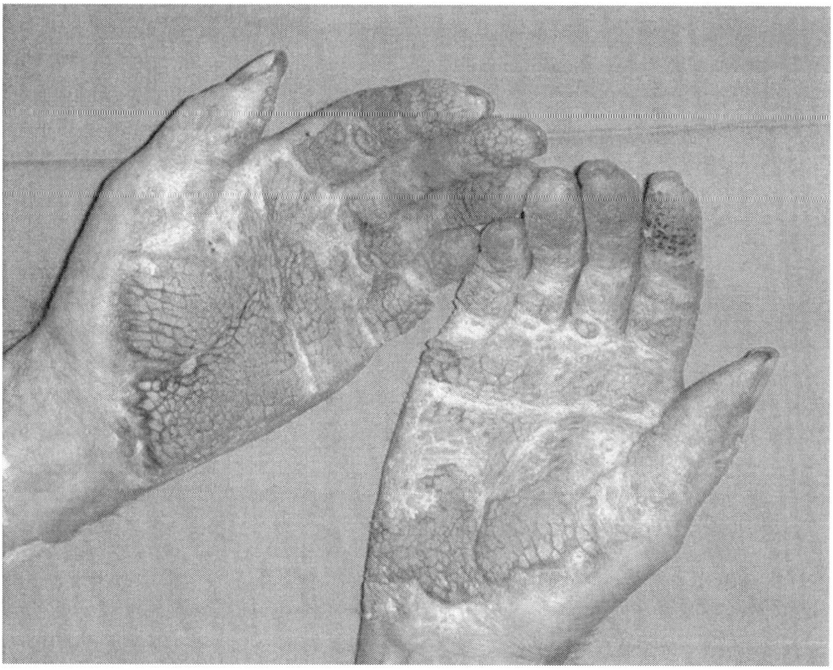

Figure 3. Acrokeratosis. (Bazex's disease)1

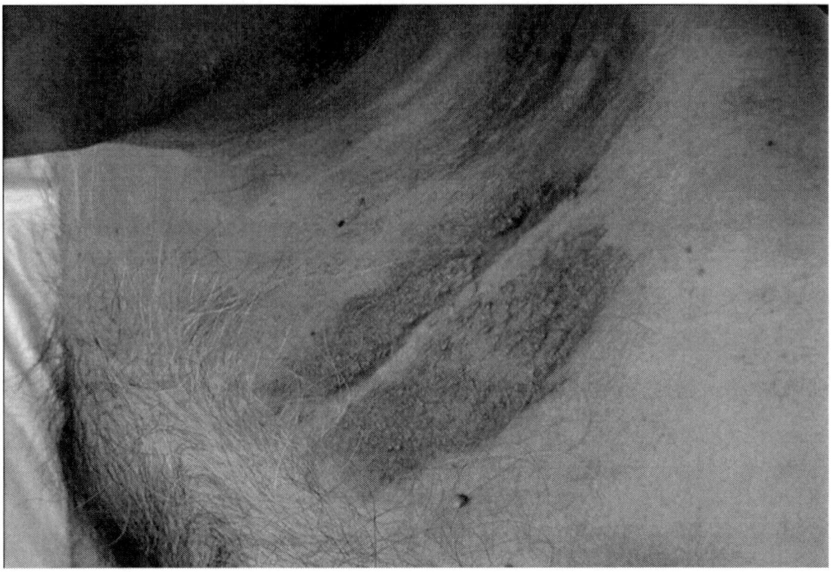

Figure 4. Acute febrile neutrophilic dermatosis (Sweet syndrome) on the neck and front chest area1.

Acute febrile neutrophilic dermatosis (Sweet syndrome) is characterized by sudden onset of painful erythematous changes on the skin of trunk, face and extremities in the form of papules, plaques and nodules, associated with systemic reactions such as fever and blood neutrophilia (Figure 4.). The syndrome occurs rarely in lung cancer, most commonly it is observed in hematologic malignancies, breast, gastrointestinal and genitourinary cancers [78, 79]. Therapy of choice is with topical and systemic corticosteroids.

Rhinophyma is recently observed and described paraneoplastic syndrome in a patient with NSCLC. The syndrome occurred prior the lung cancer diagnosis, withdrew after chemotherapy and surgical treatment, reappeared with tumor marker elevation (cyfra 21-1) and tumor mass progression; then faded again after cancer targeted therapy with epidermal growth factor receptor inhibitor - erlotinib, and raised again in the terminal stage of cancer disease [80].

Symptomatic treatment of paraneoplastic rhinophyma is insufficient, but successful management of underlying malignancy showed regression of the syndrome.

Conclusion

Paraneoplastic manifestations and syndromes occur frequently in patients with lung cancer, being either the first sign of underlying malignancy or it's recurrence, or appear in the later phase of disease and irrespectively of tumor mass. As the understanding of pathogenetic mechanisms and diagnostic methods are improving, earlier recognition of paraneoplastic syndrome may speed up the cancer diagnosis and improve survival and quality of life of these patients. The mainstay of management of paraneoplastic syndromes is treatment of underlying cancer along with specific and symptomatic therapy of particular paraneoplastic syndrome.

References

[1] Monsieur I, Meysman M, Noppen M, de Greve J, Delhove O, Velckeniers B, Jacobvitz D, Vincken W. Non-small-lung cancer with multiple paraneoplastic syndromes. *Eur Respir. J.* 1995;8:1231-4.

[2] Hansen M. Paraneoplastic syndromes and tumor markers for small-cell and non-small cell lung cancer. *Curr. Opin. Oncol.* 1990; 2: 345-51.

[3] Gandhi L, Johnson BE. Paraneoplastic syndromes associated with small cell lung cancer. *J. Natl. Compr. Canc. Netw.* 2006; 4: 631-8.

[4] Terzolo M, Reimondo G, Bovio AA, et al. Ectopic ACTH syndrome: molecular basis and clinical heterogenicity. *Ann. Oncol.* 2007; S83-7.

[5] Barbosa SL, Rodien P, Leboulleux S, et al. Ectopic adrenocorticotropic hormone-syndrome in medullary carcinoma of the thyroid: a retrospective analysis and review of literature. *Thyroid* 2005; 15. 618-23.

[6] Ellison DH, Berl T. The syndrome of inappropriate antidiuresis. *N. Engl. J. Med.* 2007; 356: 2064- 72.

[7] Patel AM, Davila DG, Peters SG. Paraneoplastic syndromes in lung cancer. *Mayo Clin. Proc.* 1993; 68: 278-87.

[8] Raftopuolos H. Diagnosis and management of hyponatriemia in cancer patients. *Support Care Cancer* 2007; 15: 1341-7.

[9] Lumachui F, Brunallo A, Roma A, Basso U. Medical treatment of malignancy-associated hypercalcemia. *Curr. Med. Chem.* 2008; 15: 415-21.

[10] Hiraki A, Ueoka H, Takata I, et al. Hypercalcemia-leukocytosis syndrome associated with lung cancer. *Lung Cancer* 1997; 43: 301-7.

[11] Scaglioti GV. Carcinoma of the lung. In: Spiro SG, ed. Carcinoma of the lung. Lund, Sweden: *European Respiratory Monograph,* 1995; 91-136.
[12] Morandi U, Casali C, Rossi G. Bronchial typical carcinoid tumors. *Semin. Thorac. Cardiovasc. Surg*. 2006; 18: 191-8.
[13] Kvols LK. Metastatic carcinoid tumor
[14] Teves DA. Clinical approach of Cushing syndrome resulting from ACTH-producing metastatic neuroendocrine tumor. *Endocrinologist* 2005; 15: 401-4.
[15] Pelesof LC, Gerber DE. Paraneoplastic syndromes: An Approach to Diagnosis and Treatment. *Mayo Clin. Proc*. 2010; 85: 838-54.
[16] Nieman LK: Medical therapy of Cushing's disease. *Pituitary* 2002; 5: 77-82.
[17] Moses AM, Scheinman SJ. Ectopic secretion of neurohypophyseal peptides in patients with malignancy. *Endocrinol. Metab. Clin. Nort. Am. 1991*; 20: 489-506.
[18] Stewart AF. Hypercalcemia associated with lung cancer. N Engl J Med 2005; 352: 373-9.
[19] Ralston SH, Gallacher SJ, Patel U, campbell J, Boyle IT. Cancer-associated hypercalcemia: morbidity and mortality. Clinical experience in 126 treated patients. *Ann. Intern. Med*. 1990; 112: 499-504.
[20] Clines GA, Guise TA. Hypercalcemia of malignancy and basic research on mechanisms responible for osteolytic and osteoblastic metastases in bone.
[21] Martin T, Molesely J, Gillespie M. Parathyroid hormone-related protein: biochemistry and molecular biology. *Crit. Rev. Biochem. Mol. Biol.* 1991; 26: 377-95.
[22] Tanaka H, Kobayashi S, Masaoka A, Honda S, Yamagushi K. Hypercalcemia induced by parathyroid hormone-realated protein from lung cancer tissue. *Chest* 1991; 100: 1451-3.
[23] Chen HL, Demiralp B, Schneider A, Koh AJ, Silve C, Wang CY, McCauley LK. Parathyroid hormone and parathyroid hormone-related protein exert both pro- and anti-apoptotic effects in mesenchymal cells. *J. Biol. Chem.* 2002; 277: 19374-81.
[24] Tomas L, Kwok Y, Edelman MJ. Management of paraneoplastic syndromes in lung cancer. *Curr. Treat. Options Oncol.* 2004; 5: 51-62.
[25] Spiro SG, Gould MK, Colice GL. Initial evaluation of the patient with lung cancer: symptoms, signs, laboratory tests, and paraneoplastic syndromes. ACCP evidence-based clinical practice guidelines (2nd edition). *Chest* 2007; 132: 149S-160S.

[26] Heineman S, Zabel P, Hauber HP. Paraneoplastic syndromes in lung cancer. Review article. *Cancer Therapy* 2008; 6: 687-98.

[27] Mollina-Garido MJ, Guillen-Ponce C, Martinet Z, Guirado-Risueno M. Diagnosis and current treatment of neurological paraneoplastic syndromes. *Clin. Transl. Oncol.* 2006; 8: 796-801.

[28] De Baukelaar JW, Sillevis Smith PA. Managing paraneoplastic neurological disorders. *Oncologist* 2006; 11: 292-305.

[29] Didelot A, Honnorat J. Update on paraneoplastic neurological syndromes. *Curr. Opin. Oncol.* 2009; 21: 566-72.

[30] Vernino S. Autoimmune and paraneoplastic channelopathies. *Neurotherapeutics* 2007; 4: 305-14.

[31] Honnorat J, Antoine JC. Paraneoplastic neurological syndromes. Orphanet J Rare Dis 2007; 2: 22.

[32] Dalmau J, Rosenfeld MR. Paraneoplastic syndromes of the CNS. *Lancet Neurol.* 2008; 7: 327-40.

[33] Pelucchi A, Ciceri E, Clementi F, Marazzini L, Foresi A, Sher E. Calcium channel autoantibodies in myastenic syndrome and small-cell lung cancer. *Am. Rev. Respir. Dis.* 1993; 147: 1229-32.

[34] Samuelsson A, Towers TL, Ravetch JV. Anti-inflammatory activity of IVIG mediated through the inhibitory Fc receptor. *Science* 2001; 291: 484-6.

[35] Kessel A, Ammuri H, Peri R, et al. Intravenous immunoglobulin therapy affects T regulatory cells by increasing their suppressive function. *J. Immunol. 2007*; 179: 5571-5.

[36] Verschuuren JJ, Wirtz PW, Titulaer MJ, Willems LN, Van Gerven J. Available treatment for management of Lambert-Eaton myasthenic syndrome. *Expert Opin. Pharmacother.* 2006; 7: 1323-36.

[37] Ibrahim RB, Liu C, Cronin SM, et al. Drug removal by plasmapheresis: an evidence based review. *Pharmacotherapy* 2007; 27: 1529-49.

[38] Dau PC, Lindstrom JM, Cassel CK, Denys EH, Shev EE, Spitler LE. Plasmapheresis and immunosuppressive drug therapy in myasthenia gravis. *N. Engl. J. Med.* 1997; 297: 1134-40.

[39] Darnell RB. Paraneoplastic neurologic disorders: window into neuronal function and tumor immunity. *Arch. Neurol.* 2004; 61: 30-2.

[40] Kummel DW, O'Neill BP, Lennon VA. Subacute sensory neuropathy associated with small-cell lung carcinoma: diagnosis aided by autoimmune serology. *Mayo Clin. Proc.* 1988; 63: 29-32.

[41] King PH, Dropcho EJ. Expression of Hel-N1 and Hel-N2 in small-cell lung carcinoma. *Ann. Neurol.* 1996; 39: 679-81.

[42] Molinuevo JL, Graus F, Serrano C, Rene R, Guerrero A, Illa I. Utility of ant-Hu antibodies in the diagnosis of paraneoplastic sensory neuropathy. *Ann. Neurol.* 1998; 44: 976-80.
[43] Rojas I, Graus F, Keime-Guibert F, et al. Long-term clinical outcome of paraneoplastic cerebellar degeneration and anti-Yo antibodies. *Neurology* 2000; 55:713.
[44] Bataller L, Graus F, Saiz A, Vilchez JJ. Clinical outcome in adult onset idiopathic or paraneoplastic opsoclonus-myoclonus. *Brain* 2001; 124: 437-43.
[45] Anderson NE, Budde-Steffen C, Rosenblum MK, Graus F;Ford D, Synek BJ, Posner JB. Opsoclonus, myoclonus, ataxia, and encephalopathy in adults with lung cancer: a distinct paraneoplastic syndrome. *Medicine* (Baltimore) 1988; 67: 100-9.
[46] Lennon VA, Sas DF, Busk MF, et al. Enteric neuronal autoantibodies in pseudo-obstruction with small-cell lung carcinom. *Gastroenterol. Assoc.* 1991; 100: 127-42.
[47] Mauricio O, Francis L, Athar U, Shah C, Chaudhary M, gajra A. Hypertrophic osteoarthropathy masquerading as a lower extremity cellulitis and response to bisphosphonates. *J. Thorac. Oncol.* 2009; 4: 260-2.
[48] Thiers BH, Sahn RE, Callen JP. Cutaneous manifestations of internal malignancy. *CA Cancer J. Clin.* 2009; 59: 73-98.
[49] Myers KA, Farquhar DRE. Does this patient have clubbing? *JAMA* 2001; 286: 341-7.
[50] Olan F, Portela M, Navarro C, gaxiola M, Silveira LH, Ruiz V, Martinez-Lavin M. Circulating vascular endothelial growth factor concentrations in a case of pulmonary hypertrophic osteoarthropathy. *J. Rheumatol.* 2004; 31: 614-6.
[51] Atkinson S, Fox SB. Vascular endothelial growth factor (VEGF)-A and platelet-derived growth factor (PDGF) play a central role in the pathogenesis of didital clubbing. *J. Pathol.* 2004; 203: 721-8.
[52] Amital H, Applbaum YH, Vasilev L, Rubinow A. Hypertrophic pulmonary osteoarthropathy: control of pain and symptoms with pamidronate. *Clin. Rheumatol.* 2004; 23: 330-2.
[53] Hill CL, Zhang Y, Sigugeirsson B, Pukkula E, Mellemkjaer L. Aririo A, Evans SR, Felson DT. Frequency of specific cancer types in dermatomyositis and polymyositis: a population-based study. *Lancet* 2001; 357: 96-100.

[54] Dalakas MC, Hohlfeld R. Polymyositis and dermatomyositis, Lancet 2003; 362: 971-82.

[55] Krathen MS, Fiorentino D, Werth VP. Dermatomyositis. *Curr. Dir. Autoimmun.* 2008; 10: 313-23.

[56] Jemeson JL, Johnson BE. Paraneoplastic syndromes: endocrinologic/hematologic. In: Fauci AS, Braunwald E, Kasper DL, Hauser SL, Longo DL, jameson JL, Loscalzo J, editors., eds. Harrison's Princiiples of Internal Medicine. 17th ed. New York, NY: McGraw Hill Medical; 2008: 617-22.

[57] Kasuga I, Makino S, Kiyokawa H, katoh H, Ebihara Y, Ohyashiki K. Tumor- related leukocytosis is linked with poor prognosis in patients with lung carcinoma. *Cancer* 2001; 92: 2399-2405.

[58] Matsuguchi T[1], Okamura S, Kawasaki C, Shimoda K, Omori F, Hayashi S, Kimura N, Niho Y. Constitutive production of granulocyte colony-stimulating factor and interleukin-6 by a human lung cancer cell line, KSNY: gene amplification and increased mRNA stability. *Eur. J. Haematol.*1991;47:128-33.

[59] Sawyers Cl, Golde DW, Quan S, Nimer SD. Production of granulocyte-macrophage colony stimulating factor in two patients with lung cancer, leukocytosis and eosinophilia. *Cancer* 1992; 69: 1342-6.

[60] Tefferi A, Patnaik MM, Pardanani A. Eosinophilia: secondary, clonal and idiopathic. *Br. J. Haematol.* 2006; 133: 468-92.

[61] Anagnostopoulos GK, Sakorafas GH, Kostopoulos P, et al. Dissminated colon cancer with severe periferal blood eosinophilia and elevated serum levels of inreleukine-2, interleukine-3, interleukone-5, and GM-CSF. *J. Surg. Oncol.* 2005; 89: 273-5.

[62] TefferiA, Gotlib J, Pardanani A. Hypereosinophilic syndrome and clonal eosinophilia: point-of-care diagnostic algorithm and treatment update. *Mayo Clin. Proc.* 2010; 85; 158-64.

[63] Aoe K, Hiraki A, Ueka H, Kiura K, Tabata M, Tanaka M, Tanimoto M. Thrombocytosis is a useful prognostic indicator in patients with lung carcinoma. *Respiration* 2004; 71: 170-3.

[64] Moller Pedersen L, Millman N. Prognostic significance of thrombocytosis in patients with primary lung cancer. *Eur. Respir. J.* 1996; 9: 1826-30.

[65] Sierko E, Wojtukiewicz MZ. Platelets and angiogenesis in malignancy. *Semin. Thromb Hemost.* 2004; 30: 95-108.

[66] Blay JY, favrot M, Rossi JF, Wijdenes J. Role of interleukin-6 in paraneoplastic thrombocytosis. *Blood* 1993; 82: 2261-2.

[67] Tesselaar ME, Osanto S. Risk of venous thromboembolism in lung cancer. *Curr. Opin. Pulm. Med.* 2007; 13: 362-7.
[68] Girard P, Rayneaud C, Meyer G, Parent F, Besse B. Thrombosis and lung cancer. *Rev. Pneumol. Clin.* 2008; 64: 85-91.
[69] Molnar S, Guglielmone H, Lavarda, Rizzi ML, Jarchum G. Procoagulant factors in pateients with cancer. *Hematology* 2007; 12. 555-9.
[70] Akl EA, Rohilla S, Barba M, Sperati F, Terrenato I, Muti P, Schunemann HJ, Anticoagulation for the long term treatment of venous thromboembolism in patients with cancer. *Cochrane Database Syst. Rev.* 2008; 16, CD006650.
[71] Enck RE. Paraneoplastic syndromes. *Am. J. Hosp. Palliat. Care* 2004, 21: 85-6.
[72] Rubinstein M, Duvic M. Cutaneous manifestation of Hodgkin's disease. *Int. J. Dermatol.* 2006; 45: 251-6.
[73] Perez NB, Bernard B, Narvaez J, et al. Erythema nodosum and lung cancer. *Joint Bone Spine* 2006; 73: 336-7.
[74] Mekhail TM, Markman M. Acanthosis nigricans with endometrial carcinoma: case report and review of the literature. *Gynecol. Oncol.* 2002;84: 332-4.
[75] Anderson SH, Hudson-Peacock M, Muller AF. Malignant acanthosis nigricans: potential role of chemotherapy. *Br. J. Dermatol.* 1999; 141: 714-6.
[76] Khachemoune A, Yalamanchili R, Rodriguez C. Bazex syndrome (paraneoplastic acrokeratosis). *Cutis* 2006; 64: 23-7.
[77] Akhyani M, Mansoori P, Taheri A, et al. Acrokeratosis paraneoplastica (Bazex syndrome) associated with breast cancer. *Clin. Exp. Dermatol.* 2004; 29: 429-30.
[78] Cohen PR. Sweet's syndrome
[79] *Raza S, Kirkland RS, Patel AA, Shortridge JR, Freter C.* Insight into Sweet's syndrome and associated-malignancy: a review of the current literature. *Int. J. Oncol.* 2013; 42:1516-22.
[80] Rakusic N, Baricevic D, Rakusic N, Samarzija M, Jakopović M, Baricevic M. Acquired rhinophyma as a paraneoplastic manifestation of non-small cell lung cancer. *Wien Klin Wochenschr.* 2012; 124: 276-7.

Reviewed by:

Prof. dr. Zoran Slobodnjak, FECTS, University Thoracic Surgery Clinic, Clinical Hospital Centre, Zagreb, Croatia

Ass. Prof. dr. Marko Jakopovic, Clinical Hospital Centre, University Hospital for Lung Diseases „Jordanovac", Zagreb, Croatia

Index

#

10q23, 86

A

acetaminophen, 115
acetic acid, 115
acetonitrile, 180
acetylcholine, 12, 121, 123, 154, 206
acid, 15, 16, 46, 47, 52, 111, 114, 138
acne, 50, 52, 58
acquired immunodeficiency syndrome, 40
acrocyanosis, 51
acromegaly, 70, 210
ACTH, 3, 5, 50, 51, 87, 108, 111, 131, 136, 138, 202, 217, 218
action potential, 11, 152
acute leukemia, 61
acute myeloblastic leukemia, 29
acute myeloid leukemia, 21, 34
acute renal failure, 111
AD, 21, 141, 160
adaptation, 168, 189
adenocarcinoma, 12, 13, 14, 15, 20, 28, 29, 37, 40, 43, 46, 60, 64, 67, 71, 73, 76, 96, 98, 101, 104, 109, 121, 130, 132, 137, 139, 144, 146, 153, 159, 206, 210, 212, 213
adenoma, 81
ADH, 4, 112, 113, 114, 136, 203, 204
adhesion, 45
adrenal gland(s), 51, 111, 125, 130, 203
adrenocorticotropic hormone, 47, 50, 51, 112, 138, 202, 203, 217
adulthood, 57, 83, 87
adults, 6, 33, 45, 121, 123, 135, 167, 210, 220
adverse effects, 207
adverse event, 4, 5
advocacy, 131
aerodigestive tract, 40
aetiology, 135
afebrile, 34
African American(s), 124
age, 26, 31, 38, 42, 52, 66, 68, 82, 83, 84, 91, 126, 129, 133, 134
aggregation, 46
alcoholic cirrhosis, 206
aldosterone, 113
algorithm, 221
alkalosis, 51
allergic reaction, 48, 118
allergy, 124
alopecia, 15, 31, 37, 45, 57, 68, 71, 91
amenorrhea, 136
amine(s), ix, 107, 108, 114, 116
amino, 38, 116
amino acid(s), 38, 116

amnesia, 119
amplitude, 11, 152
amygdala, 119
amyloidosis, 56, 57, 85, 95, 105, 128, 144
amyotrophic lateral sclerosis, 128
anaphylaxis, 53, 100
androgen(s), 52, 130, 131, 135, 138
anemia, xi, 6, 34, 37, 53, 164, 165, 166, 167, 169, 170, 171, 172, 173, 176, 178, 180, 181, 182, 185, 186, 191, 193, 194, 196, 199, 211
angioedema, 48, 50, 100
angiogenesis, 166, 187, 221
angiography, 8
angiosarcoma, 91
ankles, 73, 209
anorexia, 71, 110, 113, 127, 204, 205
antibody, xi, 20, 29, 119, 145, 159, 160, 175, 176, 201, 208, 209
anti-cancer, x, 163
anticancer activity, 179, 186, 187, 193
anticholinergic, 207
anticoagulant, 62, 212
anticoagulation, 8
antidepressant, 115
antidiuretic hormone, 112, 139, 202, 203, 204
antigen, 26, 29, 40, 67, 129, 144, 145, 156
antihistamines, 45
anti-inflammatory agents, 210
anti-inflammatory drugs, 126
antinuclear antibodies, 50
antioxidant, 178, 179, 190, 191, 197
antitumor, 165, 196
anus, 13, 17, 36
anxiety, 209
aortic valve, 212
apathy, 113
APC, 82
aplasia, 6, 18, 211
aplastic anemia, 91
apoptosis, 110, 167, 179
arginine, 112, 114, 202, 203
arrest, 124
arsenic, 42
arsenic poisoning, 42
arterioles, 46
arthralgia, 70
arthritis, 15, 31, 68, 69, 209, 210
aspartic acid, 8
assessment, 110
asthenia, 110, 122, 130
astrocytoma, 55, 91
asymmetry, 11
asymptomatic, 4, 7, 51, 84, 113, 118, 125, 129, 135, 206, 211
ataxia, 10, 11, 60, 120, 121, 123, 124, 134, 142, 145, 151, 155, 206, 209, 220
atmosphere, 168, 180, 189
atrial myxoma, 87
atrophy, 11, 61, 89, 120, 123, 210, 211
autoantibodies, 11, 12, 14, 16, 28, 50, 121, 123, 133, 157, 207, 219, 220
autoimmune disease(s), 12, 73, 156
autoimmunity, 158
autonomic neuropathy, 154, 160, 207
autopsy, 151
autosomal dominant, 17, 78, 80, 82, 83, 84, 87, 88
autosomal recessive, 89, 91
awareness, viii, 24, 25
axilla, 117, 213
axonal degeneration, 152, 154
axonal polyneuropathy, x, 150, 151, 155

B

basal cell carcinoma, 88
basement membrane, 27
basic research, 218
behavioral change, 11
beneficial effect, 124, 178
benefits, 178
benign, 12, 15, 37, 40, 42, 43, 59, 79, 84, 86, 129, 134, 135, 136
benign prostatic hyperplasia, 129
benzene, 180
bioavailability, x, 164, 179
biochemistry, 26, 30, 218
biological activity, 109, 179

biomarkers, 83
biopsy, 12, 13, 14, 15, 16, 33, 38, 40, 53, 56, 75, 131
birefringence, 56
bisphosphonate treatment, 138
bladder cancer, 109, 111, 123, 132, 133, 134, 145
bleeding, 131, 212
blood, 5, 6, 7, 8, 18, 26, 30, 34, 50, 60, 61, 63, 64, 73, 79, 113, 114, 115, 117, 127, 166, 168, 169, 172, 173, 175, 177, 181, 182, 185, 189, 193, 195, 203, 205, 216, 221
blood circulation, 203
blood clot, 63, 114
blood flow, 60
blood plasma, 168, 177
blood pressure, 79, 113
blood smear, 169
blood supply, 60
blood urea nitrogen, 205
blood vessels, 30
body weight, 181
bone(s), 3, 6, 15, 18, 47, 52, 53, 73, 79, 82, 88, 109, 110, 125, 127, 129, 130, 132, 137, 138, 167, 168, 170, 171, 172, 173, 174, 181, 183, 184, 204, 209, 210, 211, 218
bone form, 209
bone marrow, 6, 52, 53, 127, 167, 168, 170, 171, 172, 173, 174, 181, 183, 184, 211
bone marrow biopsy, 6, 53
bone resorption, 3, 110
bowel, 43, 71, 81, 83
bradykinin, 51, 114
brain, 10, 46, 47, 55, 80, 81, 82, 83, 100, 120, 123, 142, 212
brain cancer, 81
brain stem, 120
brain tumor, 46, 47
brainstem, 119, 208, 209
breakdown, 115
breast cancer, 7, 11, 14, 17, 18, 20, 26, 29, 30, 40, 44, 48, 49, 54, 60, 62, 64, 68, 73, 75, 76, 78, 79, 94, 104, 109, 111, 138, 155, 205, 222
breast carcinoma, 63, 65, 71, 76, 102, 123, 135
breast infection, 62
bronchiolitis, 28
bronchoscopy, 37
bronchus, 50, 130
buccal mucosa, 83, 86
Budd-Chiari syndrome, 101
buffalo, 50

C

cachexia, 55
caffeine, 115
calcification, 88
calcinosis, 37
calcitonin, 108, 202
calcium, 3, 12, 109, 110, 121, 123, 126, 130, 137, 204, 205, 207
cancer cells, 164, 166, 179, 190, 192, 206
carbon, 178
carbon atoms, 178
carcinoid syndrome, 16, 46, 51, 54, 100, 114, 202
carcinoid tumor, 16, 51, 53, 60, 72, 100, 114, 115, 116, 130, 218
cardiac arrhythmia, 208
cardiovascular disease, 196
carpal tunnel syndrome, 56
castration, 131, 138
Caucasian population, 124
cell cycle, 175
cell death, 198
cell line(s), 191, 221
cell size, 168
cell surface, 10, 109
cellular immunity, 206
cellulitis, 220
central nervous system, 20, 72, 119, 153, 205, 207, 208, 209
central obesity, 111
central pontine myelinolysis, 4
cerebellum, 206, 208

cerebral cortex, ix, 72, 149
cerebral edema, 64
cerebrospinal fluid, 152
cerebrum, 206
cervical cancer, 60, 69, 76, 86
cervix, 32, 45, 68, 91, 109
channel blocker, 208
cheilitis, 47
chemical, 115, 179, 199
chemotherapy, 5, 9, 40, 71, 94, 135, 140, 166, 178, 211, 216, 222
childhood, 41, 42, 45, 80, 83, 96, 109, 121
children, 28, 34, 113, 123, 167
China, 194
cholangiocarcinoma, 40, 66, 67, 103
cholestasis, 55
chromatography, 180
chromosome, 42, 79, 80, 82, 83, 84, 87, 88, 89, 136
chronic lymphocytic leukemia, 49, 50, 154
chronic myelogenous, 49
cimetidine, 141
circulation, 51, 59, 63, 131, 208
cirrhosis, 71, 210
classes, x, 164
classification, 100, 133, 159
cleft lip, 88
clinical diagnosis, 7, 13, 16
clinical oncology, 166
clinical presentation, 3, 14, 15, 28, 135, 152, 155
clinical symptoms, 122, 123
clinical syndrome, x, 2, 111, 150, 153, 155
clinical trials, 131
cloning, 137
clubbing, 51, 58, 72, 73, 76, 209, 220
clusters, 175
CNS, 9, 19, 219
CO2, 168, 180, 189
coagulopathy, ix, 149, 212
cognitive function, 119
collagen, 55, 66, 77, 118
collateral, 59, 63
colon, 14, 18, 29, 40, 45, 59, 60, 62, 65, 68, 81, 82, 83, 86, 102, 199, 221
colon cancer, 18, 81, 102, 199, 221
colonoscopy, 75, 82, 83
color, 38, 60, 71, 145
color blindness, 145
colorectal cancer, 17, 48, 49, 81, 83
coma, 4, 130, 153, 204, 205
common presenting symptoms, 71
common symptoms, 154, 204
complement, 50
complete blood count, 6, 28, 205
complications, vii, 1, 8, 31, 156, 205
composition, 169, 172, 173, 174
compounds, x, 164, 178, 196, 199
compression, 63, 126, 127, 150, 207
computed tomography, 8, 28, 112, 119, 124, 203, 207
conduction, 152, 153, 155, 159
conflict, 92
conflict of interest, 92
Congo, 56
connective tissue, 60, 209
consciousness, 204, 205
consensus, 100
constipation, 130, 154, 205, 208
consumption, 131
contact dermatitis, 74
control group, 180, 181, 184, 187
copyright, 92
correlation, 46, 59, 105, 119, 126, 167
cortex, 79, 87, 111, 119, 209
corticosteroid therapy, 118, 154
corticosteroids, 16, 26, 37, 45, 64, 110, 117, 134, 208, 211, 213, 216
corticotropin, 51, 111
cortisol, 5, 51, 111, 112, 131, 203
cost, 118
cough, 51, 63, 115
cranial nerve, 206
creatinine, 204, 205, 210
crises, 31
Croatia, 201, 222, 223
crust, 15
CSF, 7, 8, 9, 18, 117, 118, 120, 121, 152, 153, 155, 211, 221

CT, 84, 96, 112, 120, 124, 133, 152, 203, 207
CTA, 8
culture, 168
culture medium, 168
cure, 116
cutaneous lesions, viii, 17, 23, 28, 68, 80
cuticle, 73, 74
CV, 21
cyanosis, 63
cyanotic, 210
cyclophosphamide, 9, 208, 211
cyclosporine, 211
cysteine, 131
cystoscopy, 133
cytokines, viii, xi, 24, 25, 45, 53, 127, 165, 166, 179, 201, 212
cytoplasm, 13, 15, 68, 175
cytotoxic agents, 207
cytotoxicity, x, 164, 175

D

damages, 164
deaths, 124
deep venous thrombosis, 212
defecation, 13
defects, 91
deficiency, 37, 40, 173, 211
deficit, 119, 206
dehydration, 3, 55, 110, 205
delusions, 209
dementia, 119, 120, 209
demyelinating polyneuropathies, x, 150
dendritic cell, 119
deposition, 16, 128, 210, 212
deposits, 27, 37, 56, 128, 209
depression, 10, 119, 120, 203, 209
deprivation, 130
derivatives, 196
dermatitis, 27, 45, 49, 66, 141
dermatologist, 92
dermatomyositis, 21, 25, 26, 27, 93, 122, 145, 146, 210, 220, 221
dermatoses, viii, 23, 24, 93, 97
dermatosis, 33, 35, 45, 49, 66, 95, 96, 99, 103, 213, 216
dermis, 13, 15, 16, 33, 59, 68, 74
destruction, 6, 173, 204, 209
detectable, 51, 94, 152
detection, viii, 23, 40, 47, 56, 68, 123, 145, 154
developing countries, 133
developmental disorder, 91
dexamethasone suppression test, 5, 112
diabetes, 5, 38, 42, 55, 59, 71, 125
diagnostic criteria, 9, 19, 81, 88, 113, 150, 153, 160
dialysis, 4
diarrhea, 17, 37, 47, 51, 52, 53, 71
differential diagnosis, 38, 150
dilation, 167
dilutional hyponatremia, 112
diplopia, 120, 123, 207
disability, 120, 123, 153
disease progression, 130
diseases, viii, x, 2, 15, 24, 40, 44, 50, 59, 66, 73, 96, 128, 164, 207
disorder, x, 9, 15, 30, 31, 40, 43, 45, 49, 52, 53, 57, 59, 60, 73, 78, 80, 89, 91, 119, 121, 124, 131, 136, 149, 163, 191, 210
dispersion, 153
distillation, 180
distribution, 66, 111, 156, 175, 182
diuretic, 126, 204
diversity, viii, 24, 164
dizziness, 7, 10, 64
DNA, 79, 81, 89, 167
DNA repair, 90
dominance, 198
dosage, 166
down-regulation, 179
drug resistance, 168
drug therapy, 219
drug treatment, 116
drugs, x, 28, 48, 58, 60, 65, 110, 112, 115, 116, 163, 166, 178, 193, 203, 205, 206, 207
duodenum, 130
dysarthria, 10, 120, 123, 152, 207, 209

dysphagia, 10, 56, 152, 207
dysplasia, 79
dyspnea, 51, 52, 63, 211
dysuria, 133

E

ecchymosis, 60
echocardiogram, 80
eczema, 13, 39, 40, 102
edema, 14, 25, 33, 48, 51, 64
editors, 141, 199, 221
education, viii, 24, 25
elbows, 13, 38, 69
electroencephalography, 208
electrolyte, 9, 207
electromyography, 14, 123, 208
electrophoresis, 28, 50, 110
ELISA, 168
emboli, 52, 212
embolism, 8
embolization, 52, 212
EMG, 152, 153
emission, 208
emphysema, 57
encephalitis, 9, 10, 19, 20, 119, 120, 132, 135, 141, 142, 207, 208
encephalomyelitis, 10, 19, 122, 123, 134, 141, 142, 152, 156, 157, 158
encephalopathy, 119, 220
endocarditis, 131, 212
endocrine, ix, xi, 40, 53, 65, 84, 87, 105, 107, 108, 109, 111, 117, 125, 126, 128, 129, 201, 202, 210
endocrine disorders, 65, 117
endocrine glands, 87
endometrial carcinoma, 222
endoscopy, 83
endothelial cells, 29, 70
enlargement, 206
entrapment, 130
enzyme, 14, 70, 116, 175
eosinophilia, 8, 18, 45, 70, 117, 141, 211, 221
eosinophils, 7
epidemiologic, 101
epidermis, 13
epidermoid cyst, 82
epidermolysis bullosa, 71
epilepsy, 80
epithelial cells, 166
epithelium, 66, 82
erythema multiforme, 27, 71, 103
erythema nodosum, 70
erythrocyte sedimentation rate, 155
erythrocytes, 168, 173, 182, 196
erythrocytosis, 7
erythroid cells, 169, 171, 172, 173, 174, 181, 183, 184, 185
erythropoietin, 6, 126, 127, 143, 194
esophageal cancer, 41, 42, 103
esophagus, 16, 36, 40, 49, 64, 91, 210
ESR, 30
essential fatty acids, 38
ethanol, 189
ethnic groups, 2
etiology, viii, x, 7, 12, 15, 24, 54, 59, 150, 151
evidence, 51, 113, 128, 136, 137, 153, 154, 155, 197, 218, 219
evolution, 31, 123
examinations, 50, 119
excision, 52, 77, 91
exclusion, viii, 2, 7, 207
excretion, 3, 110, 113, 114, 203
exercise, 72, 207
exposure, 45, 133
extensor, 25, 40, 69, 84, 90, 91, 120
extraction, 180
extravasation, 189
eye movement, 11, 121, 123, 124

F

facial expression, 56
facies, 51, 56
family history, 17, 82
fascia, 118, 125
fasciculation, 100
fat, 50, 56, 70, 111, 118

femur, 181
ferritin, 127
fever, 10, 16, 33, 45, 70, 127, 128, 131, 197, 216
fiber(s), 11, 57, 72, 152, 210, 211
fibrin, 131, 212
fibrinogen, 212
fibrinolysis, 131, 212
fibroblast growth factor, 129
fibroblast proliferation, 209
fibroblasts, 56, 70
fibrosarcoma, 88, 91, 167
fibrosis, 15, 22, 30, 31, 56, 118
fibrous tissue, 82
filters, 189
filtration, 205
flank, 124
fluid, 4, 5, 9, 19, 110, 113, 205, 207
focal segmental glomerulosclerosis, 167
follicle, 84, 202
follicle stimulating hormone, 202
folliculitis, 58
food, 197, 205
Food and Drug Administration, 112
Ford, 220
formation, 17, 29, 45, 81, 110, 164, 167, 175, 178, 179, 180, 193
fragments, 109
friction, 37, 43
fruits, 179
fumarate hydratase, 84
funding, 92
fungal infection, 39, 178, 203

G

gait, 10
gallbladder, 114
gallium, 110
gastrointestinal tract, 52, 62, 108, 132
gene amplification, 221
genes, 79, 80, 81
genetic predisposition, 85
genitals, 12
genitourinary tract, vii, ix, 62, 107, 116
genomic instability, 90
gingival, 80, 85, 86
glial cells, 158
glioblastoma, 91
glioma, 55
glomerulonephritis, 167, 195
glossitis, 37, 47, 51
glucagon, 6, 15, 37, 38, 117, 129, 144
glucocorticoid(s), 50, 112, 118, 211
glucocorticoid receptor, 112
gluconeogenesis, 5
glucose, 5, 37, 117, 125, 128
glutamine, 168, 180, 189
gluten enteropathy, 66
gonads, 146
granulocytosis, 7, 118
granulomas, 68
Great Britain, 66
Greece, 149
growth factor, viii, ix, 12, 14, 18, 24, 25, 40, 77, 107, 117, 118, 166, 195, 210, 211, 213, 216, 220
growth hormone, 87, 117
growth rate, 176, 180
guidelines, 28, 218
Guillain-Barre syndrome, 208
gynecomastia, 135, 202, 206

H

hair, 47, 48, 50, 58, 66, 84, 86, 135, 214
hair follicle, 66, 86
hair loss, 50
hairy cell leukemia, 29
hallucinations, 119, 120, 124
Harlequin, 72
headache, 4, 7, 10, 47
health, 178
heart disease, 210
heart failure, 45, 57
heart rate, 154
hematocrit, 6, 168, 169, 170, 176, 181, 182
hematomas, 212
hematopoietic system, 167, 185
hematuria, 47

hemochromatosis, 71, 76
hemoglobin, xi, 6, 164, 166, 168, 169, 170, 172, 176, 182
hemorrhage, 212
hepatitis, 127
hepatocellular carcinoma, 28, 29, 31, 37, 40, 54, 64, 65, 66, 94
hepatomegaly, 175, 180
hepatosplenomegaly, 64, 128
hepatotoxicity, 112
hepatotoxins, 128
herpes, 75, 198
herpes simplex, 198
herpes virus, 75
hippocampus, 119
hirsutism, 52, 136
histamine, 51, 53, 54, 114, 116
histology, 15, 126, 130
history, viii, 2, 3, 9, 10, 11, 13, 26, 28, 30, 53, 59, 110, 125, 136, 202, 211
HIV, 71
HM, 20, 93
homeostasis, vii, 1, 2
hormone(s), vii, viii, xi, 1, 2, 17, 24, 25, 52, 87, 108, 114, 109, 113, 129, 143, 165, 201, 202, 203, 218
host, 25
human, 75, 111, 114, 137, 143, 146, 167, 196, 197, 202, 206, 221
human body, 114
human chorionic gonadotropin, 202, 206
human condition, 167
Hunter, 21
hybrid, 84
hydrogen, 179
hydroxyl, 179
hypercalcemia, 3, 17, 18, 109, 110, 126, 130, 134, 136, 137, 138, 140, 143, 202, 204, 205, 217, 218
hypercalciuria, 3
hyperglycaemia, 128
hyperglycemia, 51, 203
hyperhidrosis, 58, 72
hyperparathyroidism, 85, 130, 136
hyperplasia, 38, 85, 111
hypersensitivity, 65, 67
hypertelorism, 88
hypertension, viii, 2, 5, 47, 111, 126, 203
hyperthyroidism, 46
hypertonic saline, 4, 113, 204
hypertrichosis, 47, 100, 213, 214
hypertrophy, 47, 82, 122, 210
hyperuricemia, 205
hypoglycemia, 3, 5, 140
hypokalemia, 5, 203
hyponatremia, 4, 10, 18, 113, 139, 204
hypophosphatemia, 3, 130
hypoplasia, 73
hyporeflexia, 110
hypotension, 115
hypothalamus, 72, 112, 119, 203, 208
hypothermia, 45, 208
hypothyroidism, 113
hypovolemia, 113
hypoxia, 127, 195, 199

I

idiopathic, 21, 31, 33, 35, 45, 48, 52, 53, 56, 60, 72, 101, 121, 122, 132, 153, 156, 220, 221
idiopathic thrombocytopenic purpura, 60
ileum, 114
immune complexes, viii, 24, 25, 29, 50
immune response, vii, 1, 8, 40, 119, 165, 198
immune system, 8, 28, 30, 119, 128
immunity, 219
immunodeficiency, 60
immunoglobulin(s), 27, 37, 50, 142, 175, 208, 219
immunomodulation, 208
immunoprecipitation, 28
immunoreactivity, 152
immunosuppression, viii, 2
immunosuppressive therapies, 11
immunotherapy, 9, 10, 11, 12, 120, 125
impotence, 207, 208
in transition, 146

in vitro, 168, 169, 179, 180, 186, 187, 196, 199
in vivo, 168, 170, 179, 187, 196, 198
incidence, ix, 18, 41, 91, 107, 109, 111, 118, 124, 126, 128, 133, 134, 135, 142, 146, 150
individuals, 29, 37, 44, 45, 46, 64, 86, 87, 88, 136
indolent, 52, 153
induration, 68, 118
infants, 195
infection, 7, 9, 75, 118, 196, 198, 207, 211
inferior vena cava, 212
infertility, 135
inflammation, 8, 10, 16, 17, 64, 68, 96, 118, 134, 155
inflammatory bowel disease, 33, 35, 38, 210
inflammatory disease, 56
inflammatory mediators, 132
ingestion, 72
inguinal, 42, 78, 82, 136
inguinal hernia, 136
inhibition, 112, 138, 170, 174, 178, 179, 186, 187, 196, 203
inhibitor, 50, 131, 179, 216
initiation, 32, 165
injections, 116
injury, x, 63, 128, 150, 198
inoculation, 168, 169, 172, 173, 175, 177, 180, 181, 187
inositol, 137
insulin, 5, 18, 42, 111, 117, 129
insulin resistance, 111, 117
integrity, 167
intensive care unit, 4
interface, 27
interferons, 127
interleukine, 18, 221
intersex, 136
intestinal tract, 51
intestine, 61, 76, 114, 212
intoxication, 3, 113, 204
intravenous fluids, 3
involution, 180
iodine, 115
ipsilateral, 125
iron, 127, 166, 211
irritability, 113, 119, 120
ischemia, 61
Islam, 21
isolation, 62
isoniazid, 115
isotope, 115
Italy, 107
IVIg, 154

J

Japan, 168, 181
jaundice, 89, 132, 144
joint swelling, 209
joints, 210

K

Kaposi sarcoma, 40
karyotype, 136
keratin, 42, 66
keratinocyte(s), 14, 15, 16, 27, 39, 40, 43, 70, 71
keratosis, 14, 42, 43, 44, 133, 213
kidney, x, 5, 10, 40, 43, 48, 56, 57, 61, 80, 84, 97, 114, 124, 125, 132, 153, 155, 163, 165, 203, 212
kidney failure, 57, 165
kinetics, 188
knees, 13, 38, 69, 73, 90, 209

L

laboratory tests, 218
lactate dehydrogenase, 211
lactoferrin, 127
larynx, 32, 40, 45, 48, 114
lead, 10, 16, 25, 51, 53, 57, 110, 132, 135, 193, 203, 209
legs, 30, 54, 64, 69, 76, 133, 155, 209
leishmaniasis, 196
leprosy, 40, 64

lesions, viii, 14, 15, 17, 23, 24, 25, 26, 27, 28, 29, 32, 33, 34, 35, 37, 38, 40, 41, 42, 43, 44, 51, 53, 54, 57, 59, 60, 61, 64, 65, 67, 68, 69, 70, 71, 75, 77, 80, 86, 87, 89, 92, 117, 118, 119, 126, 134, 209, 214
lethargy, 113, 130, 204, 205
leukemia, 28, 29, 32, 35, 48, 49, 53, 54, 56, 59, 60, 61, 63, 64, 70, 79, 89, 91
leukocytes, 173
leukocytosis, 34, 45, 117, 118, 141, 181, 194, 211, 217, 221
leukopenia, 173
leukoplakia, 91
Lewis lung carcinoma, xi, 164, 167, 169, 176, 179, 180, 186, 187, 191, 193, 195, 196, 199
lichen, 27, 54, 55, 85, 94, 105
lichen planus, 27, 94
life expectancy, 192, 204
lifetime, 129, 173
ligand, 3, 12, 110, 138
light, 44, 56, 91, 110, 129
limbic system, 10, 119, 208
lipids, 40, 178
lipodystrophy, 111
lipoma, 85
liquid chromatography, 180
liver, x, 5, 26, 32, 38, 43, 45, 46, 51, 52, 64, 71, 76, 83, 113, 114, 125, 127, 132, 134, 163, 165, 167, 174, 175, 210
liver cancer, 76, 83
liver enzymes, 127
liver failure, 38, 46
liver function tests, 26, 125, 127
liver metastases, 127
localization, 52
loci, 79
locus, 146
loss of libido, 135
lumbar puncture, 9
lung disease, 64, 210
lung metastases, 175, 177, 181, 187, 189
Luo, 194
lupus, 31, 32, 59, 68, 95, 96
luteinizing hormone, 202
lymph, 40, 45, 52, 64, 68, 75, 77
lymph node, 40, 52, 64, 68, 75, 77
lymphadenopathy, 45
lymphatic system, 73
lymphedema, 73, 75
lymphocytes, 152, 173, 182
lymphoid, 28, 29, 30, 59, 60, 63, 64, 70, 175
lymphoid tissue, 175
lymphoma, 10, 13, 16, 28, 29, 31, 32, 35, 40, 45, 46, 48, 49, 50, 54, 56, 58, 59, 60, 61, 63, 64, 66, 67, 68, 70, 71, 72, 76, 88, 94, 95, 96, 100, 104, 153, 155, 159, 160, 212
lysis, 71

M

machinery, 108
macroglossia, 57
macrophages, 152
magnetic resonance, 80, 112, 119, 146, 203, 207
magnetic resonance imaging, 80, 112, 119, 146
majority, 81, 119, 127, 130, 135, 151, 152, 166, 192, 206, 210
malabsorption, 38, 71, 102
malaise, 127
malignant melanoma, 36, 88, 159
malignant tumors, 65, 73, 164, 191, 192
malnutrition, 40, 55, 64, 71
mammography, 62
man, 142, 145
management, viii, 2, 18, 19, 22, 93, 110, 113, 117, 124, 126, 130, 139, 140, 146, 195, 197, 211, 216, 217, 219
marrow, 47, 53, 168, 171, 174, 181, 184
Maryland, 1
mass, xi, 7, 13, 47, 124, 134, 180, 202, 216, 217
mast cells, 52, 53, 70
mastectomy, 68, 104
mastitis, 62
matrix, 209
matter, 113

MB, 98, 101, 103
measurement, 79, 110, 115
median, 109, 133, 134
medical, viii, 2, 3, 4, 5, 15, 112, 117
medication, 9, 204
medicine, 17, 19, 116
medulla, 108
medulloblastoma, 79, 91
melanin, 70
melanocyte stimulating hormone, 47
melanoma, 31, 48, 61, 71, 76, 78, 79, 88, 154, 159, 167
mellitus, 42, 59, 67
memory, 10, 119, 151, 208
memory loss, 119, 151
meningioma, 55, 86
mental retardation, 80
mental status change(s), viii, 2, 4
mesothelioma, 212
meta-analysis, 95
Metabolic, 136
metabolic alkalosis, 5, 205
metabolism, 125, 128
metastases, viii, ix, 18, 23, 24, 25, 51, 53, 58, 76, 114, 127, 130, 132, 138, 149, 175, 177, 181, 187, 189, 207, 218
metastasis, xi, 40, 47, 51, 60, 135, 137, 164, 175, 176, 177, 186, 187, 191, 198, 199, 201, 204
metastatic cancer, 130, 137
metastatic disease, 84, 119, 124, 127, 130, 134
mice, xi, 164, 167, 168, 169, 170, 171, 172, 173, 174, 175, 176, 177, 179, 180, 181, 182, 183, 184, 185, 186, 187, 189, 191, 193, 196, 198
migration, 75, 189, 190, 199
mimicry, 159
mitosis, 171
mitotic index, 172, 183, 184
model system, 179
models, 167, 180
mole, 88
molecular biology, x, 163, 178, 218
molecular weight, 8
molecules, 2, 45, 156
monoclonal antibody, 103, 111, 208
mononeuritis multiplex, 155
mood swings, 51
Moon, 197
morbidity, ix, 3, 6, 55, 134, 137, 149, 218
Morocco, 105
morphology, 129
morphometric, 172
mortality, 3, 6, 27, 134, 166, 194, 218
Moses, 218
motor neuron disease, 144, 155, 160
motor neuronopathy, x, 150, 155, 160
MR, 19, 20, 94, 95, 103, 141, 142, 152, 158, 160, 219
MRI, 9, 10, 11, 119, 120, 124, 133
mRNA, 221
mucin, 55, 56, 62
mucosa, 15, 27, 43, 83, 86, 91
mucous membrane(s), 16, 34, 70, 91
multiple myeloma, 13, 29, 36, 40, 49, 50, 56, 60, 61, 63, 64, 94, 95, 101, 103, 104
muscle biopsy, 14, 211
muscle strength, 207, 208
muscles, 25, 51, 121, 122, 123, 133, 155, 207
mutation, 80, 83, 84, 85, 86, 87, 88, 89
mutations, 78, 79, 81, 82, 83, 84, 87, 89
myasthenia gravis, 151, 207, 219
myasthenic syndrome, 20, 121, 123, 134, 142, 145, 207, 219
mycosis fungoides, 28, 39, 40, 70, 101
myelin, 154
myelodysplastic syndromes, 29, 35
myelogram, 168, 171, 174
myeloproliferative disorders, 45, 59
myoclonus, 9, 10, 11, 20, 121, 123, 207, 209, 220
myopathy, 14, 122, 133, 210
myositis, 26, 133, 145

N

nares, 55
nasopharyngeal carcinoma, 26, 58, 76

National Academy of Sciences, 137, 163
NATO, 199
natural compound, 178
nausea, viii, 2, 4, 10, 64, 71, 110, 112, 113, 130, 154, 204, 205, 209
necrosis, 15, 26, 28, 34, 38, 61, 70, 93, 128, 155, 174, 209, 210
neoplasm, x, 28, 43, 61, 80, 82, 109, 111, 126, 127, 135, 150, 151, 152, 153, 178
nephrectomy, 125, 126, 127, 128, 144, 160
nephron, 125
nephropathy, 129
nerve, x, 12, 72, 121, 128, 150, 152, 153, 155, 156, 207
nerve biopsy, 152, 153, 155
nerve fibers, 152
nervous system, ix, 10, 19, 119, 122, 123, 142, 149, 150, 156, 206
Netherlands, 199
neuroblastoma, 11, 121, 123, 152
neuroendocrine cells, 114
neuroendocrine tumors, vii, 1, 2, 51, 114, 116, 140
neurofibroma, 78
neurogenic bladder, 209
neurologic complications, 119, 135, 150
neurologic disorders, ix, 19, 20, 149, 158, 219
neurologic symptom, ix, 141, 149, 151, 207
neurological disability, 124
neurological syndromes, ix, 19, 20, 108, 132, 151, 158, 160, 206, 219
neurons, 10, 112, 121, 151, 152, 154, 156
neuropathy, viii, x, 2, 119, 120, 132, 150, 151, 152, 153, 155, 157, 159, 161, 207, 208, 209, 219, 220
neurotoxicity, 150
neutrophils, 15, 118
nevus, 88
New England, 137, 139, 142
niacin, 16, 52
niacin deficiency, 52
nicotinamide, 52
nicotinic acid, 42
NMR, 180
nodules, 15, 16, 28, 33, 57, 59, 67, 68, 69, 70, 75, 79, 80, 82, 84, 134, 181, 216
non-Hodgkin's lymphoma, 32, 89, 94, 103
non-steroidal anti-inflammatory drugs, 15
North America, 141
nuclear bone scan, 210
nuclei, 203, 209
nucleus, 13
nutrients, 178
nutritional deficiencies, 150
nutritional status, 127
nystagmus, 120, 123, 209

O

obesity, 42
obstruction, 63, 152, 154, 209, 220
obstructive lung disease, 28
occult blood, 26
oedema, 102, 113
OH, 110, 139
oil, 189
old age, 206
onycholysis, 13, 73
opioids, 55
optic glioma, 78
oral cavity, 31, 36, 75
orchidectomy, 146
organ(s), 30, 24, 51, 53, 55, 68, 75, 95, 108, 110, 112, 114, 127, 128, 130, 175, 192, 193, 198, 205, 212, 213
organism, x, 163, 164, 165, 166, 178
orthopnea, 63
orthostatic hypotension, 154, 208, 209
osmolality, 4, 113
osteoarthropathy, 58, 73, 76, 96, 98, 209, 220
osteomalacia, 132
osteoporosis, 111
ovarian cancer, 4, 7, 43, 60, 86, 98, 102, 104, 109
ovaries, 114
overlap, 87
overproduction, 3, 111, 211
oxidation, 178

oxidative stress, 90, 197
OXY, x, xi, 164, 179, 180, 181, 182, 183, 184, 185, 186, 187, 188, 189, 190, 191, 192, 193
oxygen, 60, 73, 199
oxyresveratrol, vii, x, 164, 179, 197, 198

P

pain, 45, 47, 53, 63, 122, 124, 125, 132, 151, 208, 209, 220
palate, 64, 88
palliative, 55, 125, 126
pallor, 47
palpitations, 47, 53
pancreas, 37, 48, 61, 64, 70, 76, 85, 104, 108, 114, 130, 132, 212
pancreatic cancer, 42, 62, 88, 199
pancreatitis, 205
parallel, 32, 102
paralysis, 128, 209
paralytic ileus, 110
paraneoplastic manifestations, viii, ix, 24, 108, 206
paraneoplastic phenomena, viii, 23, 24
parasites, 50
parasitic infection, 118
parathyroid, 2, 18, 85, 108, 109, 137, 140, 143, 204, 218
parathyroid glands, 85
parathyroid hormone, 2, 18, 108, 109, 137, 140, 143, 204, 218
paresthesias, 11, 151, 207, 208
Parnes, 197
paronychia, 27
parotid, 72
pathogenesis, viii, 24, 25, 29, 30, 38, 40, 42, 54, 67, 70, 94, 129, 132, 137, 150, 167, 198, 211, 212, 220
pathology, 167
pathophysiology, 14, 15, 17, 126
PCA, 10
pellagra, 51
pelvis, 28, 125, 132, 140, 210
pemphigus, 16, 27, 28, 37, 49, 67, 93, 94, 103
penis, 86
peptic ulcer, 85
peptic ulcer disease, 85
peptide(s), viii, ix, xi, 5, 17, 24, 25, 47, 107, 108, 112, 113, 117, 131, 137, 201, 218
perineum, 15, 37
peripheral blood, 18, 46, 167, 169, 171, 173, 181, 183, 185, 195
peripheral nervous system, 150, 160, 207
peripheral neuropathy, x, 56, 119, 120, 123, 141, 150, 151, 158
permeability, 48
permission, 122
pernio, 68
personality, 10, 119, 151, 206, 209
PET, 116, 119, 120, 140, 152, 158, 203, 208
PET scan, 158, 203
petechiae, 212
phalanges, 72, 209
pharmacology, 179
pharynx, 36, 133
phenol, 199
phenotype, 136
pheochromocytoma, 51, 53, 72, 85
Philadelphia, 136, 143, 156
phlebitis, 157
phlebotomy, 7
phosphate, 86, 205
phosphorus, 3, 205
photosensitivity, 89
physical activity, 62
physicochemical properties, 198
Physiological, 137
physiology, 137
pigmentation, 47, 83, 87, 105
pituitary gland, 85, 131, 203
pituitary tumors, 5
plants, x, 163, 178, 196
plaque, 33, 65, 74, 76, 78, 102
plasma cells, 119, 152
plasma levels, 52
plasmapheresis, 9, 124, 132, 219
platelet aggregation, 114, 178

platelets, xi, 7, 114, 164, 168, 212
pleuritic chest pain, 8
plexus, 63
PM, 137, 145
pneumonia, 4
PNS, vii, x, 1, 2, 6, 7, 8, 9, 10, 11, 12, 19, 118, 125, 126, 129, 132, 133, 135, 150, 163, 164, 165, 167, 174, 176, 178, 179, 186, 191, 192, 193
PNS polyneuropathies, vii
polar, 180
polycystic ovarian syndrome, 52
polycythemia, 45, 49, 63, 143
polycythemia vera, 45, 49
polydipsia, 110
polymyositis, 93, 122, 210, 220
polypeptide, viii, 24, 25, 108
polyphenols, x, 164, 178
polyps, 17, 82, 83, 85, 86, 101
polyuria, 110, 205
pools, 171, 173, 185
population, 32, 71, 78, 83, 123, 124, 152, 220
positron, 116, 158, 203, 207
positron emission tomography, 116, 158, 203, 208
potassium, 112, 204, 205, 208
precipitation, 66
precocious puberty, 135
prednisone, 3
pregnancy, 34, 46, 65
prevention, 19, 197
primary amyloidosis, 56, 57
primary hyperparathyroidism, 3, 126
primary tumor, vii, viii, xi, 1, 2, 23, 24, 25, 28, 180, 181, 186, 189, 193, 201, 203, 206
proctoscopy, 83
proctosigmoidoscopy, 75
producers, 190
progenitor cells, 118, 167
prognosis, 28, 44, 48, 57, 75, 84, 109, 117, 123, 126, 128, 130, 131, 134, 135, 143, 144, 152, 159, 166, 204, 212, 221
prolactin, 87
proliferation, 55, 56, 71, 167, 173, 179, 209
prophylactic, x, 164
prostaglandins, xi, 51, 127, 129, 201
prostate cancer, 26, 60, 104, 111, 112, 117, 118, 119, 123, 129, 130, 131, 132, 138, 139, 141, 144, 145, 210
prostate carcinoma, 129, 132
proteinase, 131
proteins, vii, 1, 2, 16, 119, 128, 133, 145, 178, 204
proto-oncogene, 85
pruritus, 51, 53, 54, 55, 64, 85, 89, 213, 214
psoriasis, 13, 38, 42, 102
psychiatric disorders, 37
psychosis, 51
PTEN, 86, 87
ptosis, 207
puberty, 42, 206
pulmonary diseases, 203
pulmonary embolism, 8, 203
pulmonary hypertrophic osteoarthropathy, 220
pulp, 175
purpura, 28, 29, 57, 59, 60, 61, 102, 212
pyoderma gangrenosum, 34, 35, 51

Q

quality of life, 192, 217
quercetin, 196

R

radiation, 116, 125, 129, 192, 207, 210, 211
radiation therapy, 125
radio, 166
radioactive tracer, 210
radiography, 50, 210
radiotherapy, 40
rash, 13, 25
RE, 17, 96, 146, 220, 222
reactant, 128
reactions, 53, 206, 216
reactive oxygen, 199

reactivity, 40, 135, 206
receptors, 8, 114, 195
recognition, x, xi, 3, 92, 149, 202, 217
rectum, 50, 91, 114
recurrence, xi, 73, 77, 111, 118, 127, 133, 202, 203, 213, 217
red blood cell indices, 170
red blood cells, 6
redistribution, 50
reflexes, 12, 119, 120, 151, 207, 208
regression, 40, 59, 216
rehydration, 110
relevance, ix, 108
relief, 13
remodelling, 109
renal cell carcinoma, ix, 7, 66, 67, 99, 103, 107, 109, 125, 126, 134, 137, 141, 142, 143, 144, 160
renal failure, 110, 131
renin, 113, 126
repair, 79, 81, 91
RES, 179
resection, 13, 51, 125, 127, 154, 155, 210
resistance, 196
resolution, 14, 110, 117, 213
respiratory distress syndrome, 212
respiratory dysfunction, 123
respiratory failure, 160
response, viii, xi, 9, 24, 25, 31, 52, 62, 92, 103, 113, 114, 121, 123, 124, 130, 132, 141, 150, 156, 159, 166, 171, 178, 201, 203, 206, 207, 213, 220
restoration, 110
resveratrol, x, 164, 179, 196, 197, 198
retinoblastoma, 79
retinopathy, 132, 157
RH, 138, 145, 146, 159
rheumatoid arthritis, 35, 37, 46, 73, 97
rheumatoid factor, 50
rhinophyma, 51, 216, 222
rings, 36
risk(s), viii, xi, 17, 24, 29, 30, 31, 32, 37, 42, 60, 62, 66, 71, 78, 81, 83, 86, 87, 88, 91, 95, 96, 125, 133, 164, 166, 186, 203, 212
rituximab, 11, 67, 103, 208
root, 119, 120, 151, 152
rosacea, 16, 51

S

sarcoidosis, 3, 40, 68, 70, 95, 203
scaling, 13, 32, 38, 41, 45, 51, 64, 65, 214
scavengers, 197
scleroderma, 16, 30, 31, 51, 55, 57, 95
sclerosis, 30, 31, 80, 81, 95
secondary sexual characteristics, 136
secrete, 114, 128, 166, 203
secretion, 7, 16, 47, 50, 51, 70, 112, 113, 114, 126, 137, 138, 139, 144, 195, 202, 203, 204, 213, 218
seed, 189
segmental glomerulosclerosis, 167
sensation, 208
sensitivity, 52, 90, 91, 187
sensory neuronopathy, x, 9, 11, 119, 150, 151, 152, 156, 157, 158
sensory symptoms, 154
serology, 207, 219
serotonin, 16, 51, 54, 108, 114, 115, 116
serum, 3, 4, 5, 7, 18, 28, 47, 50, 66, 110, 112, 113, 117, 120, 121, 126, 128, 130, 144, 154, 158, 167, 168, 175, 177, 180, 189, 203, 204, 205, 206, 209, 210, 211, 221
sex, 135, 136
sheep, 43
shortness of breath, 6, 7, 8, 16
short-term memory, 120
showing, 11, 27, 126, 129, 190, 211
SIADH, 3, 4, 112, 113, 130, 139, 202, 203, 204
side effects, ix, 8, 149, 192
signalling, 109
signs, viii, xi, 2, 16, 22, 24, 25, 47, 50, 52, 53, 54, 58, 63, 78, 80, 85, 86, 87, 92, 100, 110, 111, 118, 120, 125, 134, 143, 151, 154, 155, 176, 201, 202, 203, 209, 218
Singapore, 93

skeletal muscle, 14
skin cancer, 31, 77, 82, 89
skin tags, 84
skinfolds, 42
sleep apnea, 208
sleep disturbance, 119, 120
small intestine, 61, 82, 83
smoking, 145
social exclusion, 21, 98
sodium, 4, 113, 204
solid tumors, 32, 35, 36, 43, 45, 54, 60, 68, 76, 91, 94, 151, 155, 194, 195
solubility, x, 164, 179
solution, 4, 115, 168, 180, 204
SP, 20, 21, 102
species, 190, 199
spinal cord, 72, 206, 207, 208, 209
spleen, 52, 167, 174, 175, 212
splenomegaly, 127, 174, 175, 176, 180
spontaneous pneumothorax, 84
squamous cell, 3, 12, 13, 15, 18, 40, 65, 91, 108, 109, 140, 204, 210, 213, 214
squamous cell carcinoma, 3, 12, 13, 15, 18, 40, 65, 91, 108, 109, 204, 210, 213, 214
SS, 93, 142, 159
stability, 193, 221
stabilization, 208
stasis, 63
state(s), 8, 61, 71, 110, 111, 113, 130, 173, 205, 212
statistics, 145, 168
stem cells, 129
sterile, 131, 212
steroids, 8, 9, 11, 15, 16, 50, 52
stilbenes, x, 164, 178, 196, 197
stimulation, 121, 123, 128, 131, 186, 187, 193
stomach, 14, 32, 43, 45, 49, 60, 61, 62, 64, 68, 69, 71, 76, 82, 83, 98, 101, 130
stomatitis, 16, 27
storage, 174
stress, 72
striae, 50, 111
structure, 175, 179, 180
subacute, x, 11, 31, 32, 95, 96, 119, 120, 150, 154, 155, 158, 160, 208
substitution, 196
sulfate, 52
superior vena cava, 63
supplementation, 16
suppression, 28, 112, 167, 171, 173, 178, 179, 186, 193, 197, 203
surgical removal, 16, 47
survival, 57, 109, 124, 126, 127, 128, 189, 196, 217
survival rate, 128
susceptibility, 40
Sweden, 218
swelling, 46, 47, 49, 55, 63, 113, 118, 134, 210
symptomatic treatment, 8, 213
synthesis, 40, 112, 116, 126, 131, 202
systemic lupus erythematosus, 32, 95, 96
systemic mastocytosis, 53
systemic sclerosis, 30, 95

T

T cell, 54, 128
T regulatory cells, 219
tachycardia, 8, 47, 53
target, 105, 193
TCC, 132, 133, 134, 145
techniques, 24, 146
teeth, 82
telangiectasia, 53, 59, 60, 89, 90, 91, 111, 210
temporal arteritis, 29
temporal lobe, 10, 119, 120
tendon, 207, 208
terminals, 121
testicle, 134
testicular cancer, ix, 10, 108, 119, 120, 134, 135, 142, 146
testing, 12, 27, 28, 67, 110
testis, 120, 134, 135, 136, 146, 150, 158
TGF, 117, 126
therapeutic agents, x, 164
therapeutic approaches, 110, 192

therapeutic effects, x, 164
therapeutics, x, 163
thiazide, 205
thiazide diuretics, 205
thinning, 50, 79
thorax, 60
thrombocytopenia, 60, 101, 131
thrombocytopenic purpura, 60
thrombocytosis, 7, 18, 194, 211, 221
thrombophlebitis, 59, 62, 212
thrombosis, 62, 63, 76, 131, 212
thymoma, 6, 10, 28, 36, 49, 151, 152, 153, 158
thymus, 180, 210
thyroid, 5, 15, 32, 43, 45, 47, 49, 50, 51, 53, 59, 67, 73, 82, 83, 85, 86, 87, 108, 123, 130, 204, 210, 217
thyroid cancer, 15, 47, 49, 85, 86
thyroid gland, 108
tissue, xi, 32, 52, 56, 76, 78, 115, 116, 117, 118, 127, 129, 131, 145, 174, 181, 189, 192, 195, 201, 206, 209, 212, 218
TNF, 15, 126, 127, 179, 198
TNF-alpha, 15, 198
toxic effect, 211
toxicity, 166, 178, 181, 192, 193, 205, 207
transcription, 127
transformation, 79, 82, 129, 136
transforming growth factor, 126, 213
transfusion, 166, 195
transitional cell carcinoma, 97, 140, 142, 145
translocation, 77
transmission, 121
transplant, 71
transplantation, 168
transurethral resection, 129
trauma, 57, 62, 67, 70, 82, 84, 123
tryptophan, 51, 115
tuberculosis, 37, 64, 203
tumor cells, 3, 5, 6, 25, 29, 70, 118, 127, 131, 156, 166, 168, 179, 180, 187, 189, 190, 191, 192, 206, 212
tumor development, 165
tumor growth, xi, 38, 124, 164, 166, 168, 169, 170, 172, 173, 175, 176, 177, 181, 185, 186, 187, 189, 191, 193, 196, 199
tumor invasion, viii, 23, 24, 189
tumor metastasis, vii, 1, 2, 199
tumor necrosis factor, 53, 126, 179
tumor progression, xi, 164, 166, 186
tumours, ix, 80, 82, 84, 85, 108, 111, 114, 115, 116, 118, 119, 126, 146
turgor, 113
turnover, 110

U

Ukraine, 163
ulcerative colitis, 33, 59
ultrasonography, 119
ultrasound, 8, 64, 80, 83, 84, 156
uniform, viii, 24
United States (USA), 93, 124, 129, 133, 134, 137, 142
urea, 204, 205
ureter, 132, 139
urethra, 114, 129, 133, 136, 146
urinalysis, 26
urinary bladder, 114, 133, 140
urinary retention, 154
urinary tract, 82, 132, 133
urine, 3, 4, 5, 47, 52, 110, 112, 113, 115, 116, 133, 204
urine cytology, 133
urticaria, 28, 49, 50, 53, 100, 213
uterus, 32, 36, 43, 45, 48, 61, 136
UV, 178, 180
UV irradiation, 178

V

vacuum, 180
vagina, 32, 91
vascular diseases, 118, 207
vascular endothelial growth factor (VEGF), 126, 143, 166, 195
vascular wall, 29

vasculature, 167, 175
vasculitic neuropathy, x, 150, 161
vasculitis, 28, 29, 30, 33, 34, 92, 94, 95, 153, 155, 160
vasodilation, 114
vasomotor, 51
vasopressin, 3, 4, 112, 113, 202, 203
vasospasm, 63
VEGF expression, 126, 166
vein, 8, 62, 76, 125
ventricle, 55
vertigo, 120, 123, 209
vibration, 151
viral infection, 67
virus replication, 197
viscosity, 61, 63
vision, 10, 64, 207
vitamin A, 40
vitamin D, 3, 109, 126
vitiligo, 154
vomiting, viii, 2, 5, 10, 71, 110, 113, 204, 205, 209
vulva, 32, 86

W

walking, 60, 203
warts, 43, 44
waste, 115
water, x, 4, 113, 114, 164, 179, 180, 203, 204
weakness, viii, 2, 4, 12, 14, 25, 56, 111, 113, 119, 120, 121, 123, 128, 133, 135, 138, 152, 155, 203, 205, 206, 207, 208, 210
weight gain, 111, 113
weight loss, 17, 37, 38, 51, 71, 89, 127, 128, 132, 154
wheezing, 8, 52, 118, 211
white blood cell count, 7, 118, 211
white blood cells, 7, 173, 182
WHO, 133
wood, 36, 179, 180
wound healing, 167
wrists, 73, 209

Y

Y chromosome, 136, 146
yeast, 50
yield, 56
young people, 81

Z

zinc, 37, 38